Cross-Cultural Psychiatry

Edited by

Albert Gaw, MD

John Wright • PSG Inc
Boston   Bristol   London
1982

Library of Congress Cataloging in Publication Data

Main entry under title:

Cross-cultural psychiatry.

    Papers from a workshop held in Apr. 1979, Boston,
Mass.
    Bibliography: p.
    Includes index.
    1. Psychiatry, Transcultural--Congresses.
I. Gaw, Albert. [DNLM: 1. Cross-cultural comparison.
2. Psychiatry. WM 100 C951]
RC455.4.E8C76   616.89   80-27879

ISBN 0-88416-338-5

Published by:
John Wright • PSG Inc, 545 Great Road, Littleton,
Massachusetts 01460, U.S.A.
John Wright & Sons Ltd, 42-44 Triangle West,
Bristol BS8 1EX, England

Printed and Bound in Great Britain by
John Wright & Sons (Printing) Ltd. at The Stonebridge Press, Bristol

International Standard Book Number: 0-88416-338-5

Library of Congress Catalog Card Number: 80-27879

Dedication

To all people of all colors.

A. Anthony Arce, MD
Professor of Psychiatry
Hahnemann Medical College
  and Hospital
Philadelphia, Pennsylvania

Enrique G. Araneta, Jr., MD
Chief of Mental Hygiene Clinic
Veterans Administration Outpatient
  Clinic
Jacksonville, Florida

Robert L. Bragg, MD, MPH
Director of Psychiatric Education
  and Training
Department of Psychiatry
Associate Dean for Special Projects
University of Miami School of
  Medicine
Miami, Florida

Johanna Clevenger, MD
Chairperson
Committee of American Indian and
  Native Alaskan Psychiatrists
American Psychiatric Association
Dallas, Texas

Marlene EchoHawk, PhD
Clinical Assistant Professor
Department of Pediatrics
Children's Memorial Hospital
The University of Oklahoma
Health Sciences Center
Oklahoma City, Oklahoma

Edward F. Foulks, MD, PhD
Director of Residency Education
Hospital of the University of
  Pennsylvania
Philadelphia, Pennsylvania

Albert Gaw, MD
Assistant Professor of Psychiatry
Boston University School of Medicine
Staff Psychiatrist
Edith Nourse Rogers Memorial
  Veterans Hospital
Bedford, Massachusetts

Angel Gregorio Gómez, MD
Former Chairperson
Committee of Spanish Speaking
  Psychiatrists
American Psychiatric Association
Rio Piedras, Puerto Rico

Alexander H. Leighton, MD
National Health Scientist, Canada
Professor of Psychiatry and
  Preventive Medicine
Dalhousie University
Faculty of Medicine
Halifax, Nova Scotia, Canada
Professor Emeritus
Harvard University School
  of Public Health
Boston, Massachusetts

Tsung-yi Lin, MD
Former President, World Federation
  for Mental Health
Health Sciences Centre Hospital
University of British Columbia
Faculty of Medicine
Vancouver, BC, Canada

Charles A. Pinderhughes, MD
Professor of Psychiatry
Boston University School of Medicine
Assistant Chief, Psychiatry Service
  for Clinical Training
Edith Nourse Rogers Memorial
  Veterans Hospital
Bedford, Massachusetts

Elaine B. Pinderhughes, MSW
Associate Professor
Boston College School of
  Social Work
Chestnut Hill, Massachusetts

Pedro Ruiz, MD
Professor of Psychiatry
Baylor College of Medicine
Texas Medical Center
Houston, Texas

Lindbergh S. Sata, MD
Chairman
Department of Psychiatry
Saint Louis University School of
  Medicine
Saint Louis, Missouri

Richard I. Shader, MD
Professor and Chairman
Department of Psychiatry
Tufts University School of Medicine
New England Medical Center
  Hospital
Boston, Massachusetts

Jeanne Spurlock, MD
Deputy Medical Director
American Psychiatric Association
Washington, DC

Adela G. Wilkeson, MD
Instructor in Psychiatry
Harvard Medical School
Assistant Psychiatrist
McLean Hospital
Belmont, Massachusetts

Joe Yamamoto, MD
Professor of Psychiatry
Neuropsychiatric Institute
The Center for the Health Sciences
University of California
Los Angeles, California

CONTENTS

viii

FOREWORD

Few of the issues confronting the mental health disciplines in the 1980s are linked more directly to every facet of the mental health system than those encountered in the context of cross-cultural practice. The increasing availability and accessibility of mental health services to all segments of the population swell demands for a variety of appropriate services. The ability to provide such services is contingent upon the skill of mental health clinical personnel; and, in turn, the content of their education and training program curricula must be determined through research.

The current centrality of cross-cultural interests reflects the confluence of disparate trends in recent decades. Increasing acceptance of mental health services, a widespread ethnic and cultural awakening by large segments of the population, and demands emanating from legislative and judicial arenas, as well as from users of mental health services, all have encouraged increasing attention to cross-cultural issues in mental health.

In the late 1970s, the President's Commission on Mental Health again underscored the issue, and the unmet needs. In a concise description of the variegated U.S. population, the Task Force on Special Populations observed that we are comprised, in part, of 3 million Asian/Pacific Americans, 22 million Black Americans, 23 million Hispanic Americans, one million American Indians, and some 53 million Americans of European ethnic ancestry. These and other special populations, the Task Force stated, "are those groups who are both overrepresented in the statistics on mental health and...are clearly underserved or inappropriately served by the current mental health system in this country."[1]

In the thirty years preceding the findings of the President's Commission, the National Institute of Mental Health has striven to improve the appropriateness of our national response to the needs of all mentally ill persons. The Institute is proud to have played a role as part of that effort, in the series of events that culminated in publication of *Cross-Cultural Psychiatry*. The reader of this volume may find informative a brief review of the Institute's activities in this regard.

The Center for Minority Group Mental Health Programs (NIMH) was established in November 1970 to serve as a focal point for activities within the Institute, including research and training programs, which bear directly on meeting the mental health needs of all minority groups. In the early 1970s the Center, in collaboration with the Institute's Division of Manpower and Training Programs, let a contract to review minority content in NIMH training programs in the core mental health disciplines. What had been presumed was clarified: many programs in each of the core disciplines (social work being the predominant exception to the rule) were characterized by inadequate or nonexistent minority curriculum content. Courses relevant to minority group mental health concerns were ancillary to most programs, and minority students were underrepresented in academic training programs.

In 1973 the Institute initiated a Minority Fellowship Program to increase the number of minorities in mental health professions and to improve the quality of research and service delivery pertinent to minority group populations.

Additional activities ensued in the following years. Technical Assistance conferences were sponsored at various sites throughout the country to enhance opportunities for minority scientists to secure research support. In the late 1970s the Institute initiated two funding programs to provide greater opportunities for minority students and scientists to pursue careers in mental health research.

Concurrent with these efforts to expand the pool of qualified minority mental health investigators, the Institute continued efforts to sensitize minority and non-minority mental health clinical professionals to cultural influences in mental health care. As Dr. Gaw suggests in his preface, the Institute's efforts would not have succeeded without the enthusiastic and creative participation of individuals in academia and a variety of other government and private sector settings. This volume, of which the nucleus reports the proceedings of a conference, represents one example of such collaboration involving the NIMH, the Veterans Administration, and Dr. Gaw and his colleagues at the Edith Nourse Rogers Memorial Veterans Hospital and the Division of Psychiatry, Boston University School of Medicine.

Though it is a text intended primarily for use by psychiatric residents, *Cross-Cultural Psychiatry* will prove a valuable reference for use by clinicians in all of the core mental health disciplines as well as in the health and social service systems, and for researchers, social scientists, students, and administrators.

The contributing authors of those chapters in Sections I through IV, which deal with the cultural aspects of mental health care for Asian Americans, Hispanic Americans, Native Americans, and Black Americans, distinguish themselves not only as skilled psychiatric anthropologists but also as astute and sensitive observers of individuals living in or at the tearing edges of cultures and subcultures in contemporary America. Perhaps the essential task of the cross-cultural practitioner is to determine that often subtle point at which culture and its manifestations end, and illness begins. Such a skill cannot simply be taught, but requires a genuine appreciation of cultural influences and individual differences. That appreciation is apparent throughout this volume.

The eight chapters on cultural aspects of care for various subgroups of the population constitute the core of this book and tell us what presently can be told about providing psychiatric services cross-culturally. The comments appended to each section and the readings in Section V provide another valuable dimension to the volume. An interest in clinical aspects of cross-cultural mental health practice should lead, ideally, to a deepening interest in the bases of what we know now, and an expanding list of questions about what we ought to know. The discussants comment provocatively not only on that which has been said, but also on that which yet must be discussed: these issues lead us into considerations of basic research needed on biological and sociocultural processes; into questions about the nature of our service delivery system; and into deeper scrutiny of the manner in which we as a nation extend opportunities to recruit and educate all mental health, health, and human service professionals.

Cross-Cultural Psychiatry is an excellent contribution to a rich and exciting field and a foundation upon which others can build. We in the profession of psychiatry and the mental health field broadly are indebted to Dr. Gaw and the distinguished contributors to this volume for helping all of us become more effective professionals.

Herbert Pardes, MD
Director, National Institute of Mental Health

REFERENCE

1. President's Commission on Mental Health. *Task Panel on Special Population.* Vol. 3, page 731, Washington, D.C.: US Government Printing Office, 1978.

PREFACE

This book is the product of a two-year project by selected experts in cross-cultural psychiatry, which culminated in a research symposium and workshop held at Boston University on April 18 and 19, 1979. The project, funded by the Center for Minority Groups Mental Health Program (Minority Center) of the National Institute of Mental Health (NIMH), signifies another step in a series of programmatic developments initiated by the Minority Center in recent years to encourage the inclusion of cross-cultural content in professional mental health training programs.

In 1973 the Minority Center conducted a study that produced guidelines for the systematic evaluation of curricular content in professional mental health training programs with respect to minority concerns. This was followed in 1974 by a conference in which professionals representing the four major minority groups (Asians, Hispanics, Native Americans, and Blacks) convened with the staff college of the NIMH to address issues of curriculum development that reflect minority content. The final impetus to action occurred in 1975 at the annual meeting of the American Psychiatric Association in Toronto.

It was then that I discussed with Dr. Lindbergh Sata, who was Chairman of the Committee of Asian Psychiatrists, my desire to bring together clinicians, researchers, and teachers in the nation to examine systematically the cultural issues attending mental health care to United States minority populations. Both of us concurred strongly with the view of NIMH that the development of culturally relevant psychiatric curricula would be an effective means of increasing psychiatrists' sensitivity about cultural and ethnic issues in patient care. As a sequel to the above events, I submitted a research proposal to NIMH for a workshop to develop a model curriculum in Cross-Cultural Psychiatry, using cultural issues influencing mental health care to United States minority groups as a research and teaching paradigm.

Though cultural issues encompass a wide spectrum of topics, ranging from epidemiologic to developmental, the workshop focused on the examination of cultural issues that may influence the process of delivery of mental health care. If one were to trace the process of patients' care-seeking behavior during the course of a mental illness (from the time of the appearance of "disturbed behavior," through contacts with providers of care, until the resolution of problems), four important questions can be delineated wherein cultural issues may play a key role in shaping patients' responses. These questions are: How is mental illness expressed in the context of culture? What kind of treatments are considered by the patient to be appropriate and acceptable within his or her cultural framework? Are there variations in the patterns of family response to mental illness across ethnic groups? What are the notions of mental illness and health held by patients from different cultural backgrounds?

In order to address the above questions and compare them across US minority groups, psychiatric clinicians of Asian, Hispanic, Native American and Black background were asked to research existing published data from a variety of sources. This book is the end result of their efforts to integrate the cultural materials in a way that would be useful for the practice and training of psychiatrists. Furthermore, to stress clinical usefulness, the concept of culture and relevant generic issues in the training of cross-cultural psychiatrists was examined by an expert trained in both psychiatry and anthropology. Specific training issues in the field of cross-cultural psychiatry were examined from the perspectives of training directors and psychiatric trainees. Finally, experts outside the research group were invited to discuss the papers written by the researchers. The papers and the comments of the discussants form the substance of this book.

Because of the constraints of time, budget, and personnel, it was impossible to include in the study all the identified US minority groups. Some arbitrary selection had to be made. Hence, those groups that represent the largest population census were selected. This arbitrary selection should not be construed to mean that other groups lack data attesting to their unique cultural patterns in the seeking of mental health care; quite on the contrary, groups like the Korean Americans, Indochinese, Pacific-Islanders, Hispanics from South and Central America, Caribbean Blacks and others may have unique cultural issues that should be studied in their own right. We hope this book will spur others to pursue research in this direction.

Arrangement of the chapters is guided by content so that an easy "flow" of reading can be maintained throughout. Cultural issues attending mental health care of specific ethnic groups are presented first, in order to provide the background materials that help clarify the important concepts and training issues addressed in the latter section of this book.

This book can be used as a text for courses on cross-cultural psychiatry, a comparative system of delivery of mental health care, or ethnic and cultural aspects of mental health care, as well as a general reference text. Our teaching experience at the Boston University Psychiatric Residency Program has shown that if a clinician from the specific ethnic group being discussed participates in a seminar, it can add breadth and depth of cultural understanding by drawing on the personal, as well as the professional experiences of the clinician. We hope that this book can provide psychiatrists in training and practitioners with insights into the cultural milieu of the four minority groups mentioned.

Many individuals assisted in the planning and implementation of the workshop from which *Cross-Cultural Psychiatry* emerged. Dr. Sanford Cohen, Psychiatrist in Chief of the Division of Psychiatry of the Boston University School of Medicine and Dr. Ethan Rofman, former Chief of Psychiatry at the Edith Nourse Rogers Memorial Veterans Hospital, were both very supportive throughout this project. Dr. Charles Pinderhughes, Assistant Chief of Psychiatry for Clinical Training at our Veterans Hospital, and Dr. Jeanne Spurlock, Deputy Medical Director of the American Psychiatric Association, have been immensely helpful in providing ideas, suggestions, and support for the project and in recommending names of individuals for me to contact. Dr. Peter Knapp and Dr. Robert Goldman of Boston University assisted in the implementation of the workshop. Dr. Charles Colburn, Chief of Staff at our Veterans Hospital, provided administrative assistance. Special acknowledgement is extended to Donna Marcy, Patricia French and Marilyn Jacobs for their excellent assistance in the development of the workshop. Marilyn Jacobs has been meticulous in preparing the manuscripts for publication. I am most grateful to all faculty and discussants of the workshop for their cooperation in preparing the manuscripts. I thank the many individuals whose names cannot be mentioned due to the constraint of space, to my colleagues both at the Veterans Hospital and Boston University, each of whom, in his or her own way, gave letters of support and invaluable suggestions, comments, and moral support. I also thank all the participants in the workshop.

Last, but not least, I am most grateful to Dr. James Ralph, Chief of the Center for Minority Groups Mental Health Programs, NIMH, and members of his staff, for providing technical assistance and continuing support. His office is always accessible. Without the financial support of the Center, this workshop would not have been possible.*

It has not been easy for us as psychiatric clinicians to venture into the realm of psychiatric anthropology. I hope we have made a contribution to this subject and demonstrated that the manifestation and the cure of illness in an individual cannot be separated from cultural milieu.

This project demonstrates the feasibility of a collaborative endeavor between a private university and two federal agencies; namely, the Veterans Administration and the Center for Minority Groups Mental Health Program, National Institute of Mental Health, in the development

---

*This workshop was supported by conference Grant 1R13MH31753-01 from the National Institute of Mental Health.

of a teaching curriculum with strong emphasis on content materials relating to minority mental health care.

The workshop proved to be an exciting two days. I hope our labors together will help to bring a keener awareness of the cultural issues that influence the delivery of mental health care to both minority and non-minority patients. There is a saying in Chinese — Remember the source of the spring as you drink the water. In the truest spirit of this statement, I say, "謝謝,(*'hsieh hsieh'), thank you.*"

ACKNOWLEDGEMENTS

The author wishes to thank the Center for Minority Group Mental Health Programs, National Institute of Mental Health for funding this project. (Grant Number MH 31753-01).

The author wishes to thank copyright owners and publishers of the following writers for permission to adapt or reprint their work:

Aberle DF, Cohen AK, Davis AK, Levy MJ, Jr, Sutton FX: The functional prerequisites of a society. Reprinted from *Ethics,* 60 (January 1950), 100-111, by permission of the University of Chicago Press, © 1950, University of Chicago.

Leighton AH: The therapeutic process in cross-cultural perspective. A symposium. *American Journal of Psychiatry* 124(9):1171-1183, 1968. © 1968, the American Psychiatric Association. Reprinted by permission.

Leighton AH: The Erosion of Norms. *Australian and New Zealand Journal of Psychiatry* 8:223-227, 1974. By permission of the publisher.

Pinderhughes E: Adapted from Teaching empathy in cross-cultural social work, by Elaine Pinderhughes. *Social Work* 24(4):312-316, 1979. By permission of the publisher.

Sharp L: Steel axes for stone age Australians. From *Human Problems in Technological Change,* edited by Edward H. Spicer, © 1952 by the Russell Sage Foundation, Publishers, New York, pp 70-90, by permission of the publisher.

SECTION I
Cultural Aspects of Mental Health Care for Asian Americans

1 Chinese Americans

Albert Gaw, MD

What happens when a Chinese American* becomes mentally ill? Can he find a psychiatrist who speaks his language? Can he find a doctor, social worker, or other mental health professional who would understand his personal, family, and social life and religion and how he was raised? If he needs hospitalization, would the foods be different from those he is accustomed to? Does he understand that patients are often helped by talking regularly with a psychiatrist, nurse, or social worker? Is he able to develop enough trust in professionals to disclose his feelings, as

Supported by a Conference Grant from the National Institute of Mental Health 1 R13 MH31753-01.
*Chinese American denotes both native and foreign-born Americans of Chinese ancestry and noncitizen Chinese residing in the United States.

1

he is most likely expected to do? Can he accept the merit of having his family come in regularly to see the social worker, while he is being identified as the patient rather than in his traditional family role? Does he understand an inkblot test; can he expect a right interpretation to his answers? What association and emotional response would he have when blood is drawn from him for tests?

What are the meanings of all these experiences for a Chinese American mental patient seeking treatment in an American community mental health center? How does the health-care provider go about attempting to understand the patient's illness in the light of his cultural background as Chinese and American?

HISTORICAL BACKGROUND OF CHINESE IN AMERICA

The Chinese immigrated to the United States about 1850 and were the first Asian group from the Far East to set foot on the West Coast of America. Their immigration was prompted by the combination of a natural catastrophe and political unrest in China and the promise of opportunity in America. The occurrence of flooding and the Taiping Rebellion in China, coupled with the news of the discovery of gold and the need for cheap labor to engage in railroad construction and industrialization in America, provided powerful incentives for the seafaring coastal people of KwangTung Province in southern China to emigrate to the United States (Sung 1967). Within two years of their first arrival, the Chinese population in California swelled to 25,000 (Sung 1975). Unlike other immigrant groups, many of these early Chinese settlers were male, and the settlers came with the intention of returning home. However, their dream of seeking a better livelihood in America was shortlived. As aliens who staunchly maintained their dialects, habits, customs, and traditions and who were proud of their cultural heritage, they were slow in assimilating the American culture and slow to be accepted by the larger American society. Perhaps out of ignorance, fear, threat of competition for jobs during a period of economic depression, and a sentiment arising from a white supremacist ideology, the Chinese became an easy target for racial discrimination (Kim 1973). Quickly, anti-Chinese sentiments were enacted into a series of exclusion laws. Beginning with the Chinese Exclusion Act of 1882, at least 14 pieces of legislation were enacted by the United States Congress over the years, which virtually halted the immigration of Chinese to the United States, and the Chinese immigration quota was eventually set as a trickle of 105 per year (Sung 1975). These federal acts and similar state laws prevented Chinese from bringing over their wives and denied the right of citizenship and due process of law (Kim 1973). The total Chinese population in the United States declined from a high of 107,488 in 1880 to a low of 61,639 in 1920 (Sung 1975). By prohibiting Chinese males from bringing their wives and children, United States immigration laws were, in effect, indirectly supporting a genocidal policy that could have eliminated future generations of Chinese in the United States.

While many Chinese returned to China upon retirement, World War II and the Communist occupation of mainland China forced many who had intended to be transients in America to retire in America, without the traditional family network of support.

After World War II, United States immigration policy toward orientals became more liberal. The War Bride Act of 1946 allowed Chinese wives of American soldiers to join their husbands in the United States. Finally, the restrictive National Origins Quota System was abolished in 1965. Chinese increased in number from 77,504 in 1940 to 435,062 in 1970. More significantly, the Chinese who immigrated to the United States after World War II were predominantly female, many of whom took the first opportunity to rejoin their husbands who were already residing in the United States. Many were students, semi-skilled and skilled laborers and professionals coming from all over mainland China as well as the province of KwangTung and other Chinese communities in the Far East.

The influx of younger males as well as a large number of female immigrants is profoundly significant for the number and character of the Chinese American communities. By permitting the reestablishment of the Chinese family unit (parents and children), the liberalization of United States immigration laws appeared to have arrested the previous genocidal policy. At present the Chinese, along with Japanese and Filipinos, constitute the three largest Asian races in the United States.

LEGACY OF THE LEGISLATION

The effect of the exclusion acts was to alter profoundly the size and sex ratio of contemporary Chinese American communities. Before the liberalization of the immigration laws, there were few native-born Chinese Americans. Among the elderly Chinese, men were found to outnumber women by a ratio of more than 6 to 1 beyond 60 years old in the northeast region of the United States in 1960 (Li et al 1972). Following the repeal of the exclusion acts, a substantial number of Chinese women and families immigrated into this country. The population of native-born Chinese Americans increased considerably and by 1960, in the northeast region, the numbers of native-born Chinese Americans had grown approximately equal to the number of foreign-born Chinese Americans. However, the foreign-borns were nearly all beyond middle age, whereas over one-half of the native-born were children or young adults. This population distribution has implications for mental health:

1. The presence of a large, predominantly single, male elderly population unable to care for themselves because of the lack of traditional family support systems means that the Chinese elderly males will face increasing difficulty in coping with old age unless alternative support systems beyond the reliance on family unit in the community can be provided. The presence of increasing medical, psychiatric, social, and other problems associated with advancing age, and few community resources to provide for the needs of the elderly make the care of the elderly an important public health problem in most Chinese American communities. As will be noted later in the chapter, the suicide rate among Chinese elderly is found to be high and would need special attention from mental health professionals to overcome this problem.

2. The influx of younger immigrants and the emergence of a generation of native-born Chinese Americans create new demands for jobs, housing, education, and other human services. Many of these youths are discontented with the low status of Chinese in America, and they desire better living conditions. They are faced with the problem of having to assimilate the values of a westernized society that may be at variance with their more tradition-bound values at home. The intensification of this conflict in the process of acculturation may lead to a sense of uncertainty in the youths' own identity. Should they consider themselves Chinese, American, or both? Would they be able to achieve equal social status with youths of other ethnic backgrounds? The frustration of the young Chinese American is particularly felt among those whose family ties have been weakened by the absence from home of parents who had to work long hours for a livelihood. In recent years, juvenile delinquency, youth gangs, and school dropouts are beginning to appear in some Chinese American communities (Abbott and Abbott 1973; Berkeley 1977; Lyman 1973).

CHINESE AMERICAN COMMUNITIES

Bonded together for economic, cultural, psychological, political, social, and other reasons, Chinese enclaves became closely knit communities known as Chinatown. Due to the historical reasons previously discussed, Chinatown drew its residents mainly from KwangTung province of China, where Cantonese and Toishanese are the two main dialects spoken. At present, the Chinatowns located in San Francisco, New York, Honolulu, Los Angeles, Chicago, Boston, and Sacramento are the largest centers of Chinese population in the United States.

United States Chinese communities can further be roughly divided into subcultural groups according to spoken dialects such as Cantonese, Toishanese, Mandarin, Shanghainese, Taiwanese, Fookienese, and others. These spoken dialects, reflective of the provincial dialects spoken in China, are different one from the other in sounds and therefore cannot be used as a means of communication among the various Chinese ethnic groups. For purposes of inter-ethnic verbal and written discourse, Mandarin, which is the national language of China, is used.

There is also a growing, significant number of native-born Americans of Chinese parentage, who, with the exception of their physical appearances, speak English and share the life-style and values not different from those of many Caucasians.

MENTAL HEALTH: MYTHS AND REALITIES

The presence of highly visible Chinatown communities tends to reinforce stereotypes about Chinese. These stereotypes seem to reflect social, economic, and historic events occurring in America at the time these stereotypes occurred. For example, during the period of the enactment of the exclusion acts, Chinese were depicted as pigtailed, strange, exotic, filthy, unassimilable, immoral, treacherous, and cowardly; these negative stereotypes appeared to justify continuing discrimination and enactment of exclusion laws (Sue and Kitano 1973). During World War II, when China became an ally of the United States, these negative stereotypes gradually gave way to more positive characterizations depicting Chinese as intelligent, law-abiding, quiet, loyal, hardworking, and model Americans. Both types of stereotyping are regarded by Sue and Kitano as potentially damaging, for they tend to ignore the variation of individual and group characteristics of Chinese Americans. These stereotypes can also serve as reasons to neglect the multiple mental health needs confronting Chinese American communities.

Stereotyping also prevents accurate assessment of mental health needs of Chinese American communities. For many years, Chinese American communities were reputed to be model communities, having a low incidence of crime and mental illness, because of the theory that a strong Chinese family can act as a buffer against mental illness. Such an attitude painted an over-idealized picture of the Chinese family and lent justification for governmental and private agencies to neglect the provision of mental health programs for Chinese American communities. Glossed over was the reality of the various social forces that tend to tear the Chinese family apart.

It is not uncommon, for example, to find the male of a Chinatown family working long hours in restaurants and the mother working as a seamstress in a factory, leaving the parents with little time to attend to the care of their children. Cultural pride and unwillingness to display one's "dirty linen" also prevent many Chinatown leaders from acknowledging publicly the presence of mental health problems in Chinese communities, a necessary first step to justify seeking outside funding to establish mental health programs in the community.

The practice of keeping problems within one's community is now rapidly changing as various kinds of mental health facilities have been initiated by community members and professionals in the Chinese communities in recent years (Gaw 1975). The data now suggest a more realistic appraisal of the mental health needs of the Chinese American communities.

MENTAL HEALTH NEEDS OF CHINESE AMERICANS

Systematic surveys of rates of mental illness in Chinese American communities are not available, as is true for most United States ethnic communities. Epidemiologic data from Taiwan suggest that the rates of mental illness in their Chinese society are comparable to those of many Western countries (Lin 1953). There are limitations, however, to generalizing the findings of Taiwan studies to Chinese American communities since the Chinese American communities are comprised of more heterogeneous cultural groups, which are subjected to the social stresses of an advanced technological Western society quite unlike that of Taiwan. Data on the assessment of the mental health needs of Chinese American communities are therefore extrapolated from various sources such as the study of the hospital commitment rate, psychological testing results, the examination of patterns of use of mental health services by Chinese as compared to other Asian groups, and anecdotal experiences of mental health professionals who have worked in United States Chinatown communities.

A study of trends in Chinese American mental hospital commitment rates in California from 1855 to 1955 showed a seven-fold increase in the rate among the Chinese as compared to a two-fold increase for the general population (Jew and Brody 1967). As expected, males, the aged, and foreign born experienced substantially greater increases since there is a large male population among the Chinese.

It is not clear whether this trend reflects a real increase in the amount of mental disturbance in the Chinese American community, a reduction in cohesion in Chinese American communities, increased usage of public institutions to cope with mental problems in the Chinese community, or a reflection of discriminatory practices on the part of the larger society.

A study based on the Minnesota Multiphasic Personality Inventory Test (MMPI) administered to a mixed racial group of students seen at the Student Health Psychiatric Clinic of the University of California in Los Angeles revealed that Chinese and Japanese males exhibit more severe mental problems compared with their non-Asian counterparts (Sue and Sue 1974) Mental problems manifested as blunted affect, dependency, inferiority feelings, ruminations, somatic complaints, and lack of social skills were found to be more common among Chinese and Japanese, and pseudoneurotic schizophrenia was the most common diagnosis given.

Whether these findings reflect cultural attributes or a true decrease in mental functioning is not clear. Validity and reliability of these tests applied to Chinese populations have not been clearly established. The cultural norms for behavior among Chinese must be carefully considered before generalizing the findings to other Chinese American populations.

In a study that examined the pattern of utilization of mental health services at 17 community mental health facilities in Seattle, Washington, Sue and McKinney (1975) found that far fewer Chinese, Filipinos, and Japanese utilized these facilities than would be expected from their numbers in the communities served by these facilities, as compared with the utilization rate by white patients. The Asians had a higher proportion of individuals with a diagnosis of psychosis and were found to be older and less educated.

Sue and McKinney's data seemed to confirm the impression of mental health providers working in other Chinese communities — that Chinese patients appeared reluctant to seek mental health services in existing mental health centers without bilingual staffs. There seemed to be also a delay from the time symptoms of mental disturbance appeared in a Chinese patient to the time he sought assistance at mental health facilities, so that, compared to patients of other ethnic groups, the Chinese patient was more seriously disturbed when mental health services were finally sought. The factors that seemed to deter Chinese patients from seeking treatment early appeared related to fear of the stigma of mental illness and lack of bilingual mental health personnel who could communicate with the patients and who were sensitive to the patients' cultural background.

Statistics and service utilization rates alone cannot fully reflect the mental health needs of Chinese American communities. Chinatown communities, as enclaves of tightly knit immigrants in inner cities, are subject to all the stresses associated with features of ghetto living. Much of the housing in Chinatowns is old and dilapidated. Crowding is severe. Health and social resources are inadequate to cope with the problems associated with an elderly population, which is increasing as a percentage of the population, and youth who often rebel against established authority. The political and social structures continue to be dominated by the traditional, conservative segment of the community, which is slow to accommodate the introduction of new social programs. Many immigrants, unable to speak English, found themselves "locked in" to menial jobs and had little opportunity to become acculturated to the larger American culture.

The problems of the elderly and youth deserve special attention. Chinatown communities have been found to have a disproportionate number of elderly men. Many of these men are early transient residents who were stranded in the United States. They are faced with health, social, transportation, language, housing, economic, and legal problems; attention to the solution of these problems is complicated by the absence of the traditional family system of support. The plight of this group of Chinese elderly is just beginning to receive some attention by social groups in some Chinatowns in recent years.

There is another group of Chinese elderly whose plight in the United States is relatively unknown — immigrants from Taiwan and from other Far Eastern countries who came to the United States after World War II and who planned to retire in the United States and live with their children. The children of these Chinese elderly came to the United States earlier, during or after World War II and have now permanently settled here and may have become acculturated to the American way of life. Their parents, who have lived apart from them for years, still pretty much retain traditional Chinese values. When the elderly Chinese immigrated here, many suddenly found themselves transplanted from a social matrix of closed interpersonal contact that they were accustomed to in the Far East to one that values independence and privacy in America. If the elderly immigrants live with their children in suburban areas where public transportation is not readily accessible and are handicapped by their inability to speak English and to drive a car, they may be forced to become totally dependent on their children. Without a network of friends for social contact, the sense of extreme loneliness and helplessness that may set in among the elderly may lead to depression. Their adjustment problem may in turn create family stresses.

On the other end of the age spectrum, the recent influx of young immigrants is beginning to strain the resources in Chinese American communities, which are unprepared to absorb the increase in population. The lack of youth-oriented community resources, the poor social conditions in Chinatown, the lack of English-speaking skill and job opportunities, and the breakdown of some family systems are factors believed to be related to the appearance of petty youth gangs in Chinatown (Lyman 1973). Unfortunately, these youth gangs have been exploited for sensationalism by the media among a people otherwise noted for their social order and quiescence.

The presence of youth gangs nevertheless calls attention to a community facing rapid social change. Many Chinese youths are searching for their identity, trying to come to terms with both their Chinese cultural heritage and American value systems. It is heartening to note that an increasing number of programs being started in the Chinese communities by Chinese American groups serve as "bridges" between the Chinatown communities and the larger American societies. Chinese students in high schools and universities are beginning to demand curricular and educational experiences that they perceive will be relevant to their sociocultural experience in America. They are finding ways to synthesize their new identity as Chinese American, a blending of old and new cultures, which will equip them to adjust to a rapidly changing technological society while maintaining their cultural continuity.

CULTURAL ASPECTS OF PSYCHIATRIC PHENOMENOLOGY

There are few studies that compare psychiatric phenomenology of Chinese Americans with that of other United States ethnic groups. It is generally assumed that the expression of mental illness among Chinese Americans is generally similar to that of other United States ethnic groups of comparable age and socioeconomic background. However, among unassimilated Chinese, because of their tendency to adhere to traditional cultural beliefs toward illness, there may be significant differences in the way mental illness is expressed and mental symptomatology is interpreted, as exemplified by the following case:

An elderly Cantonese woman was experiencing the symptom of belching. An upper GI series revealed no abnormal physical findings. She was depressed and had tears in her eyes when she talked about her recently deceased husband. According to the 2nd edition of the *Diagnostic and Statistical Manual of Mental Disorders* (DSM-II) of the American Psychiatric Association, she appeared to be suffering from an acute grief reaction with features of neurotic depression.

She denied, however, a depressive affect. She was very preoccupied with the fact that while her husband was dying, she had touched him. When she found him dead a few hours after touching him she was afraid his vital energy called *chi* had entered her body. Her belching, which occurred frequently in the morning when she thought of him, was her way of expelling excessive *chi* (gas) in her body. She was given a tranquilizer in an attempt to control her symptom of belching, but developed urticaria due to the drug. She thought the urticaria was caused by the bad *chi* escaping from under her skin. In accordance with the ancient Chinese belief in *chi,* she believed *chi* or vital energy caused her illness.

Expressions of Mental Illness

Despite a dearth of controlled studies that substantiate cultural variations in psychiatric symptomatologies, studies and anecdotal reports are beginning to delineate certain cultural phenomena worthy of note. A review of the current literature on cultural aspects of psychopathology related to Chinese Americans indicates that, because of variations in Chinese cultural backgrounds and the degree of acculturation among Chinese Americans, a spectrum of responses to mental stress is found. The responses range from that of a completely westernized native-born American of Chinese parentage whose expression of illness is no different from that of any Caucasian, to the other extreme of an elderly, poorly educated, tradition-bound Chinese immigrant whose response to mental illness is based on supernatural beliefs or naturalistic interpretation of bodily phenomena.

Somatization and depression   Somatization as a cultural mode of expressing mental distress has been noted for quite some time by psychiatrists of Chinese ancestry and by psychiatrists who have compared mental illness in different cultures. One recent study supported the presence of a tendency toward somatization among Chinese depressives (Marsella, Kinzie, and Gordon 1973).

They compared 196 depressed, third-generation Chinese and Japanese Americans with a comparable Caucasian population at the University of Hawaii. The symptoms or complaints of depression were divided into four broad categories of functioning: existential, interpersonal, cognitive, and somatic. Factor analysis revealed the following:

1. Chinese exhibited depression in one existential pattern, while both Caucasian and Japanese groups had several existential patterns of depression.
2. Chinese and Japanese showed clear-cut complaints in cognitive processes, while Caucasians appeared to show complaints in this area only in association with other areas of functioning (cognitive apparatus and functioning, and existential complaints).
3. "Chinese seemed to be the only group with rather definite patterns of depression associated with somatic functioning."
4. Loss of interest in sex was found in the somatic interpersonal pattern for the Chinese and in existential patterns among Caucasians and Japanese.
5. Feelings of guilt were associated with a somatic pattern in the Chinese and an existential pattern in the Japanese, and were absent from Caucasian patterns.

6. Chinese and Japanese had more gastrointestinal complaints (poor appetite, indigestion, gas, belches), while Caucasians had a need to eat even when not hungry.

Although the findings of Marsella and co-workers reveal that somatization is prominent among Chinese depressives, it is not to be taken as the exclusive mode of the Chinese for expressing depression. Clinically, many Chinese depressed patients do have symptomatologies indistinguishable from the classic picture of neurotic or psychotic depressions. Their findings, however, suggest a more pronounced pattern of somatization among Chinese. It would be interesting to replicate this study in a hospital or in a community setting on a group of clinically depressed patients who represent different ethnic backgrounds.

The findings of Marsella et al also tended to support a hypothesis by Tseng as to why Chinese tended to somatize (Tseng 1975). Tseng cited four reasons:

1. An organ-oriented concept of pathology predominates. Traditional Chinese medicine views the human body as a microcosm of the universe. Body organs and human emotions correspond to various phases in nature. For example, the liver corresponds to spring, wood, and anger; the heart corresponds to summer, fire, and joy. With such cultural concepts of diseases, psychic distress could well be expressed through bodily organ symbols.
2. Expression of physical complaints is much more socially acceptable than expression of emotional complaints.
3. Chinese are reluctant to express openly emotion (particularly sexual or negative feelings) to others.
4. There is social reinforcement of concerns about bodily symptoms.

The presence of a tendency toward somatization has various implications for the role of the psychiatrist. At this point, it will suffice to state that somatic symptoms that represent expression of psychic distress should be carefully distinguished from symptoms arising from somatic diseases, and the psychiatrist is uniquely suited by his or her training in medicine and psychiatry to make the distinction.

Suicide   A high suicide rate has been reported in San Francisco's Chinatown community (Bourne 1973). Over a 16-year period, from 1952 through 1968, Bourne found that the suicide rate among Chinese was 27.9 per 100,000 population per annum. This rate was not significantly different from that of the entire population of San Francisco (27.5 per 100,000), but it was three times higher than the national average of 10.0 per 100,000. The Chinese rate is also substantially higher than the figure of 12.0/100,000 per annum reported by Yap for Hong Kong (Yap 1958b).

Bourne also found that the frequency of Chinese men committing suicide was four to five times more than that for Chinese women. The peak decade for suicide for both sexes was between 55 and 65 years of age. Barbiturate ingestion was noted to be the most common method of suicide for Chinese men, while hanging was the most frequent method for women. Despondency over physically ill health was found to be the most frequent cause of suicide in Chinese men. In Chinese women, interpersonal conflict, with a past history of psychiatric illness, was noted to be the most frequent cause of suicide.

From Bourne's findings, it can be concluded that lonely, single, elderly Chinese men who are poorly educated and came to America as sojourners before World War II, with few friends in their old age and despondency over physical illness, constitute a high-risk group for suicide.

The phenomenon of female suicide and attempted suicide is worthy of closer scrutiny from a cultural standpoint. Bourne's findings revealed that hanging was the most frequent method of suicide for Chinese women. Yap (1958a) has found that in Hong Kong the frequency of attempted suicide precipitated by interpersonal conflicts (recent quarrels, parental scolding, chronic family strife, desertion by a spouse, unrequited love) was 50.6/100,000 for women and 22.9/100,000 for men.

Bourne speculated that in traditional Chinese society where the role of women is subjugated to men and open expression of aggressive feelings is not tolerated, coupled with the traditional Chinese belief that the ghosts of those who died by hanging can return to torment the living, dying by hanging may be a means of achieving final and lasting vengeance.

Although this explanation has some support even in Chinese folk literature, Bourne professed that substantiating it was difficult. Still, Bourne raised the issue that a pattern of suicide behavior may be conditioned by cultural belief; this needs further exploration.

Yap borrowed Lindemann's concept of hypereridism, a term denoting a morbid state of hostile tension arising from a series of repeated provocations which might result in "explosive behavior more aggressive than is appropriate to a given set of circumstances," to explain the high frequency of interpersonal stress as a precipitating factor for unconsummated suicide among certain Hong Kong Chinese women. He asserted that because, in traditional Chinese culture, women are denied opportunities for self-assertion and are subjugated to men, interpersonal conflicts produce in susceptible individuals, a hypereridic state which exerts a prolonged, unexpressed pressure slowly leading to sorrow and despair that cannot be alleviated by threats or appeals. When a person is in such a condition, an acute quarrel or even a minor reprimand can set off an impulsive, poorly planned, or unplanned suicidal acting-out within a day. At the same time, the very nature of impulsiveness and explosiveness also tends to prevent the successful completion of a suicidal act.

Since a substantial number of Chinese American women are from Hong Kong, would not one expect to find the phenomenon of hypereridism present among this group of immigrants? We have not data to substantiate it one way or another at present, and this question awaits further study.

Schizophrenia   Phenomenologic study of schizophrenia among Chinese Americans has not been done. A study to determine the nature, course, and outcome of schizophrenia among Chinese in Hong Kong was done (Lo and Lo 1977). Of 133 Chinese schizophrenic patients first seen in 1965, the authors were able to examine 80 patients for a follow-up assessment ten years later. The course and outcome were graded into four categories. Diagnosis was based mainly on the criteria from the standard textbook of Mayer-Gross, Slater, and Roth. Of the patients evaluated for follow-up, 65% had full and lasting remission or showed no or only mild deterioration, despite some relapse. The factors associated with a favorable prognosis are female sex, a shorter duration of illness, an acute onset, presence of symptom groups other than disturbance of emotion and volition, and the presence of a supportive relative.

Alcoholism   Although no statistics are currently available on the rate of alcoholism among Chinese Americans, the general impression is that the problem of alcoholism among Chinese Americans is not prevalent. Of about 80 Chinese American mental patients treated in Boston's Chinatown over a 5-year period (1970 to 1975) by the author, only one case of alcoholism was found.

If this impression is borne out by subsequent survey data for Chinese American communities, the finding would be compatible with the low rate of alcoholism reported among Chinese and other ethnic groups in the Far and Middle Eastern countries (Chafetz 1964). Sociocultural and genetic factors were offered as possible explanations.

Sociocultural reasons (Chafetz 1964) that have been advanced to account for the low prevalence of alcoholism among Chinese in the Far East include: 1) drinking used as a means to promote social intercourse and communication, with alcoholic beverages generally consumed only at parties and during mealtime (solitary drinking for whatever reason is frowned upon); 2) a strong social sanction against drunkards and drunken behavior; 3) the presence of a strong Confucian moral ethic that prescribes proper interpersonal conduct for all ages and discourages the exhibition of any deviant behaviors including those caused by drunkenness.

Genetic reasons postulated to account for the low prevalence of alcoholism among Chinese were inferred by the presence of ethnic differences in alcohol sensitivity that suggest a probable variation in autonomic reactivity. Wolff (1972) found that Taiwanese, Japanese, and

Korean babies, after drinking amounts of alcohol that have no detectable effect on Caucasian babies, responded with marked facial flushing and mild to moderate symptoms of intoxication. He subsequently found a similar autonomic alcohol sensitivity among American-born Chinese and Japanese adults, in one tribe of North American Indians, and among hybrid offspring of Caucasian and Mongolian parents (Wolff 1973).

Comparative rates of alcohol and acetaldehyde metabolism among Chinese, Caucasians, and American Indians have also been reported. When ethanol was given by mouth to 102 healthy, young volunteers comprised of Caucasian men and women, Chinese men, and Ojibwa men, the venous blood concentrations of ethanol and acetaldehyde measured at 60, 90, 120, and 150 minutes after the end of drinking revealed the rate of ethanol metabolism to be highest in American Indians, lower in Chinese Americans, and lowest among Caucasians (Reed et al 1976). The authors felt that habitual level of alcohol consumption, proportion of body fat, and genetic factors appear to account for the group differences.

Drug abuse, personality disorders, and psychoneurosis   No data exist on the prevalence, rate, form, and expression of psychoneurosis and personality disorders among Chinese Americans. The problem of drug abuse is presumed to be present, but the extent of the problem in Chinese American communities is not clear. A low incidence of psychopathic personality disorders and obsessive-compulsive neurotic disorders has been reported by Lin in Taiwan (Lin 1953), but no comparable data exist for Chinese American communities.

Culture-Bound Syndromes

The study of the so-called culture-bound syndromes offers a unique insight into the whole interrelationship between culture and mental illness.

> Nature is nowhere accustomed more openly to display her secret mysteries than in cases where she shows traces of her workings apart from the beaten path; nor is there any better way to advance the proper practice of medicine than to give our minds to the discovery of the usual law of nature, by the careful investigation of cases of rarer forms of disease.
>
> William Harvey

Culture-bound syndromes are considered by Yap as "culture-bound in that certain systems of implicit values, social structures, and obviously shared beliefs produce unusual forms of psychopathology that are confined to special areas" (Yap 1969).

Among Far Eastern Chinese, disorders such as *koro,* (Yap 1965), *latah* (Yap 1952), *hsieh-ping* (Lin 1953), *utox* reaction (Rin and Lin 1962), and *amok* (Carr and Tan 1976) have been reported. Although these syndromes are rarely reported among Chinese Americans, the ease of international travel and migration may allow susceptible individuals to appear in Chinese American communities, as in the cases of *koro* that had appeared in Boston in recent years (A. Gaw, unpublished data, 1973).

The description of culture-bound syndromes remains unsettled, but Yap has proposed a tentative classification as follows (Yap 1969):

Paranoid syndromes
Emotional syndromes
    Depersonalization state: *koro*
    Fear-induced depressive state: *susto*
Syndrome of disordered consciousness
    Impaired consciousness: *latah*
    Turbid state: Malignant anxiety, *amok, negi-negi*
    Dissociated consciousness: *hsieh-ping, windigo* psychoses

Some may consider the above syndromes to fall under the heading of psychoses not elsewhere classified, or atypical psychosis, in the 3rd edition of the *Diagnostic and Statistical Manual of Mental Disorders* (DSM-III) of the American Psychiatric Association (American Psychiatric Association 1979).

The descriptions of some of the culture-bound syndromes more likely to be encountered by western practitioners of psychiatry are as follows:

1. *Amok.* This condition is usually reported to occur among Malayans, but may be found among Chinese (Carr and Tan 1976). The condition is described as "a furious assault commonly found in Malayan males, especially farmers and mountain dwellers, unrelated to suicide, drugs, or alcohol, but related to physical stress in the form of fright, anger, grief, or nervous depression. The attacks are preceded by vertigo ("fever") and visions ("influences"), are directed against friend and foe alike, may last a few hours, and are followed by total amnesia and deep stuporous sleep for several days.

2. *Hsieh-ping.* Lin considered *Hsieh-ping* as a possession syndrome in which a person in a trance state identifies with a deceased from the "after-life world" (Lin 1953) (see also section on Popular Medicine). The onset of the condition is often sudden and is preceded at times by heavy-headedness and numbness of extremities. The condition may last from one-half hour to many hours and is characterized by tremor, disorientation, clouding of consciousness, delirium, and visual and auditory hallucinations. The afflicted person talks in a strange tone of voice. The

contents of the speeches are religious in nature and are related to ancestor worship. The person may imitate the behavior of the deceased.

Since the Chinese regard these "spiritual seizures" as possession by ghosts or devils (*kwei*), *wu* priests who are regarded to be possesed by "*shen*," (a good spirit), may be called upon to drive out the *kwei* through exorcism.

The condition is traceable to a belief in an after-life world. Sickness and disaster of the afflicted is considered an expression of punishment by dead ancestors and is related to not offering sufficient worship to the deceased.

Lin reported five cases found in one highly religious family in Taiwan. The afflicted individuals were mostly uneducated women with hysterical personalities. The condition has not been reported to occur among Chinese Americans but should be kept in mind if a patient who believes in a supernatural cause of mental illness presents himself or herself with this symptomatology.

3. *Koro.* This refers to a state of acute anxiety associated with a belief that the genitals are shrinking into the abdomen (in males), resulting in death (Yap 1965). It is regarded by Yap as a syndrome of partial depersonalization usually induced by conflict over sexual intercourse or masturbation (Yap 1965). The syndrome is thought to be confined to Chinese in South China and in the Far Eastern countries. A *koro* epidemic has also been reported among Chinese in Singapore (Koro Study Team 1969). Sporadic cases of *koro* have been reported in North America (Lapierre 1972). I have personally treated a case of *koro* in Boston on and off for 3 years.

Koro should be distinguished from *koro*-like states, which are associated with a brain disorder (Edwards 1970) or drug intoxication (Dow and Silver 1973). In a typical attack, the patient may come to the emergency room complaining of penile shrinkage and holding onto his penis or clamping the penis with instruments.

Susceptible individuals are described by Yap to include men of poor educational background with personalities described as immature, dependent, lacking a sense of virility, and who are in conflict over expression of sexual impulses.

The cultural belief in an interchange of yin-yang during intercourse between male and female provides the background wherein the loss of yang due to excessive masturbation or sexual activity can induce a state of panic and anxiety.

Psychotropic drugs, reassurance, and support are usually sufficient to treat the illness.

Cultural Conception of Mental Illness in Traditional Chinese Medicine

It is widely recognized that a dual system of medical care exists in Chinese American communities as in most Chinese societies. This dual system of care is referred to in Chinese as western medicine as (*hsi-i,* 西医) and Chinese medicine (*chung-i* 中医).

Western medicine denotes a system of medical care based on western, European-oriented medical tradition. Insofar as our current body of psychiatric theories and diagnosis of mental illness and its treatment is based on European "scientific" tradition, our system of psychiatric care can be regarded as part of western medicine. The inherent value system is reflective of middle-American culture.

Chinese medicine denotes a system of medical care that includes a broad category of traditional healing activities handed down through the medical literati and folk practitioners in China. Such healing practices may range from diagnosis and treatment based on a traditional, highly abstract theory of cosmology to treatment by exorcism and incantation. Chinese traditional medical practitioners are called *chung-i-shih* (中医师) and may consist of herbalist, acupuncturist, bonesetter, shaman, and others. Their diagnostic tools rely chiefly on the interview, pulse diagnosis, inspection, and palpation. Their treatment repertoire ranges from use of an extensive herbal pharmacopoeia to the practice of exorcism and fortune telling. Their value systems reflect cultural sentiments of the Chinese people such as conformity, filial piety, order, and human interaction based on interdependence and reciprocity. They have their own code of professional and ethical conducts. License to practice is usually not required.

Given this dual system of medical care, a Chinese American mental patient may prefer one form of care over the other or, as in many instances, may simultaneously utilize both forms of care. Examination of the reasons that guide the decision toward the preferential usage of one form of care over the other is beyond the scope of this chapter. The thrust of this discussion is on the cultural tradition of Chinese medicine that may affect how mental illness is defined, expressed, interpreted, and reacted to by Chinese American patients.

For heuristic purposes Sivin has classified the field of Chinese medicine into two broad types — classical and popular (or folk) (N. Sivin, unpublished data, 1975).

Classical Chinese medicine   Classical Chinese medicine is built on beliefs that define health and illness according to a unitary world view of cosmology. Man is conceived to be a microcosm of the macrocosmic universe, in which the objective rhythm of the cosmos intimately affects the workings of the human body. When there are 1) a finely balanced and rhythmic working of the body, 2) a good adjustment of the body to its physical environment, and 3) a harmonious relationship between bodily functions and emotions, so that *order* is present, this state of being is regarded as *health* (Sivin). The opposite is illness. This concept of health based on theories universal in natural philosophy is emphatically ecological, dynamic, and holistic. It integrates somatic, psychologic, social, and ecologic phenomena into a unitary conceptual system. Emotions, for example, are expected not only to be appropriate in intensity and quality to specific situations, but also in harmony with the daily and seasonal cycles of nature (Sivin).

This system of theory and prescribed medical practice is best exemplified by the *Yellow Emperor's Classic of Medicine* (*Huang Ti Nei Ching Su Wen*). The theory served as a basis of medical practice among the literate minorities in China and has evolved over the centuries into a highly abstract pattern of Chinese metaphysics.

The key concepts are yin-yang, (陰陽) a bipolarity that is both opposite and complementary at the same time; five evolutive phases (五行) sometimes called the five elements; and *chí* (氣, vitality). These concepts are elaborated into a series of correspondences between the external physical environment and the internal milieu of the human body so that certain objects suggest a series of equivalent meanings (correspondences) that are easily grasped by Chinese who are brought up in this medical milieu, as illustrated by Table 1-1.

Table 1-1
Correspondences of the Five Evolutive Phases

Correspondence	Direction	Season	Organs	Orifices	Emotions	Color
Wood	East	Spring	Liver	Eyes	Anger	Green
Fire	South	Summer	Heart	Ears	Joy	Red
Earth	Middle	Late summer	Spleen	Nose	Compassion	Yellow
Metal	West	Autumn	Lungs	Mouth	Sorrow	White
Water	North	Winter	Kidney	Genitals	Fear	Black

The role of yin-yang and five evolutive phases is thought to regulate *chí*, an all-pervasive force that is believed to permeate the whole macrocosm and the human body. Man's existence is thought to be dependent on *chí*, which is the origin of all diseases.

What lets the yin and yang rise and fall is *chí*, what lets the *hsueh* flow and the pulses move is *chí*, what lets the five yin orbs and five yang orbs (*horrealis* et *aulici*) maintain the mutual relationships of production and sustenance is again *chí*. When it is decrepit, the organism is exhausted.

When it is concurring, the organism is at peace. When it is contrary, the organism suffers from disease. In sum, all these phenomena are as they are because of the (quality) of *chí*. *Chí* constitutes, of course, the root and foundation of man, but it is also the origin of all disease (Porkert 1974, p 174).

In Chinese metaphysics, many terms are concerned with functions. *chí,* originally a word for air, gases, or vapors, came to refer less to the air one breathes than to the energy that it carries. Sivin translates it to mean *vitality.*

The multiple meanings and connotations of *chí* are so pervasive that *chí* has become very much a part of present Chinese venacular. For example, when a Chinese is describing anger, it is called *sheng-chí* (生氣 , to produce *chí*). To express anger, it is *chú-chí* (出氣 , to let out). To feel righteous, it is *i-chí* (義氣 , righteous *chí*). A man with hot temper may be described as having too much *huo-chí* (火氣 , fiery *chí*). Thus, the use of this term is extremely dynamic and is defined by the function it performs. Porkert cited many uses of *chí* in traditional Chinese medical texts (Porkert 1974, pp 167–176).

The concept of *chí* extends to ancient theory of the causation of mental illness. Classical Chinese description of mental illness has long distinguished two types of deviant behavior described as *k'uang* (狂) and *tien* (癲).

A person afflicted with *k'uang* (according to *Nan Chin* classics) could be recognized by feeling sad, eating and sleeping less, developing into a megalomaniac with an exaggerated opinion of his intelligence, either scolding day and night or stopping to talk, running about restlessly, singing, behaving strangely, seeing and hearing things. This condition is attributed to excessive yang energy and *chí* disturbance. Treatment is accordingly directed to reducing food intake and the utilization of measures to restore the balance of yin and yang in the body.

Tien is a more quiet and withdrawn form of mental illness. An afflicted person will fall to the ground with eyes closed and appear asleep. This condition is thought to be due to a preponderance of yin. *Nei Ching* attributed the prenatal predisposition to *tien* to sudden fright during pregnancy resulting in an insufficiency of *chí* (氣) and *ching* (精) in the fetus.

From the perspective of present western nomenclature, *k'uang* is akin to the picture of a manic-depressive psychosis; and *tien* could be either schizophrenia or epilepsy. Other forms of psychiatric conditions that had existed in China were mentioned by Tseng (1973).

The ubiquitous concept of *chí* pervades both classical and popular medical thinking, which demonstrates the dynamic interchange of medical concepts between the classical and popular health sectors in China. These concepts (*chí,* yin-yang, five phases, and so on) provided a rational scheme that gave coherence and legitimacy to ancient diagnostic and therapeutic procedures and served to legitimate the role of classical medical practitioners as exemplified by the imperial court physician.

Popular Chinese medicine Contrary to the elaborate, highly abstract theory of medicine that characterizes the classical tradition, popular medicine is the therapy for the vast number of illiterate commoners in China (Sivin). Because of constant interchange of ideas between the popular and classical health sectors, many medical ideas that originated in the popular sector have found their ways into the medical classics, and vice versa. Many of the folk healers were poor and illiterate. They used healing practices that could be described as symbolic therapies (verbal or nonverbal procedures directed at bringing on or preventing a specific change usually having a religious significance) (Sivin). These healers ranged from shaman to magician, physiognomer, and fortune teller. Some of the ritualistic and magical cures they employed are charms, prayers, and exorcism. These popular medical theories were rooted in a folk tradition that can be traced to ancient Taoist, Buddhist, and Confucian teachings. In the villages and among the vast number of common people in China, these notions of health and illness provided meaning to the daily stresses and illnesses that confronted the common man.

Sivin points out that, in the realm of folk beliefs, the world of man is surrounded by gods and demons. A hierarchy of gods exists that could invade the human body and feed on its vital energy, causing illness, if proper rituals were not rendered. Since the daily lives and activities of the common man are thought ultimately to be involved with his celestial world, rituals and liturgies were performed to appease the gods. The common man came to be familiar with the tasks and rank order of gods within the celestial bureaucracy. He saw his gods every time he went to the temple, offered them foods on special occasions, and burned incense in front of their images at home. He could consult his gods on business matters or before making important life decisions. During illness he turned to his gods for guidance and succor. The gods also have their own arrangement of bureaucratic structure and rank orders. Sivin cited the example of the Jade Emperor who governed and superintended the operations of earth and sky and had power to judge, punish, or reward both the living and the dead. He could be appeased, pleased, angered, and sometimes even bribed just like a terrestrial officer (Sivin). Ahern has documented how Taiwanese peasants clearly understand the role of *ong-ia-kong* (a god) in their community affairs (Ahern 1975).

These gods can be further divided in two general categories according to their functions. The "good" gods are called *shen* (神), are seen arising from the yang, and are consequently responsible for all the good that befalls men. The "bad" gods are called *kwei* (鬼) and are yin demons.

Supposed to be all-pervasive in the cosmos, *shen* and *kwei* infuse the human body at birth. At death the *shen* returns to the yang of heaven and *kwei* to the yin of the earth.

The *kwei* can become a free-floating spirit called *hsieh-chi* (邪氣), which roams the earth freely. It can inflict illness on man by invading his body when human transgression occurs, such as family strife, not rendering filial obligations, interpersonal quarrels, or social decay. When this happens, a person may be invaded by *chi*, "possessed" by *kwei*, and manifests symptoms of illness.

To treat the illness, a healer, usually a medium, is summoned to "diagnose" the causes of the illness by determining which ghost in the family or in the community has been offended. In the course of investigation, the healer tries to untangle interpersonal conflicts among members of the family and even among relatives. Once the cause of disorder is diagnosed, and the offending spirit identified, it is the task of the healer to locate the superior of the offending spirit in the spiritual hierarchy and to intercede on the patient's behalf by driving the evil spirit (*kwei*) out.

Certain individuals called shamans, because of their professed ability to be possessed by the Shen spirit, were believed to be effective healers of deadly diseases inflicted by the *kwei*. Their curing rituals included exorcisms, beatings, and ceremonies to call back lost souls.

To prevent being infected by demons, a person must conduct himself with uprightness, purity, and cleanliness. Magical aids, such as charms containing the secret names of gods, certain drugs, and incantations, are used to protect the individual from harm. And of course, social order must be maintained to prevent anomalies from occurring.

Thus we see a supernatural concept of illness that weaves together illness, patient, healer, human relationships, social order, and celestial hierarchy. Disease or illness is never divorced from this cultural context. Neither is healing. Furthermore, taking the "blame" for the illness away from the offender and attributing it to *kwei* (demons), removes the stigma of illness from the afflicted individual. And in the process of healing, all parties who are involved (the individual, the family, the healer, and the gods) partake in the ritual to make the afflicted person "cured."

Family Response to Mental Illness

The Chinese American family is noted to have a high degree of tolerance in coping with and caring for its mentally ill member. Lin and Lin (1978), in a study of the pattern of help-seeking behavior among Chinese, Caucasian, and Canadian Indian mental patients in Vancouver, confirmed the widely held impression that Chinese families tend to resort to intrafamilial coping until their resources are exhausted before referring the sick member of the household to the physician for treatment or for hospitalization. This pattern of help-seeking behavior reflects genuine concern of the Chinese families for the well-being of the mentally sick member.

Paradoxically, the tendency to tolerate a mentally sick member of the family at home may at times cause unnecessary delay in seeking outside professional help. When assistance is finally sought, family resources may be depleted. In addition to this familial tolerance of deviant behavior at home, the fear of stigmatization, the avoidance of hospitalization, worry about financial expense, and the lack of bilingual mental health workers sensitive to the cultural needs of Chinese patients in mental health facilities are additional realistic factors that tend to deter Chinese from seeking outside assistance early.

This active involvement of the family members in the welfare of their sick members and their high degree of tolerance of deviant behavior can be effectively used to promote therapy within the family setting. It also implies that health centers should consider the formation of mental health teams who can visit the family to provide early intervention and treatment instead of waiting for Chinese patients to appear at the doorstep of a treatment facility and risking the patient's suffering greater morbidity due to the delay.

IMPLICATIONS FOR PSYCHIATRIC CARE OF CHINESE AMERICANS

Given a Chinese American patient seeking mental health services, what are some practical applications of this chapter? The following are some suggestions:

Overcoming the language barrier

Many non-English–speaking Chinese patients bring their own translator when appearing for mental health assistance. If the patient is unaccompanied by a translator and one is needed, it is essential to request a translator who speaks the *patient's dialect,* not just anyone who speaks Chinese. Some of the common dialects spoken by Chinese Americans are Toishanese, Cantonese, Mandarin, Taiwanese, Fookienese, Hakka, and Shanghainese.

Many established health institutions have individuals who can readily be called upon to translate; their services can be obtained by calling the hospital telephone operators. If such a pool of translators is not available, it behooves the institution to set up one in advance.

Since the sophistication of translation varies with each translator, it would be ideal if each translator were trained in the act of translating and familiarized with commonly used mental health terms. If one is uncertain about the translating skill of the translator, the following pointers can be helpful to facilitate accurate translation:

- Use simple sentences — preferable to compound-complex sentences. A sentence-by-sentence translation avoids over-burdening the translator with having to remember too many details. Technical words such as anxiety, depression, psychosomatic, conversion reaction, etc., should be avoided. Rather, those terms should be explained in simple English.
- Tell the translator to translate exactly what you mean and not to inject his own notion into the question. If the phrasing of a question is unclear to either the translator or the patient, encourage both the translator and the patient to ask questions.
- Allot enough time to conduct an interview. Conducting an interview through a translator may require twice as much time; hence the importance of apportioning enough time for the task.

Sensitivity to the Healing System to Which the Patient Subscribes

Does the patient subscribe to a modern, western system of healing as is practiced in the larger American society or does the patient believe in the traditional Chinese medical healing practices? The cultural background of the patient will provide a clue to this question. Chinese American patients, out of embarrassment, probably will not divulge this information on initial interview. However, when a doctor–patient rapport is present and the patient senses that the psychiatrist is genuinely interested in and respectful of the patient's beliefs and practices, he or she may feel freer to share the information. I found it useful to ask routinely the question: "What are your own ideas as to why you have these symptoms or problems?"

An understanding of the patient's belief system can assist the psychiatrist to appreciate the reaction of the patient to certain bodily phenomena and to explain therapeutic procedures in such a way that the patient will understand. For example, a Chinese patient and members of his family once reacted in near panic when the patient developed a contraction of leg muscles as a side effect of a medication. They attributed the muscle contraction to "possession" by evil spirit. They believed in the supernatural causation of disease. My explanation that the muscle contraction was due to a drug side effect brought quick relief of anxiety.

Approach to the Patient

The sophistication of understanding about mental health concepts and the role of the psychiatrist and allied mental health professionals vary with each individual Chinese American patient, depending on the degree of acculturation to American society, educational background, and familiarity with the western system of medical care. Many Chinese immigrants probably will have difficulty understanding the role of a "talking doctor." Furthermore, some patients may get upset with a lengthy initial interview that probes into an "embarrassing" family, social, and personal background. However, the role of a physician is still clearly understood and respected. I suggest that the psychiatrist should not hesitate to use his or her medical paraphernalia, take blood pressure, check pulses, take weight, order laboratory tests when appropriate, and conduct himself or herself in the traditional role of a physician. These are healing activities familiar to any Chinese American patient; traditional Chinese healing practices also included pulse diagnosis, palpation, and prescription writing. Furthermore, since many patients may have somatic complaints, it is important to delineate carefully the patient's symptoms in terms of the setting, quality, precipitating and alleviating factors, timing to life events, duration, and course to provide clues toward the differentiation of the nature of somatic complaints (ie, somatic, psychologic, or both). Appropriate laboratory tests can be ordered to confirm or rule out the findings.

These diagnostic activities also have symbolic value in assisting the patient to understand the role of the psychiatrist. By starting from "where the patient is," the content of the interview can gradually move from a superficial somatic level to deeper psychologic level once a rapport is established. The psychiatrist should be careful to demonstrate to the patient the relevance of each line of questioning. For example, if a physical cause of somatic complaints can be ruled out through negative findings on physical examination and laboratory tests, the psychiatrist should suggest to the patient to explore other areas such as the setting of the onset of the symptoms (eg, "You developed back pain when you quarreled with your father-in-law; what was it all about?").

When ordering blood tests, one should be alert to the sensitivity of Chinese to the notion that blood contains vital energy (*chi*) and the belief that the amount of blood loss in the body is not able to be replenished. A large quantity of blood drawn can quickly destroy a hard-earned patient-doctor rapport. If blood needs to be drawn for diagnostic purposes only, the necessary amount should be drawn after carefully explaining the reason for it and giving reassurance.

The ordering of an x-ray usually poses no problems unless elaborate preparation is necessary, such as for a barium enema. Reasons for requesting such tests should be given in simple, plain language.

If the patient does not speak English, it is best to arrange for a translator to escort the patient to and from the examining room to overcome the language barrier and reduce the patient's anxiety.

Engage the Family in the Interview and Treatment Process

Family involvement in the management of the patient's problems is natural to Chinese Americans. The psychiatrist should not hesitate to conduct family interviews, to give advice to members of the family as to how to handle the patient's problem, and to obtain feedback through periodic family interviews. If family members become too intrusive and interfere with the patient's treatment, this should be explained and appropriate limits set

If psychotherapy or psychoanalysis is to be attempted so that the technical requirement of the therapeutic process necessitates minimal or no involvement with family members, the rationale and process of treatment should be carefully explained to both patient and family members.

Use of Psychotropic Drugs and Herbal Medicines

Because of a tradition of pragmatism, some Chinese patients may simultaneously take both western and Chinese medications, consult both western physician and traditional Chinese doctor, and visit several health centers for the same complaints. Physicians should not automatically take this to mean a lack of confidence on the patient's part toward the physicians. Rather, some patients may feel that more opinions are better than one and that using both western and Chinese medications takes care of the best "of two worlds." If the physician is concerned about a drug interaction between western medication and Chinese herbs, the physician can tell the patient that mixing Chinese and western medication is not good for fear of uncertain drug side effects. If the patient insists on taking both medications, it is advisable to ask the patient not to take them simultaneously. Fortunately, many herbal medicines are harmless, but until their pharmacologic actions are ascertained, it is hard to predict what drug actions may occur.

In the use of psychotropic medications, Lin and Yamamoto have suggested using a lower therapeutic dosage of antidepressants and tranquilizers for Chinese patients (Lin and Lin 1978; Yamamoto, Chap. 3). Body build, rate of absorption, and different rates of metabolism affect the action of drugs. It is prudent not to assume that drug dosage requirement for Caucasians will also automatically apply to Chinese Americans. A more conservative titration of drug dosage may be indicated. Further research on ethnic responses to drugs is needed.

Hospitalizing a Chinese Patient

Hospitalization of a patient is usually the last resort of a Chinese family and is seen as a failure in coping. In traditional Chinese society, many still believe hospitals are places to die, not to get well. Therefore, hospitalization can be quite traumatic for both patient and family and should be resorted to only when strongly indicated. If hospitalization is necessary, adequate preparation for finances and translation service, arrangements for interview time for family members, information on how treatment decisions are made, and rationale of hospital programs and activities (occupational therapy, group therapy, electroconvulsive therapy) should be carefully explained.

If not contraindicated, bringing in Chinese food, teas, and other culturally familiar items should be encouraged to minimize the culture shock in a hospital environment. Health-care providers should be sensitive to Chinese cultural ideas that certain foods have symbolic values in addition to their nutritional values. When advising which food to take or avoid for a certain disease condition, one should consider the belief of the patient concerning the ability of the food to restore a state of balanced yin-yang. For example, nose bleeding is considered to be related to too much yang. The ingestion of "cold" foods or drinks, such as cucumber and cold tea, is believed to counteract the excessive yang. By demonstrating a sensitivity to the food beliefs of Chinese American patients, one can establish better patient–doctor rapport.

Follow-Up Care

Appointments for follow-up care should take into consideration the different working hours of Chinese American patients, particularly those who work late in restaurants. Afternoon appointments may be preferable. Also, if a translator is required, the convenience of the translator should also be considered.

Instruction on how to take medications should be carefully given. Many Chinese patients remember their medications by the colors of pills, not their names. So the psychiatrist may wish to keep a catalogue of medications with their corresponding colors handy in the office, in order to instruct the patient and check the actual dosage taken.

CONCLUSION

Chinese American communities, like many United States ethnic communities, are in a state of sociocultural transition. Mental health problems commonly associated with the impact of immigration, social change, acculturation, and racism that beset the United States minorities are also present in Chinese American communities. In a way, their problems are compounded and complicated by the tendency of Chinese Americans to keep things to themselves and by governmental neglect.

Training curricula should include culturally relevant materials that reflect the experience of Chinese in America and in the world.

BIBLIOGRAPHY

Abbott K, Abbott E: Juvenile delinquency in San Francisco's Chinese-American community: 1961-1966, in Sue S, Wagner N (eds): *Asian American Psychological Perspectives*. Ben Lomond, Calif, Science and Behavioral Books, 1973.

Ahern E: John E. Fogarty International Center. Sacred and secular medicine in a Taiwan village: A study of cosmological disorders, in Kleinman A, Kunstadter A, Alexander ER, Gale JL (eds): *Medicine in Chinese Cultures*. US Dept HEW Pub (NIH)75-653, 1975.

American Psychiatric Association: *Diagnostic and Statistical Manual of Mental Disorders,* ed 3. Washington, American Psychiatric Association, 1979.

Berkeley R: The new gangs of Chinatown. *Psychology Today,* 10 (12):60–69, May, 1977.

Bourne P: Suicide among Chinese in San Francisco. *Am J Public Health* 63(8):744–750, 1973.

Carr JE, Tan EK: In search of the true Amok: Amok as viewed within the Malay culture. *Am J Psychiatry* 133(11):1295–1299, 1976.

Chafetz ME: Consumption of alcohol in the Far and Middle East. *N Engl J Med* 271:291–301, 1964.

Dow TW, Silver D: A drug induced Koro syndrome. *J Fl Med Assoc* 60(4):32–33, 1973.

Edwards JG: The Koro pattern of depersonalization in an American schizophrenic patient. *Am J Psychiatry* 126(8):1171–1173, 1970.

Gaw A: John E. Fogarty International Center. An integrated approach in the delivery of health care to a Chinese community in America: The Boston Experience, in Kleinman A, Kunstadter A, Alexander ER, Gale JL (eds): *Medicine in Chinese Cultures.* US Dept HEW Pub (NIH)75-653, 1975.

Jew CC, Brody SA: Mental illness among the Chinese. 1. Hospitalization notes over the past century. *Compr Psychiatry* 8:129–134, 1967.

Kim BL: Asian Americans: No model minority. *Social Work* 18:44–53, May, 1973.

Kitano H, Sue S: The model minorities. *J Soc Issues* 29(2):1–9, 1973.

Koro Study Team. The Koro "epidemic" in Singapore. *Singapore Med J* 19(4):234–242, 1969.

Lapierre YD: Koro in a French Canadian. *Can Psychiatr Assoc J* 17:333–334, 1972.

Li F, Schlief Y, Chang CJ, et al: Health care for the Chinese community in Boston. *Am J Public Health* 62:536–539, 1972.

Lin T: A study of the incidence of mental disorder in Chinese and other cultures. *Psychiatry* 16:313–336, 1953.

Lin T, Lin M: Service delivery issues in Asian-North American communities. *Am J Psychiatry* 135(4):454–456, 1978.

Lo WH, Lo T: A ten-year follow-up study of Chinese schizophrenics in Hong Kong. *Br J Psychiatry* 131:63–66, 1977.

Lyman S: Red Guard on Grant Avenue: The rise of youthful rebellion in Chinatown, in Sue S, Wagner N (eds): *Asian American Psychological Perspectives*. Ben Lomond, Calif, Science and Behavioral Books, 1973.

Marsella AJ, Kinzie D, Gordon P: Ethnic variations in the expression of depression. *J Cross-Cult Psychol* 4(4):435–459, 1973.

Porkert M: *The Theoretical Foundations of Chinese Medicine*. Cambridge, MIT Press, 1974.

Reed TE, Kalant H, Gibbins RJ, et al: Alcohol and acetaldehyde metabolism in Caucasians, Chinese and Amerinds. *Can Med Assoc J* 115:851–855, 1976.

Rin H, Lin T: Mental illness among Formosan aborigines as compared with the Chinese in Taiwan. *J Ment Sci* 108:134–146, 1962.

Sue S, Kitano H: Stereotypes as a measure of success. *J Soc Issues* 29(29):83–98, 1973.

Sue S, McKinney H: Asian Americans in the community mental health care system. *Am J Orthopsychiatry* 45(1):111–118, 1975.

Sue S, Sue DW: MMPI comparisons between Asian-American and non-Asian students utilizing a student health psychiatric clinic. *J Counselling Psychol* 21(5):423–427, 1974.

Sung BL: *Chinese American Manpower and Employment*. Report to Manpower Administration, US Dept of Labor, 1975.

Sung BL: *Mountain of Gold: The Story of the Chinese in America*. New York, Macmillan, 1967.

Tseng W: The development of psychiatric concepts in traditional Chinese medicine. *Arch Gen Psychiatry* 29:569–575, 1973.

Tseng W: The nature of somatic complaints among psychiatric patients: The Chinese case. *Compr Psychiatry* 16(3):237–245, 1975.

Wolff PH: Ethnic differences in alcohol sensitivity. *Science* 175:449–450, 1972.

Wolff PH: Vasomotor sensitivity to alcohol in diverse mongoloid populations. *Am J Hum Genet* 25:193–199, 1973.

Yap PM: The Latah reaction. *J Ment Sci* 98:515–564, 1952.

Yap PM: Hypereridism and attempted suicide in Chinese. *J Nerv Ment Dis* 127:34–41, 1958a.

Yap PM: *Suicide in Hong Kong*. Hong Kong: Hong Kong University Press, 1958b.

Yap PM: Koro—a culture-bound depersonalization syndrome. *Br J Psychiatry* 111:43–50, 1965.

Yap PM: The culture-bound reactive syndrome, in Caudill W, Lin T (eds): *Mental Health Research in Asia and the Pacific*. Honolulu, East-West Center Press, 1969.

2 Japanese Americans

Joe Yamamoto, MD

The Japanese came to America with visions of golden streets and easy opportunity to earn their fortunes and then to return to their homeland. They were like the Chinese who preceded them. Because of this, they maintained their frugal ways. Belonging to visible minority groups, speaking languages that were unfamiliar and manifestly foreign to Americans, the Chinese and the Japanese were considered to be outsiders from the very beginning. The history of discrimination against minority Americans in the United States has included many phases and has varied from one part of the nation to another. Suffice it to say, where there have been minorities, there have been discriminations. Visible minorities, by which I mean those looking unlike the stereotypical European American, suffer everywhere. The sharpest discriminatory practices have been focused on varying minorities depending on religion, ethnicity, practices of the majority populations, and numbers involved in each geographic area.

One brief example of this is the experience of the Japanese on the mainland of the United States during World War II. Although the war began with the attack on Pearl Harbor in Honolulu, Hawaii, paradoxically the Japanese Americans in Hawaii were not "relocated" on a massive basis. In contrast, Japanese Americans, who comprised tiny minorities on the West Coast of the United States, were the focus of great hostility, physical abuse, and threats of all sorts. Indeed, they were relocated in the spring of 1942 to centers located in rural, isolated, desolate areas in the United States.

This experience has been told and retold with bitterness, vehemence, and more recently by the younger generation, with questions about why the relocation was not resisted (Weglyn 1976, Thomas 1952). Such a question is like asking why those who flee the onslaught of the rushing waters of the broken dam do not stay and resist. During the early part of World War II, most people on the Pacific Coast were extremely anxious about the possibility of enemy invasion, saboteurs, and destruction of vital armed force installations. Thus the smaller group on the mainland relative to the total population were evacuated to camps but those in Hawaii were not. The emotional growth of Japanese Americans in Hawaii must have taken a different turn as compared to the emotional growth of Japanese Americans on the mainland of the United States who have scars from the camp experience. The 117,000 Japanese Americans who were imprisoned in these relocation centers must have had a very special negative experience that shaped their psychosocial development, their degree of acculturation and, of course, vastly impoverished them financially (Conrat and Conrat 1972).*

The Japanese Americans have been able to enter some aspects of the mainstream of American life. A part of this has been possible because the old myth of the melting pot has been relinquished by most sophisticated Americans. Present-day awareness of the cultural pluralism of the people of the United States results in general acknowledgment that Americans come in different colors and two sexes, an awareness that has enriched the

---

*Although I have chosen to treat this experience of the Japanese Americans on the mainland of the United States in an impersonal manner, I experienced the relocation and remember what it was like. Being imprisoned for no reason other than that I was of Japanese ancestry was very trying (Yamamoto 1968). I felt depressed in being deprived of my identity as an American. It was a bad time for our entire family, including one brother who had been drafted into the American Army before World War II. Being bright and eager, he had been promoted to the equivalent of a buck sergeant's rating in the technical series. He continued with his group until the company was ready to be sent to the European theater. At that time, he was left behind, and all his colleagues were sent to fight the Germans and Italians in Europe. Later, my brother was sent to the Japanese language school and served in military intelligence until the end of the war, including service in the Pacific theater. He had been suspected of being disloyal with no evidence whatsoever. This is what all of us experienced. In fact even in the camps, Japanese Americans were asked if they were loyal or not. I will return to the effects of the relocation camp experience on the mainland Japanese Americans later in this chapter.

American vision of the ideal citizen beyond that of the past stereotype of the European American.

THE JAPANESE AMERICAN EXPERIENCE

Historical Background

Most of the large numbers of Japanese immigrated to the United States around the 1900s to both Hawaii and to the western coastal states of California, Oregon, and Washington. Like the Chinese, the Japanese also came to the United States hoping to work hard and to earn a fortune and then to return to Japan. Despite this, many of the Japanese additionally made decisions about getting married. Compared to the Chinese, a much larger percentage of the earlier pioneer Japanese immigrants married picture brides from Japan. This custom of the picture brides is interesting and is one of the many ways in which the background of the Japanese made them seem foreign compared to the Americans. The picture brides were selected by relatives at home and one chose on the basis of a photograph. What is not considered is that this social custom was within the social context of arranged marriages in Japan. The marriages of that time were arranged mainly by the parents of the bride and bridegroom with the official help of a go-between (Baishakunin). It was the go-between's responsibility to screen the prospective bride and bridegroom as to marriageability. Factors to be considered were the family backgrounds of the prospects and the potential for having healthy children. In other words, families where there were questions of hereditary illnesses, low social status, or impoverished status would be ruled out by the go-between. Viewed in this light, the custom of the picture bride does not seem quite as strange or exotic since this family orientation fits Japanese values.

The immigrants worked mostly in rural areas, being farm hands, doing the hard work that is a common lot of the most recent immigrant laborers. Both the Chinese and Japanese groups experienced considerable discrimination, prejudice, and disadvantage. For example, over the years, there were many specific laws limiting the rights of Asian Americans. These rights pertained to the numbers being permitted to come to the United States, issues such as ownership of land and areas of residence. Since in the past there was no such thing as equal housing opportunity, most of the Japanese lived in ghettos.

In Los Angeles, one such settlement was Little Tokyo. This is where I was born and raised. I remember as a child being aware of no paradoxes in growing up in a Japanese setting in the heart of Los Angeles. All of our neighbors were Japanese and indeed the students in the elementary school were at least 90% Japanese Americans. It was a rare Anglo or Hispanic student who added some ethnic difference to most classes in this setting. Indeed, to maintain the Japanese language, cultural heritage, and customs, most of the prewar Japanese students were sent to Japanese school, which supplemented the education in the regular American public school. The Japanese school was in session every afternoon after the American school, and on Saturdays for half a day. Here one learned proper Japanese manners, written and spoken Japanese, and something about the Japanese spirit.

Before the war, the Japanese were positively stereotyped by the majority of Americans. They were seen as hard working, conscientious, and clean citizens. Despite this, because of anti-Asian prejudices, it was unusual for Japanese Americans to be able to get jobs commensurate with their education. Many with college degrees worked as gardeners, clerks in fruit and vegetable stands, or in other stereotyped positions. The alternative was to work in Little Tokyo within the ethnic businesses.

Demographic Data

According to the 1970 census there were 591,290 Japanese in the United States. Most of the Japanese Americans lived in what the Census Bureau defined as the West which included the 13 western states and Hawaii. Actually, the vast majority of the 80% who lived in the "West" lived in Hawaii or California, with some in Oregon, Washington, and Colorado and relatively few elsewhere (*Pacific Citizen* 1979).

Legislative Background

The Japanese followed the Chinese to the United States. Both groups suffered the disadvantage of considerable legislative antipathy. There were acts to exclude Japanese and Chinese as immigrants to the United States. Other acts focused on preventing them from owning land. Still other legislative acts forbade interracial marriages. Indeed, the realities of the Japantowns and Chinatowns on the West Coast were dictated by legislative acts that forbade Asian residents in all but very limited residential areas. In addition these settlements also served as little islands of Asian cultures, which was positive for the residents. They served as an island of protection against discrimination.

Immigration, Adjustment, Acculturation

Most of the Japanese immigrated to the United States before 1924 when the Oriental Exclusion Act was passed. This is not to say that there have not been war brides since World War II or additional legal immigrants since the Oriental Exclusion Act was repealed, or to gainsay that there are many traders who are here on temporary visas from large Japanese corporations. The main group of Japanese Americans, those who are here in the United States to stay, had their roots before 1924. The adjustment of the first group of Japanese called the issei was quite different since most spoke very little English and maintained the culture, the customs, the values of Japan in isolated form (Yamamoto and Iga 1974). They brought over from Japan the conservative Meiji era values and because they were residentially, occupationally, and culturally isolated, their areas (for example, Little Tokyo in Los Angeles) were little islands of Japan, a conservative traditional society with little change over the decades (Yamamoto et al 1969). Here, one could live and die speaking only Japanese. Yet the Japanese did gradually acculturate. The second generation, the nisei, were educated in the American schools. This is described by Kitano (1969).

In many ways the Japanese Americans of the second generation lived two lives. First, they were expected to attend the regular American public schools. Second, the majority of students attended Japanese language schools in the afternoons and on Saturdays. In the Japanese schools, they learned the language, customs, and manners of Japan. This dual identity was a source of some conflict for the nisei since they wanted to become American and yet could not, because of the prevalent stereotype of the European American. Unconsciously, they must have strived toward Americanization and at times felt ambivalent about the Japanese heritage since this was not "American."

World War II and the incarceration of 117,000 mainland Japanese Americans in concentration camps scattered in rural areas throughout the United States changed the situation for the Japanese Americans. In these camps they had an acute identity crisis in being questioned concerning their loyalty with no realistic basis. American ideals of justice, liberty, and freedom for all were abrogated. The structure of the families changed with authority passing to those who spoke English and could deal with the heads of the wartime relocation administration. Most nisei were trying to be American but feared rejection outside of the camps.

The notable exception was a minority who because of the trauma of relocation decided to request return to Japan, described by Thomas and Nishimoto (1946). For most second-generation Japanese Americans there was no question about loyalty to the United States. It is now recognized that there were no incidents of sabotage, espionage, or disloyalty on the part of any Japanese American in Hawaii or on the mainland of the United States during World War II. The conflicts were much more subtle in trying to develop one's American identity and yet maintain the Japanese heritage—made even more difficult because the previous pattern of American public schools and Japanese schools was interrupted and eliminated. Subsequently, it was less popular to learn Japanese, and many advocated that all the Japanese Americans become "Americans," speaking only English. The third generation has thus lost much of its rich cultural heritage.

Myths and Realities – Mental Health Attitudes

After the end of World War II, James Clark Maloney (1945) went to the island of Okinawa. There, he admired the very close mother-infant interactions. The Okinawan mother carried the baby on her back with an *ombo* cloth. The baby was fed on demand, and Maloney felt that a child could not be raised in a more ideal way. On this visit to the island of Okinawa, he saw no psychotic patients. He therefore concluded that psychosis was absent in Okinawa and attributed it to the ideal mother-infant interaction. This paper was accepted and published in a major American journal. Fortunately, in subsequent years, Wedge (1952) did a study of the incidence of psychosis in Hawaii, comparing Okinawans with other ethnic groups there. He found no significant difference in the incidence of psychosis.

Thus, the idealized mother–infant interaction as viewed by Maloney was really not related to the diminution of the incidence of psychosis. This is but one example of the ways in which Asians have been stereotyped by professionals. Indeed, Tsuang (1976) points out that the incidence of schizophrenia is not that different from one part of the world to the next. Asian Americans have also been stereotyped as model minorities (Kitano and Sue 1973). It should be noted that the actual mental health of Asian Americans is a *terra incognita* because there are no good data concerning the epidemiology of psychiatric disorders among Asian Americans.

Implications for Mental Health Care

Throughout the United States, Asian Americans underutilize mental health services (Yamamoto 1978a). In the past it was assumed by the majority of professionals that Asian Americans generally did not need mental health services. More recently it has been recognized that Asian Americans who use mental health services (even when they are bilingual and bicultural) tend to be more chronically and more severely disturbed than most Americans (Kinzie 1974). Although this conclusion is not proof positive, it does suggest that this is part of the picture of underutilization of mental health services by Asian Americans. Asian Americans will not seek mental health services unless there is some acute and direct need, usually a social need, where the patient is causing trouble in the community, being aggressive toward the family, or causing a problem such as damaging property. The patients are not just psychotic, for often psychosis has been present for many years. The complaint is of unacceptable social behavior. Underutilization of mental health services must be emphasized, for where there are data about the utilization of mental health services comparing Asian Americans with most Americans, for example in Los Angeles County, the Asian Americans only use 40% of their proportion of mental health services (Mochizuki 1975). Implications are enormous and suggest that, even more so than in the majority American community, special efforts need to be undertaken to offer care for Japanese Americans and other Asians and Pacific Islanders.

MENTAL HEALTH NEEDS OF JAPANESE AMERICANS

Cross-Cultural Psychiatric Epidemiology

There are no hard data concerning the incidence of mental illness among Japanese Americans. According to the data presented in Hawaii concerning the use of mental health services, the mental health of Japanese Americans is assumed to be better than that of the rest of Americans. But this would be a gratuitous conclusion since the high stigma of mental illness has resulted in a more than usual reluctance to use mental health services. In Japan, hospitalized psychiatric patients have dramatically increased due to National Health Insurance (Yamamoto 1973). Studies of the inhabitants of midtown Manhattan by Srole et al (1975a) show that the incidence of emotional problems is high in urban settings.

Utilization of Mental Health Services by Japanese Americans

Underutilization is apparent. Recent figures from Hawaii suggest that the utilization rates there vary tremendously from one ethnic group to the next. Among the Caucasians, the utilization rate is 711 patients per 100,000 population. Among the Chinese, it is 131 per 100,000. Among the Japanese, 185 per 100,000, and Hawaiians including part-Hawaiians, 585 per 100,000. These figures illustrate underutilization of mental health services even as reported in 1977 (*Hawaii Statistical Supplement* 1977). Mochizuki (1975) also documented under-representation of Asian Americans in Los Angeles.

In reviewing the records at the Asian/Pacific Counseling and Treatment Center for a presentation at the American College of Neuropsycho-pharmacology in Maui, December 15, 1978, it was noted that of 398 patients who were seen in the first 14 months of operation of the clinic, approximately 201 were still being actively treated there. Approximately 100 of the 201 patients were Japanese or Chinese. In analyzing the medication requirements of these two ethnic groups, a review of the records shows that 33 of 100 were taking medication. There were 9 with affective disorders and 19 with functional psychoses, 4 having been diagnosed as being anxious and 1 having an organic brain syndrome. A review of the charts showed that the patients had been sick for 5 to 10 years and longer. Thus, it was evident there had been a tremendous stigmatization of mental health services and a disinclination to use the clinic services (Yamamoto et al 1978c).

Inner City Living Conditions and Mental Health

It is difficult to make definitive statements about the impact of the social ecology on mental health (Srole 1975). We must look at the advantages and disadvantages of inner city life. Indeed, the sparse data available tend to show that those who are not integrated in either community tend to be able to proceed.

Although I have no data to present, it is my impression that there is a double pressure on those who live in the Little Tokyos or Chinatowns in the United States. This pressure is related to the cultural conflicts between the Asian ways and the American ways. Despite these problems, the vast majority are able to progress. It is the person who lives on the fringes, not integrated and not part of the Japanese American community, who most often decompensates.

Implications for Mental Health Care

In the case of the Japanese Americans, it would be a tragedy to stereotype the group. There is considerable diversity beginning with the pioneers who originally came from Japan to the United States, the issei. Now, they are elderly since the last legal immigrants came to the United States in 1924. Just as among most Americans, the issei women outnumber the men in the population. In contrast to their cultural expectation of continuing care within the warmth and protection of the family, increasing numbers are being excluded and/or are living in separate quarters (see Vieth 1978 for confirming emphasis on filial piety). Examples in Los Angeles are the Little Tokyo Towers, a federally funded housing complex in the heart of Little Tokyo, where low-cost housing is available for the issei. This is an attractive new building with adequate facilities for independent living. It is a great shame that the inhabitants must lock themselves in for fear of being robbed or mistreated in some way. This is, of course, not a uniquely Japanese problem, but one faced by the elderly everywhere in the urban centers of America because of the breakdown of the respect for the elderly and the preying by the young upon the defenseless elderly. Another example in Los Angeles is the former Jewish Home for the Aged which was bought by the community and is now the Japanese Retirement Home. Here also, elderly Japanese live in a group situation where they can receive care for their basic needs and have meals together, but it is not the most cheery situation for all.

Many of the nisei have been able to achieve in terms of education and occupational advancement (Breslow and Klein 1971). The third generation, the sansei, pose different problems. They have become more Americanized and so suffer the problems that most young Americans do. Planning programs for individuals and for communities among the Japanese requires a thoughtful consideration of the different needs depending on generation, social class, geographic data, diagnostic situation, and so on. (Yamamoto 1978b).

First, let us consider the issue of individual therapy for Japanese patients. In 1966 I had the opportunity to observe how Japanese psychiatrists in Tokyo see their patients. I was fascinated by the interactions, for almost invariably the patients came with a relative. This troubled the Japanese psychiatrist not a whit! He bowed cursorily, and the patient bowed much more formally, acknowledging his subordinate position. Communications were directed to both the patient and the relative. The assumption was that the patient and the relative worked together. In contrast, most American psychiatrists have been taught to deal with the views only for special indications. Benedict (1946) pointed out this cultural difference eloquently: "Many attempts to understand the Japanese must begin with their version of what it means to 'take one's proper station.'" She felt that their emphasis on order and hierarchy and the contrasting emphasis in the United States on freedom and equality are polar opposites. She described how the Confucian emphasis on filial piety imported from China (a combination of Chinese Buddhism and Confuscian ethics was altered to fit into the emphasis of the Japanese on the family). Thus, in China, according to Benedict, the loyalty is to one's vast extended clan. This may number into the hundreds and thousands of people. The loyalty in Japan is to a more limited family, albeit not the nuclear family prevalent in 20th century America. Emphasis in Japan on the hierarchy is illustrated by Benedict's comments:

> Even today a father of grown sons, if his own father has not retired, puts through no transaction without having it approved by the old grand-

father. Parents make and break their children's marriages even when the children are thirty and forty years old. The father as male head of the household is served first at meals, goes first to the family bath, and receives with a nod the deep bows of his family.

In postwar Japan the customs have changed, but among the first generation issei the old customs live on. Benedict notes a "popular riddle in Japan which might be translated into our conundrum form: 'Why is a son who wants to offer advice to his parents like a Buddhist priest who wants to have hair on the top of his head?' [Buddhist priest had a tonsure]. The answer is, 'However much he wants to do it, he can't."

Now, given the different socialization of the Japanese in Japan, programs of mental health and individual therapy for Japanese Americans must focus on whether the individual being treated is mainly Japanese in values and thus needs to be viewed, from the standpoint of interdependencies, as a family member. The Japanese socialization practices are very clearly decribed by Lebra (1976).

The emphasis is on social interactions, interdependency, hierarchical relationships, and empathy (*omoiyari*). All of this is so different from the American emphasis on democracy and individuality that it would be difficult to understand a person from Japan without considerable cultural education, personal experience, and orientation.

In contrast, a second generation Japanese American or nisei has been socialized first with Japanese cultural values and second also with American values, thus having a combination of both Japanese and American cultures; the nisei would not view individual therapy as quite so alien. However, there are various issues that need to be considered, including the high stigma of mental illness. The concern about gossip in the community is great so that a Japanese person may be afraid to apply to a designated mental health service for fear of being labeled a mentally ill person. Despite this, depending on the social class and degree of education and sophistication, second-generation Japanese Americans are more likely to seek mental health services for less severe and less chronic conditions. A vast majority of second-generation Japanese Americans do speak English and can avail themselves of mental health services in the majority centers and also, if they are economically advantaged, from private practitioners.

The third generation (sansei) are more acculturated Japanese Americans and have essentially American views of life. Indeed, if you look at the data about the out-marriages in this generation, it is apparent on the mainland that most marry spouses who are not Japanese (Kikumura and Kitano 1973).

In Hawaii, out-marriages occur less often, perhaps because of the different experiences of the Japanese Americans there, who were not placed in concentration camps, and who do not experience the identity diffusion of a tiny minority population. Since Asian Americans are still in the majority there, the percentage of out-marriages is only 38.6% (Hawaii Statistical Report 1977).

The fourth generation yonsei have essentially acculturated so that they marry people outside of the ethnic group and identify with the majority of Americans. Their problems thus will be more similar to those prevalent in the majority of Americans. Examples are drug abuse, delinquency, personality disorders, and the usual neuroses and psychoses seen more proportionately. Here, the individual treatment program more often resembles that prescribed for the majority of Americans. Thus, what is needed is a very flexible and specific program depending on the ethnicity generation and social class (Gordon 1964).

Specific programs for those who are not acculturated and who do not speak English fluently must be planned. Here, due recognition of the high stigma of mental illness and the reluctance to use mental health services must be paramount. To overcome the high stigma, a consistent and effective program of community information is important. Areas such as Los Angeles, which have concentrations of Japanese Americans, have the advantage of the public media, including ethnic newspapers, radio stations, and television programs. All must be involved in the educational campaign to reduce stigma and facilitate mental health services. In addition, since the unacculturated Japanese Americans often have children or grandchildren who are acculturated, the majority media can also be used to publicize the mental health needs and the importance of overcoming the reluctance to use services in the community. Mental health professionals must reach out in the community and cannot maintain the static stance of waiting for patients to apply for mental health services in the clinic or hospital. Services must be available in outreach programs in the community in addition to the clinic. The promulgation of mental health services must be acceptable to Japanese Americans; thus, the emphasis must not be on mental illness labeling, but on self-improvement, tension reduction, and relief of psychosomatic symptoms, insomnia, and depression.

CULTURAL ASPECTS OF MENTAL HEALTH CARE

Cultural Aspects of Psychopathology

Among Japanese Americans in the more acculturated group, the expression of mental illness is similar to that of the majority of Americans. Among the issei and those who are not acculturated, there are some significant differences that may pose diagnostic problems. For example, the Japanese person, when confronted by an authority figure such as a psychiatrist, has been socialized to behave in a respectful, proper, deferential manner. Because of this, overt behavior may not fit the behavior commonly associated with patients who are, for example, depressed and have an agitated depression. Many years ago, I saw a patient who was 55 years old. She had been referred by a Japanese internist, and in her very deferential Japanese, she described having difficulty with insomnia. I spent perhaps 30 minutes interviewing this patient and could not get a better picture. She sat very quietly and comfortably in my office and was not at all complaining. (At that time, I saw patients without their families, as I had been trained.) Since the expected psychopathologic disorder was not apparent, I asked to get further information from her daughter. Only then did I realize that the patient suffered from all the signs and symptoms I had associated with agitated depression among most Americans. Having seen many such patients, I was surprised to find that this patient also had a similar syndrome, but her Japanese socialization had been such that in the presence of an authority figure she sat quietly, did not complain, and revealed very little of the signs and symptoms from which she suffered.

The unacculturated Japanese patient is likely to have been sick for a long period of time. Durations of illness of 5 to 10 years are not at all uncommon, and the patient may not be brought in unless he or she is causing a social disturbance. In addition, the patient may have suffered the social breakdown syndrome due to lack of social stimulation at home. It is less likely that the Japanese patient will be brought to mental health professionals for hospital care. Thus, even when chronically and seriously disordered, the patient may not have a history of recurrent hospitalizations.

Cultural factors may of course affect the symptoms. For example, a paranoid psychotic woman presented herself and insisted that she had been impregnated by an ancestor of the Emperor of Japan, the father of all the Japanese, but an ancestor! Affective disorders do occur among Japanese Americans and are a fairly common reason for first generation Japanese Americans to seek treatment, that is to say for severe depression or manic depressive disorders (Yamamoto et al 1969). In the treatment of Japanese Americans, relatives will be more frequently available to act as part of the treatment team. Especially in outpatient care, remember to involve them actively, advising them as to the do's and don'ts in helping the patient toward recovery.

Neuroses and psychosomatic illnesses are common in Japan. In fact, since mental illness is stigmatized, it is much more common to have a psychosomatic disorder with somatic symptoms or tension. Although there has been considerable concern in the Japanese American community in Southern California about the increasing incidence of drug abuse, it is significantly less than among the majority of Americans because drug abuse tends to be associated with marginality either in terms of socioeconomic status, or marginality in terms of one's position vis-a-vis others in the community.

The incidence of alcoholism is less than among the majority of communities as far as is known. Again, epidemiologic data are not available. The Hawaii *Statistical Report* (1977) shows fewer Japanese hospitalized for alcoholism. However, there is some evidence to suggest that Japanese Americans have a higher prevalence of allergic reactions to alcohol. It is not at all unusual to see Japanese Americans have one sip of a drink, turn beet red, and appear acutely uncomfortable. And if you would inquire, the symptoms may be dyspnea, tachycardia, nasal congestion, and subjective discomfort.

Special consideration of suicide in the Japanese community is warranted because of the long history of suicide as an acceptable way out. In the history of Japan, there are many examples of heroic suicide. Two hundred years ago, there were 47 *ronin* (masterless samurai) who established themselves as national heroes in avenging their lord and then committing suicide to atone for their misbehavior in the eyes of the Emperor. Thus, they exemplified the Japanese virtues of loyalty to the lord and also obedience to the Emperor. However, despite this and many other instances of heroic suicide in Japan, studies of suicide in Los Angeles have not shown that the Japanese commit suicide more often than others (Kitano 1969, Yamamoto 1973). When they do commit suicide, the unacculturated Japanese use Japanese methods—hanging, cutting, drowning, suffocating, jumping. The more acculturated Japanese Americans use the American ways of suicide—gunshot wounds, drug overdoses.

Kitano points out that the most common diagnosis of Japanese patients is schizophrenia, but he himself points out that the funneling effect occurs in mental health as in most social situations. He quotes from Cressey (1961), "The funneling effect through which the vast majority of people are screened so that what is observed is only the tip of the funnel which may or may not reflect the actual incidence of deviant behavior." At any rate, Kitano points out that schizophrenia is the most common diagnosis.

With current diagnostic techniques, there are many questions related to misdiagnoses of affective disorders as schizophrenia by American physicians in the first place. Second, there are language problems that compound the situation, and misdiagnoses must occur very often indeed. I observed a young Chinese woman who had been diagnosed schizophrenic and was prescribed fluphenazine enanthate at one of the California state hospitals. Even though I do not speak Chinese, a brief review of the history suggested the possibility of an affective disorder. I arranged for a Chinese doctor to interview the patient in Cantonese and it turned out the symptoms were mainly those suggestive of a severe depression with insomnia, guilt feelings, and so on. The fluphenazine was discontinued, and the patient was given a tricyclic antidepressant. She responded very well with symptomatic relief.

In addition to the potential for misdiagnosis by people who do not speak the language, the other aspect is that, until they are a great social problem, patients may not seek mental health services — part of the funnel effect. Thus we see only a small percentage of those who might seek services, and the ones we see may be those who are the most chronically and seriously disordered. Certainly this is in evidence in clinical practice among Asian Americans.

Among private patients, the frequency of psychotic depressions is impressive. Perhaps this is partly related to social class factors. This certainly needs to be kept in mind, in order to prescribe adequate treatment. There are reports from Japan that smaller doses of tricyclics are effective, possibly due to smaller body size or other physiologic factors.

Cultural Aspects of Family Response to Mental Illness

Among Japanese and Japanese Americans, the family response to mental illness is catastrophic. In Japan the picture of a marriageable family is one without the stigma of mental illness; therefore, the mentally ill are secluded and hidden away from society generally (Veith 1978). Only when they cause problems are they hospitalized. This is how it used to be in the past, but the number of inpatients in Japanese hospitals has risen dramatically during the last 15 years. At present, the Japanese have more people in psychiatric hospitals relative to their population than we do in the United States. Their population is 120 million and they have some 289,000 hospitalized patients (M. Kato, personal communication, 1979). In the United States, with a population of 220 million, the hospitalized population is approximately 125,000. As a generalization, the Japanese American family is more cohesive and therefore willing to help in any treatment plan advised that makes sense to them. Naturally, should the complaint be inappropriate to social behavior, this will be the top priority objective for the family. Even for severely psychotic patients, the family will attempt to cooperate in a program of outpatient treatment to try to obviate inpatient care. This applies both to patients who have been previously admitted and also to those who have never been admitted for inpatient care. Goldstein et al (1978) recommended family crisis therapy, which should be studied. The availability of support from the Japanese American social system is in great contrast to the picture with the majority of American patients seen in mental health services in California, where our patients are not only socially isolated from the general population but lack social supports generally, even from their own families.

PRACTICAL GUIDES IN THE CARE
OF JAPANESE AMERICAN PATIENTS

Overcoming the Stigma Barrier

Much has been written about the Japanese Americans and Chinese Americans as the model minority. Indeed, Kitano (1969) points out that Japanese Americans are under-represented in terms of social deviance and mental illness. However, he is aware that this may be related to the funnel effect and may represent a distorted view of all those in the community who might need care. Thus, priority for the treatment of Japanese Americans is a good educational campaign. That the response can change is evidenced in what had happened in Japan. There, national health insurance covers hospitalization. Most of the hospitals are private and relatively low-cost compared to American hospitals. There, patients stay a long time, much as they used to in American psychiatric hospitals 20 years ago. It is no wonder then, with the financing of national health insurance, that the number of beds has increased tenfold in the last 15 years so that there are now 289,000 inpatients in Japan with a population of only 120 million.

These data illustrate that usage patterns can be facilitated by national health insurance coverage and by acceptance of available inpatient services. In the United States, with the emphasis on community mental health, we will emphasize outpatient care, which is much more culturally syntonic. Education and promulgation of the availability of services of professionals (physicians, clergy, health care providers such as nurses, psychologists, social workers) are all important.

Flexibility in offering the services is also a paramount issue, since not everyone will come to a designated mental health clinic. In every instance where Asian populations including Japanese Americans are served, we have to expand our outreach efforts in locales where Japanese Americans are served; for example, in physicians' offices, community centers, or low-cost housing centers for the elderly. Certainly, outreach should be offered in services helping the elderly since they often have problems with transportation. In Los Angeles there are facilities at Little Tokyo Towers and the Japanese Retirement Home. A nursing home offers more intensive care for those who are bedridden or less ambulatory. In all of these settings, elderly people need help. However, we should be careful to destigmatize the services offered. For example, classes in memory training were offered to the elderly at the retirement home. This was a scientific study, (Yamamoto et al, unpublished research, 1979), but also offered something to the participants — many of whom were retired women, and some elderly men, whose average age was about 80 years. The research staff was especially cognizant of the importance of destigmatizing the services while trying to reinforce the efforts of the aged. The staff created a graduation ceremony, served cake and punch, and made certificates of accomplishment upon completion of the memory training course and the control group's completion of the relaxation training (Yamamoto et al 1977). Other efforts include community lectures about relaxation training and other ways of reducing hypertension. We need to take the lead in trying to teach the community how to cope with anxiety and depression and not to fear getting help for appropriate mental health needs.

Flexibility in offering services is something that must be faced, for just as some people from the majority community will not seek treatment, many Japanese will also avoid treatment (Yamamoto 1978c; Reiger et al 1978). Some sociologists might counter this by saying that these people do not suffer the stigma of mental illness labeling nor the dreaded social breakdown syndrome (which they assumed occurred only in hospitals), and that there is no such thing as mental illness.

However, with the available present knowledge, some patients who have not been treated might be helped through systematic efforts in offering psychotropic drugs and family counseling.

Overcoming the stigma will take a long time because it is also prevalent in the majority society, as can be seen by what happened to Senator Eagleton during his campaign for vice presidency. Mrs. Rosalyn Carter's heroic efforts toward reducing the stigma were shown in her testimony to Senator Edward Kennedy's Health Committee in 1979.

Overcoming the Language Barrier

This is a specific problem related to the unacculturated first-generation Japanese. In these instances, even those professionals who speak some Japanese may find it difficult to interview the patient because of the propensity to speak in a dignified, deferential and formal way, acknowledging the patient's subservience to the authority figure, the physician. When the mental health professionals do not speak Japanese, helpful diagnostic techniques have been developed. For example, the Psychiatric Status Schedule of Spitzer, Endicott, and Cohen has been translated into six different Asian languages, including Japanese. In addition, an audio-visual version is available with photographs illustrating the topic question. The patient may be asked questions about appetite and the photograph may have the word "appetite" in Japanese on top of a photograph of a plate of food. The voice on the audio tape asks in Japanese, "How is your appetite?" A volunteer can be trained to score the responses on the standard answer sheet, which can then be superimposed on the English answer key so that the mental health professional can tell the responses "true" or "false" for 320 items relevant to the mental status examination.

Should this be too cumbersome, there are other techniques, for example the Minnesota Multiphasic Personality Inventory (MMPI), which has been translated into Japanese, Chinese, and Korean. However, the norms are different. In the Japanese population, the normal population scores two standard deviations above the norm on the MMPI for Americans on the depression scale. Therefore, experience with this population is necessary for the MMPI to be used in a way that makes sense. In Japan, of course, they have their own version called the Tokyo Psychological Inventory.

In addition, for rough screening purposes, translations of the Symptom Check List 90 R (SCL-90 R) developed by Derogatis (1973) has been translated into six different Asian languages—including Chinese, Japanese, Korean, Samoan, Filipino, and Vietnamese. As yet, we do not have sufficient data with normal populations and with patient populations on the SCL-90 R to be able to do other than compare with the norms Derogatis has developed using 1000 psychiatric clinic outpatients and also 1000 normal subjects for comparison purposes. Since the SCL-90 R is based on symptoms commonly observed in nine categories (somatization, obsessive-compulsive, interpersonal sensitivity, depression, anxiety, hostility, phobic anxiety, paranoid ideation, psychoticism), it has some face validity. At any rate, it would be better than not being able to ask these questions in Japanese. Thus, having established something of the history through interpreters and through help of a family, and in addition, having these psychological test and interview data available, the language barrier can be overcome even by non-Japanese-speaking mental health professionals.

Establishing a Therapeutic Alliance

This is a very important issue with Japanese American patients, and again the generation and other factors must be considered. By this, we mean the degree of acculturation, education, and social class of the patient.

We must not stereotype all Japanese and offer a standard model of treatment for them. This would be a catastrophic mistake. Indeed, the unacculturated Japanese typically will come with a relative, and it would be a mistake for the mental health professional to act as if this is an American patient and insist upon seeing the patient individually. For the issei, the alliance is between the mental health professional and the family as a unit. With the therapist coaching, the family unit will act as a team toward the recovery of the patient.

As part of establishing an alliance, it is important to realize that the unacculturated Japanese have been socialized with nondemocratic social values; that is, they have learned the importance of hierarchical relationships, "knowing one's place" (Benedict 1946). Thus, the mental health professional must be flexible enough to be able to take over the role of someone who is authoritarian and directive and able to guide the family team toward therapeutic benefit. Nothing will make the Japanese family more insecure than a professional's hedging, hemming, and hawing and appearing insecure and unsure about the problem. Thus, for the benefit of the patient and the family, omnipotence in demeanor is sometimes indicated. (We really are not omnipotent, but sometimes we behave as if we were for the benefit of the patient.)

Engaging the Family

For the unacculturated patient, the family is the treatment unit. As we move to second-generation and the more acculturated third- and fourth-generation Japanese Americans, we must shift toward a more American and democratic emphasis on independence. Thus the interaction of the family will vary depending on the extent of acculturation and the specific family's needs from one end of the spectrum, a recognition of family interdependency, to the other extreme of American independency. All of this needs to be taken into account for therapy to be effective.

Psychotropic Drugs

Psychotropic drugs are an important issue. Through empirical practice, I have established that Japanese American patients do very well on levels of lithium 0.5 to 0.6 mEq in contrast to the commonly recommended levels of 0.7 to 1.2 mEq. It should be known that this has also been reported from psychiatrists in Japan (Takahashi 1978). Similarly, at the meeting in Maui, Hawaii, of the American College of Neuropsychopharmacology in 1978, there was a session discussing psychopharmacology in Japan and among Asian Americans in the United States. Here, experts in psychopharmacology attending the meeting also pointed out that the former levels recommended for serum lithium were too rigid (0.7 to 1.2), recommending more flexibility even among the majority of American patients.

Experience both in private clinical practice and in the Asian/Pacific Counseling and Treatment Center have shown that Asian American patients generally need less medication (Yamamoto et al 1979). For the same condition (whether depression, or mania, or psychosis) the amount of drugs prescribed is commonly much less than for the majority of Americans. Again, even in prescribing psychotropic drugs, it is important to consider the degree of acculturation and importance of primary family involvement, especially in the unacculturated Japanese family.

Hospitalizing a Japanese Patient

Shakespeare immortalized the phrase "To be or not to be, that is the question." In considering hospitalization of Japanese patients, we must ask: "To hospitalize or not to hospitalize." There are two issues to be considered: 1) the stigma of mental illness may result in avoidance of professional care so that even patients unable to care for themselves may be kept at home; 2) with the cohesive and caring attitudes of the majority of families, alternative care may be considered unless the patient may be dangerous to himself or to others. The stigma of mental illness is very real and may be avoidable if the family helps by seeing that the patient attends appointments, takes medication, engages in constructive daily activities, and if the family provides the necessary supervision of the patient. (Vaughn's findings will be considered for Japanese patients in the future.)

Not enough has been written to describe the trauma experienced by the family in having a member be admitted to a psychiatric unit in a general hospital and (commonly in California and all other states) then be sent on to a state hospital, where mental health professionals who speak Asian languages are not so available. Thus, hospitalization is viewed as a last resort, when it is a question of life or death as indicated by serious suicidal trends, serious homicidal trends, or incapacity to care for oneself.

A great deal of work needs to be done with the family, since the custom in Japan has been that even patients who are admitted to hospitals do not lose contact with their families (Veith 1978). In the past, they did not have the American custom of limiting visitations, or trying to cut the ties with the family in the case of psychiatric hospitalization. Ilza Veith (1978) explains this in the American custom of blaming the family. The custom in Japan is to maintain contact. There, in the medical wards, it is common to have some family member have a bed in the room to sleep with the patient. This may sound strange to Americans but follows the Japanese customs where the families do sleep together. The family member prepares food that is familiar to the patient so that even though the patient is hospitalized, the close family ties are maintained at a different site. Since language may pose a problem, it is important to obtain the help of either mental health professionals or volunteers who speak the language. Certainly, the feeling of isolation and loneliness for a Japanese person to be in a hospital with no one who speaks the language cannot be overemphasized. The experience can be extremely anxiety-provoking and stressful.

Prescribing Culturally Relevant Treatment

With Japanese patients, especially those who are not acculturated to American society, we need to consider important contributions by Japanese psychiatrists. For example, Shoma Morita originated a form of Japanese psychotherapy for patients who have psychasthenia, which the Japanese call *shinkeishitsu* (Reynolds and Yamamoto 1973), a form of compulsive neurosis with aspects of neurasthenia. Morita initiated this form of therapy over 50 years ago in Tokyo. It was inpatient treatment in which the patient was isolated from his or her family. This phase lasted perhaps a week or two and in our view was a source of motivation toward therapeutic change, for never before had the Japanese patient been so socially isolated. Always he had grown up in a family context, first at home, then later in school, and subsequently at work. Morita and his therapy advocated that the Japanese patient be aware that one's feelings are the same as the Japanese sky and instantly changeable. One cannot be responsible for how one feels, but one is responsible for what one does. This emphasis on achievement fits the Japanese cultural values. Thus at the end of therapy, the patient focuses more on what is being done and less upon one's inner feelings, symptoms, concerns, or obsessive thoughts. Subsequent to the treatment phase in the hospital the patient becomes a part of the Morita family and attends group sessions on Sundays. The reason for the meetings on Sundays is that in Japan, the custom is to work six days a week including Saturdays.

Morita therapy is mentioned briefly as a form of treatment that fits the cultural values. How can we do this with patients who are Japanese Americans and more acculturated? The principal issues are related to Japanese families with interdependency. Even among the acculturated, this is more of an issue than among the majority of Americans and less than among the unacculturated Japanese Americans. Close family ties and interdependency are important issues. One would think carefully before recommending the American standards of independency for Japanese Americans except for those who have become fully acculturated. One therefore must use a combination of the use of psychodynamic understanding, supportive psychotherapy, and also an understanding of the needs for an authoritarian, omnipotent, and directive therapist. These are generalizations; one may adopt the opposite extreme of relatively passive, neutral, nonjudgmental, noncritical therapy for a specific Japanese American patient. Certainly in long-term relationships, the giving of gifts to authority figures is culturally sanctioned. It would be offensive not to accept a gift in this context. In addition, greeting cards for the seasons are an acknowledged part of the custom to maintain the relationship over the years.

It is important to remember William Caudill's observations of the socialization of Japanese babies (Caudill 1969). Caudill studied Japanese mothers and infants and compared the behavior of these middle-class pairs with American middle-class mothers and infants. Interestingly, he learned that the Japanese child is socialized to be quiet and contented. The American baby on the contrary is encouraged to be active, happy, and vocal. The relevance of these anthropologic observations is that some Japanese patients may not come to therapy with the idea of a talking cure. Indeed, for some, this notion may seem strange. Therefore, we must offer all sorts of treatments that make sense to us including, for example, biofeedback, a technological adaptation of the laying on of hands encountered in many of the indigenous therapies in Japan. The mode used at the Asian/Pacific Counseling and Treatment Center is electromyogram biofeedback for the relief of muscle tension symptoms. In addition, relaxation tapes have been translated into Japanese so that patients can borrow the tapes and use them for a modification of the relaxation therapy advocated by Wolpe and others.

Because of the importance of acupuncture, we proposed a study of acupuncture on neurotic Asian outpatients, but it was disapproved (which may be due to a lack of cultural sensitivity on the part of the reviewing committee). This came at a time when a report by Kane and De Scipio (1977) reported on acupuncture in the treatment of schizophrenia. Rather than to get on a discussion on the merits of acupuncture, we must realize that it is a culturally accepted form of therapy. I am delighted to be able to report that Sanford Tom, MD, in San Francisco has received a state-assisted grant to offer acupuncture in his Chinatown Acupuncture Mental Health Clinic. I believe that acupuncture needs to be offered in a setting like the Asian/Pacific Counseling and Treatment Center to encourage patients to come in for appropriate help. In the future, perhaps scientific studies will be done to establish the indications for acupuncture in psychiatry.

Follow-Up Care

The care of Japanese American patients is quite diverse. Some maintain a continuity either by mail or contact indirectly over many years. Those who need continuing care, of course, may be seen at progressively increasing intervals. Now with the findings of Brown, Birley, Wing (1972), and others about the importance of family social setting for the precipitation of recurrent schizophrenic and affective symptoms, we must be aware that in offering follow-up care the family is important even for the acculturated patient. For the latter, it is not necessarily in terms of the family team as a treatment unit, but we must show sensitivity about the possible tension-producing effects of a highly emotional family member interacting with a patient. Crisis therapy helps families to help the members who are patients.

The author gratefully acknowledges the technical assistance of William Liu, PhD, Director, Asian American Mental Health Research and Development Center, and Freda Cheung, PhD, Center for Minority Group Mental Health Programs, National Institute of Mental Health. Supported in part by UCLA Biomedical Research Support Grant, Reliability of the Psychiatric Status Schedule in Japanese, and National Institute of Mental Health Grant, Psychiatric Status Schedule in Asian/Pacific Languages.

BIBLIOGRAPHY

Benedict R: *The Chrysanthemum and the Sword*. Cambridge, Mass, Riverside, 1946.

Breslow L, Klein B: Health and race in California. *Am J Public Health* 61:736–775, 1971.

Brown GW, Birley JLT, Wing JK: Influence of family life on the course of schizophrenic disorders: A replication. *Br J Psychiatry* 58:121–124, 1972.

Caudill W, Weinstein H: Maternal care and infant behavior in Japan and America. *Psychiatry* 32:12–43, 1969.

Conrat R, Conrat M: *Executive Order 9066: The Internment of 110,000 Japanese Americans*. Los Angeles, Anderson, Ritchie & Simon, 1972.

Cressey D: Crime, in Merton, R Nisbet R (eds): *Contemporary Social Problems*. New York, Harcourt, Brace and World, 1961, pp 21–26.

Derogatis L, Lipman R, Covi L: SCL-90: An outpatient psychiatric rating scale. *Psychopharmacol Bull* 9(1):13–28, 1973.

Goldstein MJ, Rodnick EH, Evans JR, et al: Drug and family therapy in aftercare of acute schizophrenics. *Arch Gen Psychiatry* 35(10):1169–1177, 1978.

Gordon M: *Assimilation in American Life*. New York, Oxford University Press, 1964.

Hawaii Dept of Health: *Statistical Report Supplement*. Department of Health, State of Hawaii, Table 7, 1977.

Hawaii Dept of Health *Statistical Report*. Department of Health, State of Hawaii, 1977.

Kane J, and De Scipio WJ: Acupuncture treatment of schizophrenia: Report on three cases. *Am J Psychiatry* 136:297–302, 1977.

Kawaguchi P, Nishi S, Schmitt R: *Population Characteristics of Hawaii 1977*. Honolulu, Hawaii State Department of Health and Department of Planning and Economic Development, January 1979.

Kikumura A, Kitano HHL: Interracial marriage: A picture of Japanese Americans. *J Soc Issues* 29:67–81, 1973.

Kinzie JD: A summary of literature on epidemiology of mental illness in Hawaii, in Tseng WS, McDermott J, Jr, Maretzki T (eds): *People and Cultures of Hawaii.* Honolulu, Department of Psychiatry, University of Hawaii School of Medicine, 1974.

Kitano HHL: *Japanese Americans: The Evolution of a Subculture.* Englewood Cliffs, NJ, Prentice-Hall, 1969.

Kitano HHL, Sue S: Model minorities. *J Soc Issues* 29(2):pp 1-9, 1973.

Lebra TS: *Japanese Patterns of Behavior.* Honolulu, University Press of Hawaii, 1976.

Maloney JC: The psychology of the Okinawan. *Psychiatry* 8:391, 1945.

Mochizuki M: Discharges and units of service by ethnic origin: Fiscal year 1973-1974. County of Los Angeles Mental Health Service, Research and Information Section, *E & R Rows and Columns* 3(11):1-15, 1975.

Reiger DA, Goldberg ID, Taube CA: The de facto U.S. mental health services system: A public health perspective. *Arch Gen Psychiatry* 35(6):685-693, 1978.

Reynolds D: *Morita Psychotherapy.* Berkeley, University of California Press, 1976.

Reynolds D, Yamamoto J: East meets West: Moritist and Freudian psychotherapies, in Masserman JH (ed): *Research and Relevance, vol 21. Science and Psychoanalysis.* New York, Grune & Stratton, 1972.

Reynolds D, Yamamoto J: Morita psychotherapy in Japan, in Masserman JH (ed): *Current Psychiatric Therapies,* vol 13. New York, Grune & Stratton, 1973.

Srole L: Measurement and classification in social psychiatric epidemiology: Midtown Manhattan study (1954) and midtown re-study II (1974). *J Health Soc Behavior* 16:347-364, 1975a.

Srole L: *Mental Health in the Metropolis.* New York, Harper & Row, 1975b.

Takahashi R: Lithium treatment of affective disorders in therapeutic plasma levels. Presented at American College of Neuropsychopharmacology, Maui, Hawaii, December, 1978.

Thomas D: *The Salvage.* Los Angeles, University of California Press, 1952.

Thomas D, Nishimoto R: *The Spoilage.* Los Angeles, University of California Press, 1946.

Tsuang M: Schizophrenia around the world. *Compr Psychiatry* 17:477-481, 1976.

Veith I: Psychiatric foundations in the Far East. *Psychiatr Ann* 8(6):12-41, 1978.

Wedge B: Occurrence of psychosis among Okinawans in Hawaii. *Am J Psychiatry* 109:255, 1952.

Weglyn M: *Years of Infamy: The Untold Story of America's Concentration Camps.* New York, William Morrow, 1976.

Yamamoto J: Japanese-American identity crises, in Brody EW (ed): *Minority Group Adolescents.* Baltimore, Williams & Wilkins, 1968.

Yamamoto J: Psychiatry in Japan—a transcultural evaluation. *Psychiatric Opinion* 10(4):15-17, 1973.

Yamamoto J: Research priorities in Asian American mental health delivery. *Am J Psychiatry* 135(4):457-458, 1978a.

Yamamoto J: Therapy for Asian Americans. *J Natl Med Assoc* 70(4):267-270, 1978b.

Yamamoto J: Mental Health Needs of Asian Americans and Pacific Islanders. Presented to Task Force on Health and Mental Health of Asian Americans and Pacific Islanders, Advisory to the Asian American Mental Health Research Center, Chicago, November 1978c.

Yamamoto J, Fung D, Lo S, et al: Psychopharmacology for Asian Americans and Pacific Islanders. *Psychopharmacol Bull* 15:29–31, 1979.

Yamamoto J, Iga M: Japanese enterprise and American middle-class values. *Am J Psychiatry* 131(5):577–579, 1974.

Yamamoto J, Okonogi K, Iwasaki T, et al: Mourning in Japan. *Am J Psychiatry* 125(12):74–79, 1969.

Yamamoto J, Reece S, Ishikawa T: Memory Training for the Japanese Elderly. Unpublished research, 1977.

Yamashita I, Asano Y: Tricyclic antidepressants: Therapeutic plasma level. Presented at the American College of Neuropsychopharmacology Meeting, Maui, Hawaii, 1978.

3 Filipino Americans

Enrique G. Araneta, Jr, MD

THE FILIPINO IMMIGRANT

Racial and Cultural Roots

To understand properly the Filipino immigrant it is necessary to be acquainted with the Filipino: where he comes from, his historical background, and his racial and cultural heritage. The Philippine Archipelago consists of more than 7000 islands, and over 87 different dialects are spoken throughout this archipelago (Bram et al 1977). Indeed, it was not until the advent of colonization by Spain and the United States that a sense of national identity and unity developed among the people of this archipelago. Before the onset of western rule each island and region in the Philippines had its own clans and tribes with their own languages and customs. Since the major dialects are of Malayan and Polynesian derivation, the popular assumption is that these people made up the dominant group from whom most Filipinos are descended (Bram et al 1977). There were, however, other groups.

Scholars of Asian history and anthropology generally agree that the original settlers of the Philippine Archipelago were Negritos. They were believed to have come some 25,000 years B.C. by way of a land bridge that extended from the Asian continent. These people have similar physical characteristics to the pygmies of Africa, and have managed to live a nomadic existence in small tribes up to the present time. (They now provide instruction to United States airmen on jungle survival techniques.) The next wave of settlers, made up of Mongoloid tribes from Southeast Asia, arrived about 15,000 B.C. or 10,000 years after the Negritos. Larger groups of settlers from present-day China and Viet Nam arrived about 7000 and 2000 B.C. However, the largest group of settlers was made up of successive waves of invaders from the islands of Indonesia and the Malay Peninsula around the second and third century B.C. (Bram et al 1977). It is from these groups that most of present-day Filipinos are supposed to have descended.

The islands were discovered for Spain in 1521 by the Portuguese navigator Magellan. An intensive campaign to control the archipelago was forged by Spain and effected successfully by the Catholic missionaries. It was through a brand of Catholicism that reinforced dependence, conformity, and fear that Spanish rule was successfully effected and western Christian values inculcated. Spanish rule extended more than 300 years, during which time the history of the Philippines closely resembled that of the other Spanish colonies of the Caribbean and Mexico. Indeed, most Filipinos have Spanish names, and many Spanish traditions have become incorporated as customs in what present-day Filipinos like to think of as part of their cultural heritage (Bram et al 1977).

The acquisition of the islands by the United States through the Treaty of Paris added still another dimension to the evolution of the Filipino character and culture. Although a participatory democracy was introduced, promising eventual individual and national freedom, nonetheless the economic impositions wielded by America reinforced the attitude of dependence and subservience that is popularly referred to as the colonial mentality (Lott 1976). The establishment of a public school system with English as the medium of instruction and a curriculum utilizing American textbooks conspired to establish an American ego ideal in the evolving Filipino identity. Thus we see that the Filipino comes from a diversity of racial stock and represents a diversity of influences from the cultural standpoint, incorporating both oriental and occidental ideals. Also, by virtue of the separateness of the various islands that make up the archipelago, we find a regional differentiation that has been influenced by the acculturation process peculiar to and related to the economic involvement of the particular region. We find certain regions that manifest more Spanish influence, other regions that show more American influence, and still others that show more Chinese influence, and so on. Despite this diversity of cultural, economic, and regional groupings, there are common traditional beliefs and attitudes that seem to transcend these regional differences (Lott 1976). Among these are:

1. A strong kinship that extends and embraces distant relations, *parientes,* and even religiously defined relationships such as compadres, hijados, and padrinos. These strong bonds among extended family members are probably reflective of the old clan system that formed the basis of the original social organization before colonization.
2. A spirit of mutuality and togetherness among members of communities. This tradition is referred to as *bayanihan* or *pagkikisama.*
3. *Utangnaloob,* meaning a deep sense of gratitude, a need for reciprocity of favors.
4. Respect and reverence for elders (Filipino words *taha* or *respeto*). This tradition probably traces back to the Chinese and is further reinforced by the Roman Catholic Church. The next tradition is closely related.
5. A strong supernatural orientation, a strong faith in divine justice, the inevitability of retribution (Filipino saying, "Man proposes, God disposes").
6. *Hiya,* which, although it translates to the term shame, is really a much more intense and well-defined emotional experience with tremendous social implications, so that when one is referred to as *walanghiya* it means that the person is without shame, lacks the capacity to be socialized, and therefore deserves isolation and exclusion (Marsella 1974).

According to Marsella,

> One interpretation of this is that the name may be used as a technique of social control more often in Oriental societies, and children consequently learn to read the organismic and situational cues more readily. Another interpretation is that Oriental groups may be better able to read somatic cues associated with shame and thus experience it more clearly. In addition, shame may be more of an all-or-none phenomenon among Orientals. The situations in which it can occur may be more clearly identifiable, and the consequences of its occurrence may be more severe.

These traditions emphasize interdependence and conformity to normative ideals. They emphasize, and seem to be productive of, a collective rather than an individual consciousness, and have resulted in what Bulatao (1964) refers to as "the unindividuated ego of the Filipino."

Filipino Immigration to the United States

The first group of Filipino immigrants to the United States were farm laborers with little or no education. Between 1907 and 1926 the Hawaiian Sugar Planters Association brought 100,000 Filipinos to Hawaii (Amaranto et al 1978). In addition, many Filipinos were brought to the farmlands of California and the fisheries of Alaska (Kim 1973). They provided a cheap source of labor much needed at that time, since formal slavery had been abolished. These immigrants were motivated to get out from the oppressive feudal system in the Philippines. They were lured by the promise of democracy and equal opportunity and the hope of finding social and financial advancement.

As citizens of a United States territory, the Filipinos were referred to as nationals (Kim 1973). This ambiguous status technically conferred upon them the rights and privileges of citizens, except for the right to vote, the right to own property, and the right to marry a white woman. The absence of voting rights prevented the Filipino from participating in political decisions affecting himself (Kim 1973, Lott 1976). Consequently, unlike European immigrants, the Filipino found little incentive to assimilate into American society or learn the American political system (Lott 1976). This, coupled with the lack of means to acquire citizenship, reinforced the sense of being transients, sojourners, unfit for assimilation into American society. The fact that he could not own property and start a family (because of the miscegenation laws) precluded the development of a stable Filipino community. The young, single, mobile-employment males of this group, having no sense of permanence, were therefore not able to establish a stable social organization as did the Japanese and Chinese. Most of the immigrants in this group found their way into the edge of low-income, nonwhite neighborhoods, or in red-light districts (Lott 1976). This wave of immigration came to an abrupt end in 1935, when deferred independence was granted to the Philippines and immigration was restricted to 50 annually (Amaranto 1978).

The second wave of immigrants came between 1935 and 1956. They consisted of farm laborers, recruits to the U.S. Navy during the Cold War of the early 1950s, and students seeking higher education after World War II (Amaranto 1978). This latter group, having been schooled in American-established public schools, were more conversant with American customs and, as a group, had better command of the English language.

The third wave of Filipino immigration started in the late 1950s and escalated by 1965 as a result of legislation relaxing immigration quotas among Asians. This group filled the need for trained professional manpower (Amaranto 1978).

The Filipino Community in the United States

Except for the latest group of immigrants, about 25,000, most Filipinos have settled at the urban ports of entry of the first generation immigrants and near the fields where they toil. The largest concentrations are in Hawaii and San Francisco. According to Lott (1976):

> Conditions in the present community are not greatly different from conditions extant at the time of the first generation....The ratio of males to females is 10 to 9. Among the elderly the ratio is 4.5 to 1. This ratio probably can be accounted for by the non-quota migration of wives after World War II which increased the women and, of course, the subsequent generation of Filipinos.
>
> On the mainland, 36% are children 18 and under. In Hawaii, children of these ages are at a high of 42%. In female-headed families the proportion reaches 69%.
>
> The Filipino families tend to be larger than total United States families and other Asian families, with over one-third of Filipino families containing five or more members. The ratio of extended families in the Filipino community is also greater than total United States families and other Asian families. The ratio of interracial marriage is high for both Filipino men and women, 33% and 28% respectively.
>
> Educational characteristics of the Filipino community can be described only in terms of three population groups: first generation — among Filipinos 65 years old and over, the median years of completed schooling is 5.4 (not even completion of elementary school); the second and third generations — among Filipinos 18 to 24 years old, college enrollment is below the United States population average, 28% for Filipino men as opposed to 37% for U.S. men, and 23% for Filipino women as opposed to 27% for U.S. women.

Two-fifths of all employed Filipino men are in low-skilled, low-paying jobs, twice the rate of the total United States male population. From 1960 to 1970, labor force participation of married Filipino women jumped from 6% to 46%.

With 40% of Filipino men earning less than $4000 a year, their income level is less than the average for the total United States population. In female-headed families of the Filipino community, 46% have incomes of less than $4000. Income levels have not kept up with the educational attainment of the Filipino community. Of all Filipino elderly, 25% live in poverty.

Over a quarter of Filipino households are substandard. In Hawaii and San Francisco, where they can be found in large concentrations, Filipinos reside in dwellings of which 40% and 30% respectively are substandard.

Unlike other communities, in which only the new immigrants must start from the lower levels, in the Filipino community social and economic advancement and high educational attainment have been achieved solely by the new immigrants. The second and third generations are merely a cut above the first generation. Perhaps this is to be expected in a population group in which the immigrants comprise more than half the population, and which has no stable American-born and -reared community. Yet this can only be a partial reason.

These conditions do not paint a pretty picture of the Filipino community. Filipinos have been in the United States for at least three-quarters of a century, yet overall conditions are not greatly different from conditions at the time of the first generation. So writes Lott (1976), and she concludes, "The Filipino community still is a low-income, low-achievement group."

ACCULTURATION DIFFICULTIES

Westernization of Philippine Society

To evaluate properly the acculturation process undergone by the Filipino immigrant, it is necessary to understand the social dynamics existing in the Philippines. The Filipinos have for 400 years been monitoring their lives in accordance with behaviors and attitudes shown them by western colonial masters (Rizal 1950). Spanish colonization was characterized by authoritarianism and possessiveness directed toward shaping the Filipinos as obedient children or servants (Rizal 1950). Indeed, the term *Filipino* was coined originally to denote a person of Spanish descent born in the Philippines (Bram et al 1977). History attests to the valiant effort on the part of the colonizers to propagate Filipinos, or *mestizos,* as they are now called.

Meanwhile, as the term *Filipino* expanded its meaning to include other members of the population who did not trace genetically to the Spanish colonists, nonetheless, Spanish names were given to these people. Only the very remote villages escaped this extremely incorporative colonization process. What resulted (as described in Rizal's many books) was that a national identity was being shaped by the Spanish colonizers for the Philippines. The inhabitants suffered from a sense of personal ambiguity that was for the most part resolved by the adoption of the "Little Brown Brother identity" (Amaranto 1978), reflecting what is popularly referred to as the colonial mentality (Lott 1976). This mentality is characterized by an effort to imitate and assume the characteristics of the colonial master, while simultaneously resenting his authority and its symbols (Singer and Araneta 1967). The institution of the feudal system in the development of the agrarian economy of the Philippines resulted in a power structure that accentuated the sociocultural differentiation between the westernized urban dweller and the more traditional remote villagers. American control of the island further accentuated this urban-rural dichotomy in acculturation to western social and institutional patterns.

As industrialization progressed, western values became increasingly more relevant to the problems of living in the urban area. The result has been the incorporation of more western values, ideals, and style of interrelating in the urban Philippine culture (Marsella et al 1972). Meanwhile, the rural dwellers became the subject of the colonization process by the urban Filipinos and the American masters. Thus, we find that, even before the start of the immigration of the first group to this country, there existed in the Philippines a social continuum that ranged from the highly westernized, socioeconomically advantaged group to a traditional, unwesternized, economically deprived group. Simultaneously, we find a process of emergence from the colonial mentality of the latter group toward an unintegrated westernized pragmatic view of the more economically advantaged group.

From the standpoint of acculturation, it is not difficult to understand why the first group of immigrants, which consisted mainly of farm laborers, would encounter great problems, while the more recent, mostly urban professional immigrant group would have the least difficulty (Smith, Kline, and French 1978).

The study of Amaranto (1978) on the mental health of Filipinos in the New York metropolitan area, involving mainly recent immigrants, shows that on the basis of questionnaires and interviews their "findings are well within the norm compared to figures from prevalent studies of mental illness in the general population." According to the conclusion of the study, these immigrants ranked their problems as "1) loneliness and homesickness; 2) language difficulty; 3) work accessibility; 4) racial discrimination." In their list of perceived problems, "adjustment to the American way of life" ranked only fifth. The others are attributable to spatial dislocation and political issues of discrimination, showing that acculturation demands do not constitute the major difficulty for this group. However, in the case of the first group of immigrants, the problem of acculturation has been a particularly stressful and, at times, overwhelming experience. Since this group traced back to a less educated socioeconomically disadvantaged sector of Philippine society, they were least westernized in their views and were least prepared for assimilation into United States society (Lott 1976; Marsella and Gordon 1973). Faced with the discriminatory legislation imposed on them, they were torn between retreat to "cultural persistence" or submission to the colonized role. The conflict is reflected in the "high rate of confusional states" reported by Opler (1956) who writes, "High rates in lower-class Filipinos of affective disorders and catatonic confusional states were present among Hawaiians hospitalized."

Cultural Factors Influencing Difficulties in Acculturation

Some culturally-determined factors that predisposed this group to psychiatric difficulties include:

1. As a result of strong family ties and strong reliance on interdependence within the kinship structure, members of this group were not prepared to establish other forms of social organizations in the absence of a family patriarch. This resulted in loss of sentiment for obtaining social order, love, a feeling of belongingness, and physical security, and resulted in culturally incongruent acting-out behaviors and in affective disorders (Marsella and Gordon 1973).

2. As a result of long years of subservience and conformity to the omnipotent powers (God and the white man), a passive personality pattern characterized this group, thus interfering with their securing recognition for economic security or effective expression of hostility (Marsella and Gordon 1973). This could have been a big factor in the high incidence of "catatonic confusional states and depression" (Opler 1956).

3. As a result of conditioning to a social control by the experience of a deep sense of shame, *hiya* (Marsella et al 1974) members of this group experienced failures more keenly and were driven to suicide, or amok behaviors, otherwise referred to as *juramentado*. This is characterized by a person who has been shamed, running wild and killing people who may have contributed to his having been reduced to this position of shame, expecting to get killed in the process. Although this behavior was once thought to be a culture-bound phenomenon, occurring only among Malayans, especially among the Moslem group, we know that this behavior results from a feeling of desperation as has been recently, quite frequently, noted in this country, as in the case of the " Texas gunman" and a number of other desperate people.

4. Also, because of the strong interdependence that characterizes family members, Filipinos have been described to have a collective rather than individuated ego (Marsella et al 1974). In the face of a highly individualistic culture one can readily see that members of this group found a lack of opportunity to experience sentiments of belongingness, especially to a moral order where sentiments of unselfishness can be rewarded. Such a situation could not afford a better opportunity for an identity crisis (Marsella et al 1972).

5. Because members of the first immigrant group were faced with the legislation against cohabiting with white women and living in Hawaii or the West Coast, where opportunity for mating with other women was

greatly restricted; this situation afforded these people very little opportunity for seeking sexual satisfaction (Kim 1973).

Mental Health Problems of Special Groups

In addition to the acculturation problems of the transplanted traditional Filipino villager and the urban professional, there are specialized acculturation problems that face certain groups. One of these is the second or following generation, the Filipino adolescent. He has the special problem of forming an identity, a problem that involves a conflict between school and peer influence against family and tradition, and a struggle between individual autonomy (a characteristic of this culture) as opposed to a definition of self in terms of membership in a greater social group or family. Contrary to the previous observations that Asian adolescents are in general conforming, respectful of authority, and generally docile, rebellious and disruptive behaviors are now being observed quite frequently (Kim 1973).

Another group with specialized mental health problems involves those who contracted interracial marriages. Their major problem centers on differing sex-role expectations. For example, a Filipino husband is likely to appreciate his wife's devotion if she makes housekeeping and child-rearing her primary concern. On the other hand, if she sought a job to meet more effectively the needs of the family, which is financial relief, the husband could very well feel offended. In the case of a Filipina married to a white man the reverse would be true—that is, if her husband allowed her to work she might feel that her husband did not care enough to keep her completely to himself by keeping her at home. These differences in sex-role expectation become especially crucial because of the extended family's expectations that their attitudes be considered by the interracial couple.

Still another problem is the case of the old and married farm worker when he is no longer effective at work and must move to the city to be near medical and social facilities that would be of help to him (Kim 1973). He faces the problem of adjusting to an urban culture, which usually is much more impersonal and where his status takes a decided drop.

THE MENTAL HEALTH OF THE FILIPINO AMERICAN

Incidence and Special Problems of Diagnosis

Data on the prevalence of mental illness among Filipino Americans are woefully inadequate. It is generally accepted that the morbidity for psychotic and neurotic disorders is probably comparable with the rate of the general population (Opler 1956), or possibly even higher, as in the case of the other economically disadvantaged minorities. However, recent studies show that the percentage of identified cases fall short of the average for the general population. Two factors have been advanced to explain this finding: 1) the reluctance of Filipinos to get help or even be recognized as having mental disorders; and 2) difficulty in recognizing these disorders when they are present. In any event, early treatment of psychiatric disorders among Filipinos is seldom effected, with consequent tendencies toward chronicity. Studies of Yamamoto in Los Angeles indicate gross underutilization of mental health facilities by Asian Americans as a group, including the Filipinos (Personal Communication).

Conceptualization of Mental Illness

Conceptualization of mental illness varies considerably between the traditional and the more sophisticated groups of Filipino Americans. To the traditionalist, mental illness is seen as some form of penalty for misdeeds of the patient or members of his family. The illness, therefore, is a form of spiritual unrest meted out to the individual through the agency of God or some malevolent, vengeful spirit (Kim 1973; Smith, Kline, and French 1978; Tseng and McDermott 1975; and Wittkower and Warnes 1974). Many forms of spirit possession characterize the beliefs of various religions. Still another way in which mental illness is conceptualized is hereditary weakness (Singer and Araneta 1967). The assumption here is that in certain families persons reaching a certain age and having to assume certain responsibilities will start to weaken and develop hypochondriacal symptoms. A third way in which mental illness is conceptualized is physical and emotional strain and exhaustion. In many parts of the Philippines, as well as in some groups here in the United States, the belief exists that mental illness comes about from physical strain. As a consequence, rest cure is a frequently prescribed treatment for mental illness (Wittkower and Warnes 1974).

Another way in which mental illness is conceptualized as a manifestation of physical disease, especially brain disorder (probably reflective of the relationship between psychiatric symptoms and syphilis of the brain), menstrual disorders, and diseases of the liver. Still another way in which mental illness is conceptualized is that it is a result of sexual frustration, sexual excess, or unrequited love.

Among the more sophisticated or westernized group, mental illness is usually conceptualized in terms of the depiction coming from Hollywood movies or from the magazine section of the Sunday paper. In any event, in conformity with their self-concept and adherence to the cult of western rationalism, this group conceptualizes disordered behavior as being in the realm of a specialized field of medicine (Amaranto 1978). Despite this westernized outlook, however, the occurrence of mental illness among members of the family still brings feelings of guilt because of the lingering feeling that psychiatric illness, or disturbance of the spirit, is the penalty for misdeeds.

Family Response and Help-Seeking Behavior

Among the more westernized groups, the occurrence of mental illness still evokes some sense of guilt, which is often rationalized as being related to the understanding that rearing at home has a lot to do with personality development and psychological weakness. However, in most cases the guilt is still traceable to the feeling of illness being meted out as a penalty for misdeeds (Tseng and McDermott 1975). Although the patient is generally referred to the family physician, and eventually to the psychiatrist, the recognized head of the extended family is usually consulted before the referral.

Among the more traditional Filipino Americans, their feeling of guilt associated with the occurrence of the illness tends to make the family secretive about the existence of the illness (Marsella et al 1972). Indeed, they would tend to hide the occurrence from members of the family outside of the immediate household. Association of mental illness with hereditary weakness or sexual frustration or excess seems to encourage this type of behavior. Consequently, mental illness is looked upon as a source of shame and a potential deterrent to a favorable marriage contract by members of the family.

Frequently, the family will consult a priest or a spiritual healer (often a spiritist). The basis for this step is that the spiritual disturbance of the patient has resulted from the influence of malevolent spirits. Prayers, exorcism, or other forms of rituals are initiated at this time (Tseng and McDermott 1975; Waxler 1976; Wittkower and Warnes 1974). If no significant result is observed a rest treatment may be tried on the basis of the concept that emotional and physical exhaustion lead to mental illness. During this period, if problems of unrequited love are discovered, arrangements may be made to provide some form of sexual outlet. It is only when most of these measures have been tried that medical referral is seriously considered, usually after consultation with the recognized leader of the extended family. Referral would mean making public the existence of mental illness in the family, and could obstruct or hinder marriage opportunities of other members of the clan (Singer and Araneta 1967). Furthermore, psychiatric referral is used as a last resort because of the impression that hospitalization in a psychiatric hospital is permanent, and constitutes a final break between the patient and the rest of the family.

CULTURALLY RELEVANT APPROACH TO THERAPY

Integrating Function of Cultural Reinforcement

Many of the attitudes and values that characterize the world view of the traditional Filipino American derive from his long reliance on a feudalistic agrarian economy and long years of colonization. Faced with the rapidly changing demands of industrialization and urbanization, many have withdrawn to the more familiar traditional ways. This "culture shock" response, though not a progressive step, has nonetheless served as an effective defense against sociocultural disintegration. The strong reliance of Filipinos on interdependence and their lack of individuation make them vulnerable to the stresses of a highly competitive and impersonal technologic and object-oriented host culture (Wittkower and Warnes 1974).

In dealing with psychiatric casualties from this group, therefore, it is necessary to take into account that culturally reinforcing behaviors, such as seeking counsel from elders, increased participation in religious rituals, seeking help from traditional healers, and doing penance, although apparently regressive, are actually probably more integrative. Thus, therapeutic efforts that would include the participation of the family, religious leaders, and traditional healers would be more likely to be accepted and effective (Marsella and Gordon 1973; and Marsella et al 1972).

Using Traditional Institutions for Therapy and Cultural Growth

It may be argued that, although in keeping with the principles of psychotherapy advocated by Frank (1972) and supported by the findings of Wittkower and Warnes (1974), and Waxler (1976, this approach is supportive of dependency on authority and thus would perpetuate the colonial status and mentality of this group. Further, this step would detract from the much needed change in the manipulation of political power for the socioeconomic advancement of this group and its effective acculturation. Indeed, the effect would be to further accentuate the frustrating social, economic, and other environmental conditions that predisposed to the psychiatric difficulties in the first place.

I would question this assumption, since all cultures, except those that have been completely isolated, have managed to evolve (Araneta 1976). It appears that the crucial issue in cultural growth is contact versus isolation, when the members seek their identity and fulfillment within their cultural boundaries. By implementing cultural psychotherapy in collaboration with the traditional healers, exchange of views and expansion of horizons are more likely to occur than by avoidance, repudiation, and isolation. Indeed, this collaboration can very well be the entry through which community development efforts can be effected (Araneta et al 1976). It must always be borne in mind that in psychotherapy, as in community development, the one most knowledgeable about the culture can be the most effective (Araneta 1976).

With regards to the westernized, more recent Filipino immigrants, they have, for the most part, incorporated the values and institutions of the host culture and have integrated into the existential stage of suburbia. They therefore share the problems of this subculture.

CONCLUSION

The diversity of Filipinos in terms of their cultural and racial heritage has resulted in factionalism and in differing acculturation styles with differing susceptibility to environmental and psychological stress. The first immigrants share many of the traditional values and problems of other Asian Americans. They have also been subjected to the most severe discriminatory political, economic, and social regulations imposed by the host country. They experienced the greater culture shock that has resulted in "culture lag." To effectively serve this group, a culturally congruent approach in collaboration with traditional healers is advocated. With the establishment of this collaborative relationship, community development efforts can be more easily effected to overcome the culture lag through the process of "incorporation" (Araneta 1976).

BIBLIOGRAPHY

Amaranto EA: *Mental Health Studies of Filipino Immigrants in the New York Metropolitan Area,* report. Chicago, Asian-American Mental Health Research Center, 1978.

Araneta E, Jr: Scientific psychiatry and "Community Healers." *The Conch* 8:65–76, 1976.

Bram LL, Phillips RS, Dickey N: *Funk and Wagnalls New Encyclopedia,* vol 19. New York, Crowell, 1977, pp 23-24.

Bulatao J: Hiya. *Philippine Studies.* 12:424–438, 1964.

Frank JD: Common features of psychotherapy. *Aust NZ J Psychiatry* 6(1):30, 1972.

Kim BLC: Asian-Americans: No model minority. *Soc Work* 18:44–53, 1973.

Lott JT: Migration of a mentality: The Filipino community. *Soc Case Work* 57:165–172, 1976.

Marsella AJ, Gordon P: Ethnic variations in the expression of depression. *J Cross Cult Psychol* 4:435–459, 1973.

Marsella AJ, Escudero M, Gordon P: Stresses, resources and symptom patterns in urban Filipino men, in Lebra WP (ed): *Transcultural Research in Mental Health.* Honolulu, University of Hawaii Press, 1972.

Marsella AJ, Murray D, Golden C: Ethnic variations in the phenomenology of emotions — shame. *J Cross Cult Psychol* 5:312-327, 1974.

Opler MK: *Culture, Psychiatry and Human Values — The Methods and Values of Social Psychiatry*. Springfield, Ill. Thomas, 1956.

Rizal J: *Noli Me Tangere,* Tablan AA, Veloro AT (trans). Manila, Philippine Book, 1950, pp 295.

Singer P, Araneta E: Hinduization and creolization in Guyana. *Soc Econ Stud* 16:221-236, 1967.

Smith, Kline, and French: *The Asian-Pacific American, Cultural Issues in Contemporary Psychiatry*. Philadelphia, Smith, Kline & French, 1978.

Tseng W, McDermott JF: Psychotherapy: Historical roots, universal elements and cultural variations. *Am J Psychiatry* 132:378-384, 1975.

Waxler N: Culture and mental illness: A social labeling perspective. *J Nerv Ment Dis* 159:349-395, 1976.

Wittkower ED, Warnes H: Cultural aspects of psychotherapy. *Am J Psychotherapy* 28:566-573, 1974.

4 Discussion: Cultural Aspects of Mental Health Care For Asian Americans

Tsung-yi Lin, MD

Cultural psychiatry has been treated as a stepchild of psychiatry for a long time. Yet it can be fun and very interesting. Dr. Gaw demonstrated this very clearly in discussing the case of *koro*.

The three psychiatrists presented their views on their own peoples' mental illnesses, based on personal observations. They emphasized the characteristic features of illness and the specific ways in which their respective cultures view them. Evidently there are different features in each of the three ethnic groups in North America. Yet among these three groups, the Chinese, the Japanese, and the Filipinos, regardless of how far or when they came from their original countries to this new continent, two features stand out: 1) the important role of the family in caring for the mentally sick, including the responsibility of selecting the treatment modality; and 2) the term *somatization* occurring in all three presentations. It seems quite oriental to explain the nature of mental illness in somatic terms and offer a cure for mental illness by somatic means.

The task of Asian psychiatrists to treat the high-risk groups is real and urgent. First, there is a group of old, single, male, first-generation immigrants who are lonely, not knowing how to cope with themselves and their lives. Second, there is a group of young who are suffering from an identity crisis and rebelling against the older generations. For example, I once received an urgent call from a PhD candidate at the University of British Columbia whom I had never met. He said: "Dr. Lin, can I see you today?"

I said: "Why?"

"This is the last day of my school and I'm leaving Vancouver. I must have a talk with you. It is something very important."

He is a second-generation Chinese, a seemingly bright young man. He has been living as a Canadian and exclusively with Canadians. He has no girlfriend and he does not speak a word of Cantonese or Mandarin. But now that he is finishing his PhD in Psychology, he finds himself not belonging to either group. This was an example of the identity problem many Chinese youth have to resolve in living and growing in a North American society. We have to concern ourselves with this kind of problem with our children's growing up. All the three papers made mention of this issue as an important area of concern. I fully support them.

In addition to discussing the plight of the old, the plight of the young people and the plight of women, there is another important group of people with whom we should be seriously concerned: the Asian psychiatrists. This issue is central to the future of cultural psychiatry in North America, as the major work will have to be done by Asian psychiatrists who are bilingual or bicultural. A large portion of them come from the minority or foreign background and yet, the contribution from them toward the understanding of cultural issues in psychiatry has so far not been very remarkable.

Why so? There are several important sociocultural problems related to the plight of Asian psychiatrists in this North American society. First, in spite of a rich Asian heritage, little systematic knowledge or skills in psychiatry have been transmitted to them. Mental illness or psychiatry was much ignored in medical classics: only a few books are devoted to the concept, manifestation, or causes of mental illness, and they are surprisingly sketchy and incomplete compared to the western literature on mental illness. We must admit our hereditary weakness in this regard.

Second, we seem to have inherited a tremendous amount of stigma attached to mental illness, which has spread over to those working for the mentally ill. Just an example out of my own personal experience: when I decided to enter psychiatry for specialist training, I wrote to my folks. The confusion and shock generated among my family and the whole Taiwan medical community was something! I was the first psychiatrist to be trained in Taiwan, a country of 6 million people. Many people asked me: "Why, are you crazy yourself?" "You're not too stupid, why don't you become an internist?" Since then I have seen many bright young doctors who have been dissuaded from becoming psychiatrists by their families or friends because of the stigma. It is not an overstatement to say that many working in this field have still been regarded, to some extent, as crazy, stupid, or eccentric by the community.

Third, not all Asian psychiatrists have an adequate knowledge of their own cultures. I wonder, for instance, how many Japanese psychiatrists in Los Angeles, or how many Chinese psychiatrists in Vancouver have real knowledge of Japanese or Chinese culture, including some of the classics in literature, philosophy, the interpersonal relationship pattern as prescribed by Confucian teaching, or the theories on causes of mental illness recorded in classic medicine? Unfortunately, some have no clear understanding of their own cultures. Some of them do not even speak their own language. How, then, can they really function as bilingual and bicultural psychiatrists capable of assessing and treating Asian patients living in North America, who are caught in the cultural conflicts? It is a tragic social-cultural dilemma many Asian psychiatrists face today.

Fourth, Asian patients usually come to the attention of the psychiatric profession or mental health profession very late. This means that the Asian psychiatrists are only asked to see the chronically ill, "incurable" patients. In addition, when the patients come, they or their families come with a feeling of hopelessness. What the psychiatrists or mental health workers are dealing with are the chronic schizophrenic or chronic organic brain syndromes, not many depressed, neurotic, or acute schizophrenic patients. The latter types of patients usually go to other people – physicians, priests, or other healers. Then, how do the Asian psychiatrists learn to develop skills in dealing with such Asian patients? So, here we are, being handicapped in functioning as well-rounded, fully-trained psychiatrists.

Fifth, almost nothing is taught about cultural psychiatry in most residency training programs. The deficiency of didactic teaching theories on cultural psychiatry is compounded by a paucity of clinical experience with Asian patients. Not many Asian psychiatric trainees see more than one or two Asian patients during their three years of training. There is the added problem of adequate supervision by teacher(s) who are interested or well versed in cultural psychiatry. This was also true during my own experience in Boston. Although I was lucky to have had the world's greatest analysts as my supervisors, my initial confusion and difficulty in tuning into American culture, in understanding the doctor-patient relationship and in setting up the treatment goals, were matched by my supervisor's difficulty in handling my culture shock. It was only through my perseverance and the warm, supportive guidance of my teachers, especially Harry Solomon and Milton Greenblatt, that it was possible for me to learn western psychiatry and to grow with daily experiences. I wish many more foreign trainees were as fortunate as I in having good teachers. They are the key to the success of cross-cultural training.

Last, I would like to comment on the issue of "culturally relevant therapy" to which all the three authors made reference. We often hear such statements as: "western psychotherapeutic approach is not applicable to Asian patients," or "Asians are not psychotherapeutically oriented," etc. The question of relevance of western-style psychotherapy to non-western culture and the issue of developing culturally relevant treatments for Asians urgently require our major attention and effort. I believe that the future of cross-cultural psychiatry depends largely on the ability of the mental health profession to come up with a set of effective treatments or interventions relevant to each specific culture. The intellectual curiosity about differential prevalence rates of mental disorders or culture-bound syndromes in specific cultures should be complemented by an emphasis on a search for relevancy in the intervention. This would involve an intensive effort in understanding the concept of illness, the explanatory model, the image of doctors and psychiatrists, the doctor-patient relationship, the responses of the family to mental illness, and the community attitude toward the mentally ill in each culture. Based on such understanding, a truly therapeutic relationship of trust might develop between the therapist and the patient, and an effective communication, using common language would become possible. For Asian patients, the involvement of the family in the therapeutic endeavor is essential, and the importance of developing relevant family therapy for Asians cannot be too strongly emphasized.

I wish to share with you some of my thoughts regarding concrete steps one might take to explore the development of culturally relevant psychiatric treatment. The obvious would be to look into traditional healing practices. The recent increase of interest in this area is encouraging. I wish to see more specific treatment modalities like Morita therapy become a part of Asian psychiatry. One should not, however, forget that Morita therapy is practiced by only a small group of Japanese psychiatrists on a very limited number of patients suffering from a characteristic set of symptoms called *shinkeishitsu*.

Two avenues would seem most useful in the search for culturally relevant treatments. One is a collection of detailed case histories with a clear description of the process of therapist–patient interaction using standardized format. Compilation and discussion of such records would enable cross-cultural psychiatrists to conceptualize characteristic features of therapy interaction relevant to the culture. This approach, simple as it may seem, is as basic to the future of cross-cultural psychiatry, I believe, as it has been to the birth and growth of western psychiatry.

The other avenue is to study the pathways of help-seeking of patients with psychiatric problems. This would consist of a detailed analysis of the interaction of the patient's psychiatric problems with his family and society. By recording the perception of a problem by the patient and his family, their emotional, and social responses, the mode of intervention, and the result of each intervention from the onset to the time of seeing a psychiatrist or even after, one can understand more clearly the socio-cultural factors, beneficial or harmful, that influence the illness process. In our study in Vancouver, Canada, the help-seeking of the Chinese was found to show a distinct pattern, markedly different from that of Caucasians, European immigrants, or Indians. We have also learned a great deal from this study as to how we can best provide mental health services to the Chinese in Vancouver. (Lin et al, 1978, Lin and Lin 1978, 1981)

One additional important issue in cross-cultural psychiatry presents a touchy but important problem to American psychiatry: the great number of foreign medical graduates (FMGs) now working in mental hospitals. They have not been given sufficient instruction in "intercultural skills" to help American patients. David Lewis calls it, "treating the alienated by the alienated." I see no reason or justification for letting the present condition continue. We should make use of cultural psychiatric skills in helping these FMGs to be more effective in caring for the sick in these institutions. The plight of FMGs should not be swept under the carpet.

BIBLIOGRAPHY

Lin TY, Lin MC: Love, denial and rejection: Responses of Chinese families to mental illness, in Kleinman A, Lin TY (eds): *Normal and Abnormal Behavior in Chinese Culture.* Holland, Reidel, 1981.

Lin TY, Lin MC: Service delivery issues in Asian-North American communities. *Am J Psychiatry* 135(9): 454–456, 1978.

Lin TY, Tardiff K, Connetz G, et al: Ethnicity and patterns of help-seeking. *Cult, Med and Psychiatry* 2: 3-13, 1978.

SECTION II
Cultural Aspects of Mental Health Care for Hispanic Americans

5 Cuban Americans

Pedro Ruiz, MD

The United States has always attracted Spanish speaking immigrants from Central and South America, who see coming to this land as an opportunity for the economic advancement that is difficult to achieve in their native countries. As a result of this immigration process, close to 200,000 Cubans had settled in the United States before the establishment in Cuba of Fidel Castro's socialist regime on January 1, 1959. This immigrant group was composed largely of three social classes. The largest group consisted of unskilled workers mainly from the rural areas of Cuba who, as a result of their lack of education and technical preparation, found serious difficulties in securing good job opportunities on the island. The second, although small, was composed of professionals, mainly from the health care sector, who decided to come to the United States to obtain specialized training or financial security—difficult to obtain in Cuba because of the large concentration of professionals in the urban sectors of the island at that time. The third class of considerable size was composed mainly of workers from the tobacco industry who settled in the United States during the Cuban War of Independence in the last part of the 19th century.

After January 1, 1959, the nature and type of Cuban immigration to the United States altered rapidly, mainly as a consequence of the profound political changes in Cuba during the 1960s and 1970s; the result was the arrival of close to 700,000 Cubans, for the most part political refugees. This immigrant group is composed mainly of middle-class families, particularly professionals and technicians. Now, with the offspring of Cubans living in the United States, as well as the close to 130,000 who arrived in mid 1980, one could easily say that close to 1,000,000 Cubans are residing in this country. They are concentrated in Florida, with substantial numbers also in the Northeast, particularly in New York and New Jersey, and in southern California.

Cuban immigration brought with it not only the hopes and aspirations related to the historic situation surrounding their arrival in the United States, but also a set of specific cultural characteristics – values, norms, customs, belief systems – which are at the heart of Cuban society. An occupational survey (Cuban Planning Council 1974) of the Cubans living in the Miami area showed results illustrative of the socioeconomic status of the Cubans in the United States:

Professionals and technicians	13.5%
Clericals and salesmen	24.6%
Skilled labor	17.3%
Unskilled labor	44.6%

This occupational analysis does not reflect the previous socioeconomic characteristics of the Cuban immigrants when they were in Cuba, and therefore might very well reflect the tremendous impact of different language, culture, and socioeconomic structure on an immigrant minority group already experiencing the pressures imposed by the mere fact of having to leave its native land.

MENTAL HEALTH CARE CONSIDERATIONS

From a mental health care point of view, two major points must be taken into consideration before one tries to conceptualize mental health problems confronted by Cubans living in the United States:

1. The conflicts from culture shock, language barrier, socioeconomic oppression, and guilt are compounded by pressures imposed by the

Anglo population of the United States, which tries to influence the recent immigrants toward a rapid assimilation of the majority culture's values and characteristics. This factor, although of great importance, will not be discussed at length in this chapter. It is similar to the ones confronted by many other immigrant groups that have previously arrived in this country, and which have already been described in the mental health care literature (Sue 1977; Padilla et al 1975; Hollingshead and Redlick 1958; Ruiz 1979; Alvarez et al 1976; Kosa et al 1969; and Thomas and Sillen 1974).

2. Cuban attitudes toward mental illness are largely a reflection of class, originating in Cuba before the immigration process took place. This background is not well known to the professional sector of the United States and should be analyzed. We must look at the expression of mental health problems not as manifestation of an illness, but as the result of the influence of the native culture on the illness itself and on the Cuban society at large. Two major characteristics are highly influential in any cultural phenomenon observed among Cubans. The first has to do with the ethnic composition of the Cubans on the island. Out of an estimated 9,000,000 Cubans, 73% are white, mainly representing the Spanish colonizers of Cuba, and 27% are either Black or mulatto, mainly representing the slavery process which originated from West Africa during the colonization period. The second is the large proportion of the rural population in Cuba. In 1962, 42% of the labor force was dedicated to agriculture, while only 18% was dedicated to industry (Navarro 1972).

The way in which mental illness is expressed, and the process of seeking and complying with mental health care is directly related to social class. The mental health care practices in Cuba before January 1, 1959, still apply to most Cubans now living in the United States.

Forms of Mental Health Care

There were three major subdivisions in the mental health care seeking behavior among the population of Cuba.

Upper class   The first was represented by a small number there, but considerably larger among the population now living in this country, and is composed of upper-class Cubans. In this country, this group represents the upper and middle classes, who in general have all kinds of opportunities for the best private care either in Cuba or in the United States. It was common practice for them to come to the United States to secure the best treatment available—a result of the extensive influence of the United States on the Cuban upper class during the neocolonialist years of the pre-Castro period. Thus, this class has looked to the United States as a powerful country in every aspect of technical and modern life, including health care services.

Another alternative for this group was to seek mental health care among private specialists or private clinics in Havana. These private providers of services were usually trained, as far as specialization goes, in the United States or in Europe, thus offering the same type of service image as that of the United States. Havana, the capital of the country, was the only place in Cuba that offered this type of service delivery to this small but wealthy class of Cubans. For this sector, classical one-to-one, long-term therapy or short-term hospitalization in the United States were the most common. This subgroup of the Cuban population in the United States still has the same style of mental health care seeking behavior, the only difference being that the long-term therapeutic individual approach is now more mixed with short-term therapeutic treatment, since the financial capability of this group diminished after leaving Cuba.

Middle and lower-middle classes   The second subdivision observed in Cuba before Castro was represented by middle and lower-middle classes, which, although not so large in Cuba, comprise the majority of the Cuban population now living in the United States. This group, while in Cuba, sought mental health services according to geographic location. If urban, for instance, their mental health services depended a great deal on the mutualist clinics that existed in Cuba at that time. These clinics operated on a prepaid basis, with a family financial quota, thus offering unlimited health care services to members. Social and recreational services were also provided, thus giving additional incentive for participation, These social and recreational services were in a way an imitation, on a small scale, of the large private clubs that prevailed at that time in Cuba for the exclusive benefit of the wealthy. Those who did not belong to these mutualist clinics sought services from private providers on a crisis intervention basis or for short-term therapy as outpatients or inpatients. The latter created, on occasion, severe financial hardship for those of the lower middle class, resulting in many instances in financial bankruptcy. These conditions were similar to the ones observed in the United States for those facing major catastrophic illness. Mutualist clinics, in a way, represented an advanced step toward socialized medicine. For those Cubans now living in the United States, a similar treatment pattern prevails, the only difference being that many lower class Cubans have joined the numerous mutualist clinics that now flourish in Miami, either because it is financially advantageous to them, or because they are attempting to reinforce and preserve their cultural identification and heritage. In this regard, many middle-class Cubans living in the United States also join these clinics, since mental health services in this country are far more expensive than they were in Cuba.

Lower class   The third subdivision was represented in Cuba by the lower class group, which for the most part was composed of the rural population. This large population sector in Cuba was also affected by all the ills resulting from the socioeconomic oppression in Cuba at that time. This group not only had limited access to appropriate, quality health care in the cities, but was also afflicted by lack of education, poor sanitation and housing, and high unemployment. There were only four alternatives available to this group: 1) tolerance of deviant behavior; 2) provision of mental health services based on available family resources, often resulting in the locking up of afflicted relatives in their homes to receive only minimal care during the period of illness, which occasionally lasted for life; 3) hospitalization, in most instances for life, of those afflicted by severe mental illness, in the state hospital at Havana (where conditions were the most inhumane and tragic that one could imagine); 4) folk healing resources scattered throughout the island. The folk practices of *santeria* and *brujeria* were transported to Cuba by the slaves during the colonization period, and were widespread among the large Black and mulatto population of Cuba. However, as the result of the inner forces of these ritualistic practices, and the lack of professional manpower and the socioeconomic oppression during the neocolonialist period, such practices were also widespread among the white population. In terms of the lower-class Cubans now living in the United States, a similar pattern prevails, particularly in relation to folk healing, since this practice offers a good opportunity to maintain fiercely anything that represents, culturally and socially, the Cuban tradition.

CLINICAL MANIFESTATIONS OF MENTAL ILLNESS

Cubans in the United States are affected, as any other ethnic group living in this country, by all of the classical mental illnesses and syndromes commonly described in any psychiatric textbook. However, as in any other ethnic subgroup, Cubans also have some specific characteristics in relation to the manner in which such illnesses and syndromes are manifested.

These characteristics are more relevant than the illnesses themselves because 1) the majority of Cubans living in the United States have been here for fewer than 20 years; 2) very little research has been conducted in regard to this subgroup; and 3) the medical literature (even on an empirical basis) is limited insofar as the mental health care of Cubans living in the United States is concerned. My own clinical observations come from my years of psychiatric training at the University of Miami School of Medicine, 1965-1968, and from private practice in New York City from 1969-1973. I have treated many Cubans of both sexes, and all ages and social classes, and I have had the opportunity on many occasions to share my clinical experiences informally with other Cuban mental health professionals.

Transient Paranoia

Cubans often display paranoid feelings that are generally associated with the political climate characterized by the ups and downs of the political relations between Cuba and the United States. In general, these paranoid feelings are mild and do not generally require chemotherapeutic or somatic treatment. The most beneficial treatment for this condition is an appropriate understanding, by the therapist, of the heavily ingrained political environment that prevails among the Cuban population in the United States. In general, the paranoid trends are transient and usually reappear according to the political mood prevailing in the Cuban population of the United States. These clinical manifestations of paranoia are quite often found during the period following arrival in this country. A recognition of the clinical manifestations is important in order to avoid using unnecessary psychiatric services, particularly hospitalizaiton.

Adaptational Anxiety

During the period of settlement in this country, many cubans suffer from a sense of despair and anxiety, which usually is concomitant with the loss of status, prestige, loved ones, and country, and the conflict arising from exposure to new value systems and financial insecurities. These manifestations of anxiety are more often found in those Cubans who migrated to the United States during the 1960's, since they were more affected by such losses. On occasion, this type of anxiety reappears during periods of relocation to other places in the United States. In these cases, it is more important not to apply therapeutic approaches based on classical psychoanalytic or psychoanalytically oriented models, since the result might be more harmful than beneficial. It is more appropriate to intervene actively with manipulation of the social structures surrounding the patient, to assure full utilization of all socioeconomic potentials within the patient. Once dignity and respect are restored in the patient, the anxiety symptoms rapidly disappear. Classical analytic approaches should be kept for those few who do not respond. Manifestation of anxiety is often expressed in terms of personality maladaptations, which, although having similar characteristics to the classical personality deviances, are not lifelong processes, but rather recent and transient in nature.

Depressive Reactions Secondary to Diaspora

Although similar to most reactive depressive reactions, the various degrees of depression that affect Cubans are directly related to the political mood prevailing in the Cuban society of the United States. These depressive manifestations are often found among recent arrivals, are usually temporary, and require only supportive measures, particularly through the full utilization of the rich extended family network system that Cubans possess (Rumbaut and Rumbaut 1976). However, these clinical manifestations are severe among the elderly, who have little hope of returning to Cuba. In this group, particularly if they lose their self-respect, dignity, and love, suicide attempts are common. Appropriate treatment should be rapidly instituted, including chemotherapy, somatic approaches, and, if necessary, hospitalization. Of great benefit to these patients are the group approach, in which ethnic identity is reinforced, and relocation to Miami (for those who happen to live in other parts of the United States). Cubans, in general, are sensitive to isolation and loss of self-esteem resulting from threats to their dignity and self-respect.

Intrafamilial Role Identification Crisis

One of the greatest conflicts experienced by Cubans of both sexes, when arriving in this country, is exposure to the different value systems in which Americans live. Cuban males, in many instances, perceive American males as being less masculine than themselves. Many American males share some of the domestic roles of their spouses, which Cuban males have not been exposed to during their formative years. Concomitantly, Cuban females perceive American women in general to be more independent and liberated. While these standards are better tolerated by young Cubans, they cause major intrafamily conflicts for the older ones, particularly for the women, who in many cases are forced by the socioeconomic system to work and become self-sufficient, thus causing Cuban women to feel a great deal of guilt, fear, and anger. While it is most important that progress be secured for both men and women in this area, it is also important to be sensitive to those who have major problems in becoming assimilated into the American model of life. In these cases, family and group therapy approaches are beneficial, particularly if appropriate role models and intensive educational processes are used. When patients in this category are treated by an Anglo therapist, who, although well intentioned, seeks as a goal the liberalization of previously held sex role values, the consequences can be tragic. It is not uncommon to find total destruction of the family structure—a more serious problem than those intended to be solved in the first place.

Specific Behavioral Patterns

Cubans living in the United States differ markedly from other Anglo ethnic groups in certain patterns of behavior.

Substance abuse   In general, the pattern of substance abuse among Cubans is less pronounced. More important, in most cases of Cubans suffering from substance abuse one finds a major family breakdown rather than socioeconomic pressures (Szapocżnik et al 1978). Also, while Cubans like to drink socially, their pride, self-respect, and dignity tend to minimize their becoming pathologically alcoholic.

Homosexual behavior   In general, Cuban homosexual males are more at risk than their counterparts in the Anglo society in terms of freedom from guilt and normal adaptation to life. Cuban fathers, as a result of their strong male chauvinistic tendencies, do not tolerate homosexual behavior among their male offspring. It is not uncommon to see Cuban fathers telling their sons during their formative years that they would prefer to see them dead rather than become homosexual. In many instances, Cuban homosexuals tend to migrate to large cities, such as New York, Los Angeles, and Washington, where their behavior in this regard can be better disguised and tolerated. Therapists must be sensitive to the cases in which social and family pressures result in inner conflicts and even manifested depressions.

FOLK HEALING

The use of folk healing practices among Cubans living in the United States deserves special attention since it constitutes a health and mental health seeking behavior not well known to most of the mental health professionals now practicing in the United States. From another angle, the knowledge of a given culture, in this instance the Cuban subculture, is of great importance in psychiatry as demonstrated by the recent growth and development of psychiatric literature on this subject (Everett et al 1976; Foulks et al 1977; Ruiz and Langrod 1976a). Even Freud (1955) and Jung (1967) focused on the need to understand cultural manifestations when treating psychiatric patients. Some authors (Chapple 1970; Damon 1975) have even suggested that culture may influence the human biological process.

As far as Cubans are concerned, the most widespread and common folk healing practice is that of the Lucumi religion, which was innate to many of the Black slaves brought to Cuba during the colonization period from different regions of West Africa, but particularly from Nigeria, Congo, and Guinea (Cabrera 1971). As practiced in Africa, the Lucumi religious ceremonies were held in the Yoruba dialect, which predominated in these African regions. In the beginning, this cult practice was strictly confined to the Black slaves of Cuba in what was called the secret society of *Abakua* (Cabrera 1970), while later on it spread out across all classes and races of Cuba, but particularly to the lower class, both rural and urban. Since the Spanish colonizers of Cuba persecuted and prohibited the practice of the *Lucumi* religion among the Black slaves during the colonization period, the slaves substituted their African religious effigies, which represented their gods, for those that resembled them in the Catholic religion. As a result of this action, the name of *santeria* became synonymous with *lucumi* (since in the Catholic religion gods are *Santos*). Furthermore, this substitution protected the religious practice from extinction and total destruction during this period of persecution. This image substitution led to the eventual identification of many African gods (*ochas*) with their counterparts in the Catholic religion (Table 5-1). In addition to this sample of those most commonly used and venerated in this practice, of special interest is Orunmila, which, although not commonly known, represents the power of wisdom and mental illness.

Table 5-1
Lucumi Gods and Their Catholic Counterparts

African Gods (*Ochas*)	African Representation	Catholic Saints (*Santos*).
Babalu-Aye	Infections, skin lesions	San Lazaro
Ochun	Money, love, genitals, lower abdomen	La Caridad del Cobre
Obatala	Body, paralysis	Las Mercedes
Yemaya	Intestines, sea	Regla
Eleggua	Accidents, messengers	San Roque, San Antonio, San Pedro, San Pablo
Oggun	War	San Juan, San Pedro
Chango	Fire	Santa Barbara
Olofi	Well-being	Dios (Jesus)
Alosi	Evil	Diablo

As practiced by Cubans, *santeria* not only has healing powers but also harming qualities as well. Among the different groups of followers of *santeria* most respected, in terms of being able to produce harm to people, were the Ñañigos, who were believed to have originated in Congo, Africa. This group was highly feared because of its aggressiveness. They were also felt to be *brujos* (sorcerers, witches), leading to the use of the word *brujeria* (witchcraft), which is synonymous with, or a variant of, *santeria*. In accordance with *santeria,* illnesses, regardless of whether they are physical or mental, can be caused by either natural or supernatural phenomena, and the symptomatology for physical illness is the same, whether the origin be natural or supernatural.

However, for mental illness, a different concept prevails. While symptoms of mental illness are usually perceived by classical mental health professionals as synonymous with a pathologic disorder, and every attempt is therefore made to eradicate them, the *santeria* practice views mental symptoms in general as a sign of positive strength, as well as an expression of quality on the part of the patient—thus the widespread acceptance of *santeria* by its followers (Ruiz and Langrod 1976b). Another important factor in a positive identification with this type of practice had to do with the dichotomy between the natural and supernatural causes of illnesses. While medical doctors always explain the cause of illness in terms of natural factors, thus easily rejected by many believers of *santeria,* folk healers use natural or supernatural explanations, depending on the case in question (Ruiz 1976). The modes of actions of the supernatural forces are generally attributed to 1) entry into the body, either through drink or food, of a given substance prepared by the *santero* (medium), with the express purpose of making the individual sick; 2) possession of the body by an evil spirit, which has usually been directed against a person by a *santero* or *brujero,* who dedicate their work not only to help people, but on occasion to harm them as well; 3) molesting effect of the spirit of a dead relative who gets angry as the result of his being forgotten by the relative in question; 4) loss of protection of the guardian angel (spirit protector), as a result of the person's deviance from what was expected from him while on earth (*santeria* believes in reincarnation); 5) effect of the *mal de ojo* (evil eye), as a result of envy and jealousy directed at the afflicted person; and 6) expression of folk healing powers by the afflicted person.

The *santeros* in their day-to-day practice most commonly use animal sacrifices, special baths, perfumes, oils, candles, fruits, religious prayers, herbs, weeds, and plants. The special necklaces have the faculty of protecting the person from evil influences. Dreams are perceived in the practice of *santeria* as indicators of the future.

In the United States, the use of *santeria* has been mixed with other cult practices such as spiritism, voodoo, and curanderism (Ruiz and Langrod 1977). In general, *santeria* is quite flexible and therefore incorporates in its ritual practices anything that might lead to a better result. *Santeria* has grown rather than diminished among Cubans now living in the United States (Sandoval 1977). This growth has been attributed to factors such as the following: 1) lower-class Cubans have gained socioeconomic power in the United States; 2) *Santeria* is a past-oriented religion, as well as a present-oriented system and thus is well accepted by Cubans in the United States; and 3) the Catholic religion has lost considerable prestige among Cubans in the United States.

In addition, any cult practice, in this case *santeria,* permits Cuban migrants to close ranks with their cultural values and heritage, as well as promote ethnic group cohesiveness at a time when the native values of Cubans are primarily threatened by the influence of the American culture toward a more rapid assimilation.

CONCLUSION

Culturally speaking, we are not one world. Furthermore, in understanding how to successfully diagnose and treat people from a cultural dimension different from one's own, theoretical concepts and experience must be supplemented by an awareness and appreciation of the patient's cultural conditioning. This is not easy to do, but if professionals in the field do not understand the deeply held values of normative perceptions that make up the Cuban world view, they are stretching the Cuban population now living in the United States on the mental health criteria of the Anglo culture. The results can be failure and frustration for both patient and therapist and, worse, lack of adequate understanding can do harm.

BIBLIOGRAPHY

Alvarez R, Batson RM, Carr AK, et al: *Racism, Elitism, Professionalism: Barriers to Community Mental Health.* New York, Aronson, 1976.

Cabrera L: *La Sociedad Secreta Abakua.* Miami, Coleccion del Chichereku, 1970.

Cabrera L: *El Monte.* Miami, Coleccion del Chichereku, 1971.

Chapple ED: *Culture and Biological Man.* New York, Holt, Rinehart and Winston, 1970.

Cuban Planning Council: Cuban Minority in the United States: Fiscal Report on the Need Identification and Program Evaluation. Washington, 1974.

Damon A: *Physiological Anthropology.* New York, Oxford University Press, 1975.

Everett MW, Waddell JP, Heath DB: *Crosscultural Approaches to Study of Alcohol.* Chicago, Aldine, 1976.

Foulks E, Wintrob R, Westermeyer J, et al: *Current Perspectives in Cultural Psychiatry.* New York, Spectrum, 1977.

Freud S: Totem and taboo and other works, in *The Standard Edition of the Complete Psychological Works of Sigmund Freud,* vol 13. London, Hogarth, 1955, pp 1–161.

Hollingshead AB, Redlich FC: *Social Class and Mental Illness.* New York, Wiley, 1958.

Jung CG: *Symbols of Transformation, Collected Works,* ed 2, *Bollingen Series,* vol 5. Princeton, Princeton University Press, 1967.

Kosa J, Antonovsky A, Zola IK: *Poverty and Health: A Sociological Analysis.* Cambridge, Harvard University Press, 1969.

Navarro V: Health, health services and health planning in Cuba. *Int J Health Serv* 2(3):397–432, 1972.

Padilla AM, Ruiz RA, Alvarez R: Community mental health services for the Spanish-speaking surnamed population. *Am Psychol* 30(9):892–905, 1975.

Ruiz P: Folk healers as associate therapists, in Masserman J (ed): *Curr Psychiatr Ther* New York, Grune & Stratton, 1976, pp 269–275.

Ruiz P: The fiscal crisis in New York City: Effects on the mental health care of minority populations. *Am J Psychiatry* 136(1):93–96, 1979.

Ruiz P, Langrod J: Psychiatry and folk healing: A dichotomy? *Am J Psychiatry* 133(1):95–97, 1976a.

Ruiz P, Langrod J: The role of folk healers in community mental health services. *Community Ment Health J* 12(4):392–398, 1976b.

Ruiz P, Langrod J: The ancient art of folk healers: African influence in a New York City community mental health center, in Singer P (ed): *Traditional Healing: New Science or New Colonialism?* New York, Conch Magazine Ltd, 1977, pp 80–95.

Rumbaut RD, Rumbaut RG: The family in exile: Cuban expatriates in the United States. *Am J Psychiatry* 133(4):395–399, 1976.

Sandoval M: Santeria: Afro-Cuban concepts of disease and its treatment in Miami. *J Operational Psychiatry* 8(2):52–63, 1977.

Sue S: Community mental health services to minority groups: Some optimism, some pessimism. *Am Psychol* 32(8):616–624, 1977.

Szapocznik J, Scopetta MA, King OE: Theory and practice in matching treatment to the special characteristics and problems of Cuban immigrants. *J Community Psychol* 6:112–122, 1978.

Thomas A, Sillen S: *Racism and Psychiatry*. Secaucus, NJ, Citadel, 1974.

6 Mexican Americans

Adela G. Wilkeson

The 1978 President's Commission on Mental Health sub-panel on Hispanics estimated that there are currently 23,000,000 Hispanic Americans (Report to the President's Commission on Mental Health, 1978). Mexican Americans, who reside predominantly in the Southwest, make up 60% of this rapidly growing minority group. Distinctive aspects of Mexican American history and culture are relevant to mental health care providers. Important questions include how do Mexican Americans conceptualize disease (particularly mental illness), and how do cultural attitudes and expectations influence the manifestations of psychic distress, health care seeking behavior, acceptance, and response to treatment? These questions can be only partially answered because the extant mental health literature is still limited (Padilla 1978). This limitation is due in part to the fact that most Mexican Americans remain among the lower socioeconomic classes and have only begun to have mental health care provided in any systematic way since the Community Mental Health system was established in the 1960s. In addition, data regarding ethnic background have not been accurately recorded, and Mexican Americans remain under-represented in the various mental health professions. Ethnocentric biases have also influenced much of the existing psychiatric and anthropologic literature (Montiel 1973; Romano 1960; Romano 1971).

Even a cursory knowledge of Mexican and Mexican American history should offset some of the prejudicial conceptions of Mexicans being passive and indolent people (McWilliams 1968). The history of Mexican Americans in the United States is varied. Mexicans populated the Southwest, living in haciendas (large ranches) where the level of economic achievement and cultural activity paralleled that of Europe, long before Anglo-Americans moved West. Many contemporary Mexican Americans however, have immigrated to the United States in recent years. These immigrants came mainly from the mestizo population of Mexico. Mestizos are individuals of combined European (usually Spanish) and Indian blood. They are the largest Mexican social class, of low social economic status, and from a relatively agrarian background.

Kiev (1968) notes that the mestizo agrarian background includes an orientation of cooperation and subordination of the individual to the community as a whole, which is quite distinctive from the individualistic, competitive orientation of Anglo-Americans. Murillo (1971) contrasts the attitudes of Mexican Americans and Anglo-Americans toward material possessions. He notes that the acquisition of material belongings is experienced as a necessity for Mexican Americans, not as an end in itself. Mexicans and Mexican Americans also value work predominantly as it represents a contribution to the family rather than something that is of primary importance to an individual's self-esteem. The experience of life in the present and the sharing of the emotional aspects of life with others is valued far more than work accomplishments. Thus philosophers, musicians, artists, and poets are often more renowned in Mexico than businessmen or financiers. Interpersonal relationships, particularly within the family, are also highly valued. There is a genuine willingness to share life's burdens and a concern for the emotional experience (and physical well-being) of others. Murillo attributes this in part to the Indian concept of limited good; that is, that there is only so much good in the world and only so much good possible in any one person's life. Thus the usual greeting of Mexican Americans, even with strangers, includes sayings like *a sus ordenes* (at your command) and *para servirle* (to serve you). There are numerous Spanish words that convey affection for others that are not easily translatable — eg, *simpatico* (someone who is particularly nice and a pleasure to be with); *cariño* (a special fondness or caring for another person). Respect of other persons' feelings as well as of authority figures contributes to a style of diplomatic, tactful expression and reticence to be too frank or to disagree openly. Overall, Mexicans and Mexican Americans are individuals who embrace life and who embrace one another. Good times are enhanced with music, bright colors, fiestas (parties). Bad times are shared, lightening the burden for any one individual.

THE MEXICAN AND MEXICAN AMERICAN FAMILY

Two mid-1950s papers by Diaz-Guerrero (1955) and Ramirez and Parres (1957) respectively are most often referenced as descriptions of "prototype Mexican families." As Ramirez and Parres note, the prototype Mexican families belong to the numerically superior but economically impoverished mestizo class. Only a very small percentage of Mexican people belong to what would be the equivalent of the middle class of the United States. The other significant but numerically small Mexican societal class is the wealthy population which is predominantly creole (born in Mexico from foreign parents, usually Spanish).

Ramirez and Parres cite data from two sources as the basis of their comments on dynamic patterns in the Mexican family. Psychosocial data were obtained from 500 families randomly selected from 10,000 records of individuals treated at the Hospital Infantil in Mexico City (Children's Hospital: a large government funded hospital serving predominantly the mestizo population in Mexico City but also the most medically advanced and central referral hospital for all of Mexico). The more in-depth psychological patterns described were based as well on the analytic treatment of 11 patients considered typically Mexican by the two authors. The demographic data obtained revealed that 65% of the families were formed by a biosocial unit involving the father, mother, and offspring. The remaining families included this unit plus some relatives: relatives of the mother (usually the grandmother) in 65%, relatives of the father in 12%, and other individuals who are not blood relatives (compadres; godparents) in 22 percent. It was also noted that in 32% of the cases, the father was absolutely absent from the family: 7% of the time because of death and 25% because of abandonment. Further investigation revealed that in 70% of the cases of abandonment the husband left during the months of his wife's pregnancy, 20% occurred before the child reached age 1 and only 10% seemed related to motives other than psychological reaction to an infant, such as social or economic factors. Ramirez and Parres argue that these facts corroborate their impressions of the powerful role of the maternal woman as an idealized central figure in the Mexican family and individual dynamics.

Diaz-Guerrero's descriptive article (which refers to some questionnaire data on 294 Mexico City residents plus the author's experience as a psychotherapist) describes the female role as one of abnegation and self-sacrifice. The female child is taught that her destiny includes three areas:

superlative femininity, the home, and maternity. The young woman's femininity is admired and reinforced only in the years before marriage. Once married, she assumes a maternal and subservient role. "The culture and the social group overevaluate the feminine relation in its maternal aspects and devaluate the emotional and sexual living with the husband." Diaz-Guerrero describes the male role within the family as one of provider and authority figure who is to be granted absolute supremacy but is generally distant and uninvolved with the children. Masculinity for the Mexican male is primarily associated with sexual prowess. The masculine self-image is maintained by ongoing participation in group activities with males outside the family plus frequent involvement in sexual experiences outside the marital relationship. (These behaviors are what is referred to by the term *machismo*.)

The expected self-sacrificing role of the woman and the limited sexual relationship available with her husband are two factors both Diaz-Guerrero and Ramirez and Parres cite as influencing a particularly intense maternal-child bond which persists until the birth of the subsequent child. Again Ramirez and Parres note, "Statistically we have found in our material that 94% of the mothers breast feed their children. The feeding is done without schedule and is regulated by the demands of the baby. Every single frustration or anxiety of the child is calmed by giving of the breast." With the birth of the next sibling the older child is abruptly cut off from this totally symbiotic relationship with the mother. This is due in part to economic conditions necessitating breast feeding by the mother, but is also a repetition of a generational pattern of early parenting experience. This abrupt separation is seen as preconditioning the subsequent pattern of male abandonment during the wife's pregnancy as well as the female abandoning the male by turning her attention more exclusively to the child and not continuing to reinforce, by her behavior or appearance, the sexual and intimate aspects of her marital relationship. The significant number of maternal grandmothers in these nuclear family units may be further evidence of the Mexican woman's continued desire for the intense symbiotic relationship with an infant. Ramirez and Parres suggest that competition between mothers and grandmothers occurs in this area rather than the areas of femininity and relationships with men. Finally, Ramirez and Parres argue that apparent male dominance of Mexican families as well as machismo attitudes in fact represent a reaction formation against the father's lack of real importance in the family organization as well as an "excessive feminine identification" and/or dependent character traits.

Maccoby (1971) also writes about Mexican American families and general Mexican character traits. He notes in his introductory criticism of Mexican psychoanalytic literature (including the papers of Ramirez and Parres and Diaz-Guerrero) and a number of Mexican intellectuals a particularly negative and demoralized portrayal of Mexican people. He provides data from an anthropologic study of an entire Mexican village that documents that only 11% of the men demonstrate any significant pattern of compulsive "masculine" behavior while 30% showed some "machismo" traits. He further describes an absence of markedly neurotic traits in these people noting that "many villagers are well adjusted...loving and productive...interested in their families and their work."

Murillo's (1971) description of the Mexican American family reflects cognizance of the aforementioned limitations of existing knowledge. His description of Mexican American family structure is one of the most sensitive and accurate portrayals currently available. Initially he emphasizes the diversity of the background of Mexican American people:

> The reality is that there is no Mexican American family "type." Instead there are literally thousands of Mexican American families all different significantly from one another along a variety of dimensions. There are significant regional, historical, political, social, economic, acculturational and assimilation factors...there are families where Spanish is the exclusive language spoken in the home and others in which it is never spoken. There are families who trace their ancestry back to their Spanish forefathers and others who trace their ancestry back to their Mayan, Zapotec, Toltec or Aztec forefathers. Some families were living on the land which is now the Southwestern part of the U.S. before the Pilgrims landed at Plymouth Rock while others have immigrated to the U.S. in recent years.

Murillo also emphasizes the highly important role of the family and the extended family for Mexican Americans. Psychologically an individual's identification as part of a given family has greater importance than his individual identity. The family provides emotional and material support for all its members including *compadres* (unrelated godparents of each child). Respect and obedience for elders and male dominance are main characteristics cited as well as a child-centered home environment during the early years of a child's growth. The fathers are described as warm and permissive toward their children until puberty and thereafter they are distant and authoritarian. The father's authority in the family is not questioned, but his male or masculine image in the community is based in part on his fairness and justice in the authority role. The wife-mother has a subservient, though highly-respected role and continues to be giving to all family members, even when the children have reached adulthood. Distinctive roles and responsibilities are taught to boys and girls, though all children are given tasks which are valued functions for the entire family from an early age. In adolescence there is an expectation that young men gain worldly knowledge through experience while young women are expected to remain close to their mothers and have few social contacts beyond the family.

Goodman's and Bemin's well-designed study of children in a typical

Mexican American barrio (neighborhood) (1971) substantiates a number of the same familial and cultural values. Grade school children were interviewed. Fathers are authority figures, they have final disciplinary say, and they work to earn money for the family. Boy children experienced their fathers as less available than mothers to respond to questions or emotional needs. Girl children experience both parents as equally available. Mother's primary activity is in the domestic role (even if she works). She disciplines children with regard to daily routine, sibling quarrels, etc. She is valued, seen as good, pretty, fun, and experienced with feelings of warmth and closeness. Grandparents and older people are most respected and treated with deference. Family relationships with parents, grandparents, siblings, uncles, aunts, more distant relatives and compadres are valued and are more important than friendships outside the family. This is noted to be quite distinctive from similar studies of Anglo and negro children who value relationships with peers more than familial ties. These Mexican American children further relate that "the good thing to do is also the pleasurable thing to do." Thus work is valued but it is valued particularly as it is experienced as participating in and contributing to the family. A concern for *los de mas* (others) is also associated with what is good and pleasurable: "this (others) orientation is a matter of concern for and sensitivity to the feelings and wishes of people who are important to the ego."

ACCULTURATION, ASSIMILATION, AND DISCRIMINATION

The distinction between assimilation and acculturation is of considerable importance in understanding a number of specific stresses experienced by Mexican American individuals. *Assimilation* refers to the process of successful adaptation to the predominant culture without necessarily relinquishing or changing cultural attitudes and value identifications. The term *acculturation* is used to describe the process of changing value orientations (that is, substituting and adhering to Anglo-American values and attitudes rather than Mexican American cultural norms). Even the use of the term acculturation conveys a subtle bias, a bias that equates adopting Anglo ways with the acquisition of "culture." The recent Chicano movement (Martinez 1973) resists this prejudicial attitude and emphasizes the maintenance of pride in Mexican American cultural heritage.

It is clear that all immigrant people have had to struggle with adapting to a foreign culture. The dream of America as a melting pot where equal opportunity exists for all, initially fosters a willingness in some individuals to use anglicized names and to emulate American life-styles. A majority of Mexican Americans have not readily acculturated but have instead continued to live in Mexican American barrios. In the barrios Spanish is the primary language. There are stores that sell foods otherwise found only in Mexico; pharmacies sell traditional folk medicine, herbs, and ointments; and newsstands sell Mexican newspapers and periodicals. Low socioeconomic status, limited education, and limited facility with and/or confidence in speaking English clearly are factors that reinforce continued life within the barrio. In addition, the proximity of Mexico facilitates ongoing immigration and frequent return visits both of which processes further adherence to a Mexican life-style.

Coexisting forces of discrimination and prejudice that resist bilingual education and discriminate against Mexican Americans who seek entrance into more remunerative employment and/or institutions of higher education are equal factors that maintain life within the *barrios*. Dworkin's studies (1965, 1971) of foreign-born and native-born Mexican American self-images document part of the devastating effect of this discrimination. He showed that foreign-born Mexican Americans have a much more positive self-image than Mexican Americans born in this country. In addition, he documented that the self-images of foreign-born Mexican Americans who have lived in this country for a long time, are similar (much more negative) to those of American-born Mexican Americans. A study of the perception of prejudice in Mexican American preschool children also points to the devaluation of dark-haired, dark-skinned dolls beginning when the children enter school and are exposed for the first time to the Anglo cultural attitudes (Werner and Evans 1971).

Simmons (1971) notes a similar tendency of Mexican Americans in a Texas border town to define themselves as inferior to Anglo Americans. The stereotypic perceptions described by Simmons are based on interviews of representative Mexican and Anglo Americans in this town. Familiarization with these stereotypic perceptions is important for clinicians both to enhance awareness of the internalized devaluations Mexican American patients struggle with as well as the negative, prejudicial expectations Mexican Americans may have of Anglo American professionals. It is noted that Anglo Americans in border cities have a dualistic perception of Mexican Americans. On the one hand they present a belief that Mexican Americans should be fully assimilated and indicate a willingness to accept any Mexican Americans who have both achieved a certain level of occupational and financial success and demonstrate an adherence to Anglo life-styles. Simultaneously, however, Mexican Americans are also conceived of as basically inferior and therefore innately deserving of their poor social class. Stereotypic notions that are incorporated in this perception of inferiority include childlike, indolent, undependable, irresponsible, and imprudent traits: uncleanliness, drunkenness, criminality, low morality, mysteriousness, unpredictability, and hostility. The somewhat favorable stereotypes such as liking fiestas, and music; and romantic as opposed to realistic inclinations also reflect the alleged childlike and irresponsible nature. Stereotypes of Anglo Americans held by Mexican Americans include some favorable traits such as initiative, ambition, and industriousness but mainly negative traits including being cold, mercenary, exploitative, stolid, phlegmatic, boastful, conceited, inconstant, and insincere.

Casavantes (1971) describes how biases equating Mexican American culture with "the culture of poverty" have compromised many existing studies of acculturation. Padilla (1977) has recently developed a scale that assesses acculturation with questions involving six main categories: language familiarity and usage, cultural heritage (awareness and loyalty), ethnic interaction, ethnic pride and identity, ethnic distance, and perceived discrimination and generational proximity to Mexico. He illustrates the development and use of this scale with five clinical vignettes that demonstrate the complexity and diversity of personal backgrounds and styles of adapting to the issues of personal and cultural identity. Finally, Fabrega and Wallace (1968) found that transition from one set of values to another (the process of acculturation) was more characteristic of a group of outpatients while nonpatient controls either had firm traditional (Mexican) or nontraditional (Anglo) value identifications.

Consideration of the stresses of acculturation leads to the prediction that both adolescent and elderly Mexican Americans may be at high risk for increased psychic stress and mental illness. Unfortunately there is yet no reliable information on either of these subgroups. As long as acculturation is resisted, elderly Mexican Americans will most likely continue to receive the respect, deference, and familial support afforded them in Mexico. If this pattern changes, however, they may be even less prepared to deal with the problems of aging than their Anglo counterparts. Identity crisis and rebellion against familial norms is characteristic of adolescent years and certainly could be exacerbated by the contrasting cultural norms Mexican American youths experience at home and at school. Female adolescents might be particularly at risk considering the cultural expectations of their remaining close to the family, maintaining virginity, and preparing for a domestic role in adult life. Ramirez (1969) did note some increased parameters of distress in 10 Mexican American adolescents compared with 10 Anglo American controls. Matched groups of 152 Mexican American children and 152 Anglo children at a child guidance clinic were studied by Stoker and Meadow (1974). They found that a significantly high percentage of Mexican American females came in between the ages of 16 and 18 and that 49% of these young women were the oldest daughters in their families. They also reported more aggressive acting out and more need for institutionalization among the male Mexican Americans. However, they did not comment on the clinic's referral sources or on the ethnic background of the staff, which may have biased the selection or perception of these difficulties. One study that provides evidence against the stereotypic conceptions of Mexican Americans being delinquent or criminally inclined is Gossett's survey of illicit drug use among high school students in the Dallas public school system (1971). Questionnaires administered to all 56,745 students in grades 7 to 12 showed a much higher rate of drug abuse among middle- and upper-class Anglo students than by either Mexican American or Black youths.

CONCEPTS OF ILLNESS AND FOLK DISEASE

The existence and preservation of many folk beliefs regarding folk disease and folk healing practices among Mexican Americans has received considerable attention from psychiatrists and anthropologists. The current prevalence of folk beliefs and use of *curanderos* (folk healers) is not well established, partly because Mexican Americans are reluctant to reveal their beliefs to Anglos for fear of ridicule, and a desire not to expose *curanderos* whose practices are considered illegal in the United States. Existing studies are somewhat contradictory, but they do suggest considerable maintenance of these belief systems in some areas. In 1966 Martinez and Martin reported the results of their interviews of 75 housewives in a Mexican American *barrio* of a large Texas city. They found that 97% of these women were familiar with the most common folk disease concepts of *mal ojo, empacho, caida de mollera, susto,* and *mal puesto*. With the exception of *mal puesto,* 85% of the women reported one or more instances of these illnesses in themselves, a family member, or an acquaintance. One local *curandero* and eight *señoras* (older women known to specialize in the treatment of folk diseases) were well known to this population. Creson (1969) reports that of 25 consecutive Mexican American patients visiting a general hospital outpatient clinic (also in Texas), 12 (48%) had either sought the services of a *curandero* or had a family member that had seen a native healer. In addition 80% of these were quite familiar with the common folk diseases and remedies. Only four local faith healers were identified by these subjects, and they were apparently considered to be somewhat exploitative and commercial. Martinez and Martin further indicated that 80% of their subjects also sought medical attention from physicians or medical clinics. Edgerton et al (1970) reported a much diminished role of faith healers in East Los Angeles noting that in extensive interviews of 400 Mexican Americans regarding concepts of emotional and psychiatric disturbances, fewer than 1% of the responses regarding treatment included mention of folk healers. Padilla et al (1976) similarly found that only 2% of 666 subjects surveyed in three Southern California communities have sought the assistance of a *curandero*.

Certainly any medical or mental health professional working with Mexican American people should be familiar with folk disease concepts, as it is likely that the less acculturated portion of the Mexican American population will continue to maintain these beliefs. Rubel (1960) has proposed that these beliefs persist because of their supportive relationship to certain core values and behaviors in the Mexican American community. Similarly, Kiev (1968) suggested that *curanderismo* is maintained because it is a functional healing system that reinforces culturally established value systems and accepted psychological defense mechanisms. Kiev, however, does not provide any data for his hypothesis that *curanderos* function as folk psychiatrists. The subsequent study of Alegria et al (1977) involving extensive interviews of 16 *curanderos* shows that they treat a variety of predominantly medical illnesses and function quite like medical general practitioners. The folk diseases described here and psychiatric difficulties involve only a minority of the complaints brought to them. Alegria (1977) and Hamburger (1978) both found that *curanderos* are generally older individuals who practice in their homes. They are highly religious, charge minimal fees, and often refer patients to medical clinics and physicians. A number of mental health professionals have reciprocally reported considerable value in incorporating *curanderos* and folk methods in the treatment of severely disturbed Mexican American patients (Casper and Philippus 1975; Kreisman 1975, 1977a; Ruiz 1976; Ruiz and Langrod 1976).

Kiev (1968) provides a comprehensive history of the evolution of Mexican disease concepts with their combined medieval, Spanish, Catholic, and Mexican Indian roots. The initially Hellenic concept of disease's being due to a lack of harmony with nature is prominent. There are many thoughts regarding the importance of balanced diet, adequate water and air, and prophylactic and therapeutic efforts to maintain a balance of internal humors. Emotionally stressful events are also considered related to disease. An excessive accumulation of strong feelings affects physical health by causing an imbalance of humors. The Catholic belief, that all men are born sinners and that men are expected to share the joys and sorrows of their fellow men, makes illness something to be unquestionably accepted as part of God's plan for the universe. Since the ability to suffer is considered a measure of an individual's faith, *curanderos* see their major task as helping the patient accept suffering as his or her share of the burden of the world's sin and ignorance.

Kiev reports that mental illness is associated with three main factors: heredity, a preoccupation with sexual activity, and *pica* (*cometierra*). It is particularly important for psychiatrists to be aware of *pica* which means eating earth and is literally characterized by individuals eating dirt including pieces of pottery and chips of old paint. Lead poisoning is a frequent consequence.

Several authors (Clark 1959; Martinez and Martin 1966; Rubel 1960; Saunders 1958) have provided descriptions of the main Mexican American folk diseases and usual folk remedies. Mexicans do not dichotomize or separate psychic and emotional illness from somatic disease. *Caida de Mollera* (fallen fontanelle) affects only infants. It is believed to be caused by an infant falling or by the nipple being pulled away from the infant too abruptly. The result is caving in of the anterior fontanelle and symptoms of the baby being unable to grasp the nipple to feed, plus crying, vomiting, diarrhea, and sunken eyes. Individuals with "light blood" which include children and more often women than men, are more susceptible to *mal ojo* (evil eye). Particularly strong individuals in the community are considered capable of bringing on this affliction by looking at the victim with excessive attention or in a covetous fashion. The symptoms are mainly fever and vomiting, although crying and restlessness are also reported. *Empacho* (surfeit) is caused by a bolus of poorly digested food sticking to the wall of the stomach, causing pain, lack of appetite, diarrhea, and vomiting. Although this is a manifectly physiological illness, there are emotional facets to its cause. *Susto* (fright) is usually the result of a sudden dramatic experience, which may be anything from witnessing a death to a simple scare at night. It is a magical state of fright or soul loss. It is a state of anxiety and fear, which in some cases involves catatonic symptoms; other associated symptoms may be anorexia, insomnia, hallucinations, weakness, and various painful sensations.

Rubel (1960) notes that the above four illnesses are *males naturales,* that is, sicknesses of natural causes which are considered to be in the realm of God. *Mal puesto,* on the other hand, is a *mal artificial* (artificial ill), an illness outside the realm of God, that is to say the work of the devil. *Mal puesto* literally means an evil or illness put on someone willfully by another (sorcery, a hex). The symptoms described vary considerably but do seem to include mainly psychotic behavior: uncontrolled urination, sudden attacks of screaming, crying, and singing, and in some instances, bodily exposure and convulsions. Martinez (1966) reports that the dynamic of the hex almost always involves the victim's being the object of jealousy by in-laws or other relatives.

With regard to the specific concepts and attitudes toward mental health, two studies exist. Fabrega and Metzger's (1968) paper involves conceptions of mental illness as reported by representative members of a small Mexican village. The words *loco* (mad or crazy), *locurá* (madness) and *esta afuera de mentá* (is outside his mind) are used to describe individuals with clearly bizarre psychotic symptomatology. In the most virulent forms of *locurá,* the person is said to be *endiablado* (possessed by the devil). Factors that contribute to mental difficulties are numerous and interrelated. Predominantly physical causes include 1) head trauma, 2) hereditary defects, 3) birth trauma, 4) inadequate diet, 5) excessive intake of heavy food, 6) exposure to cold air drafts, and 7) excessive exercise. Psychological factors include insufficient or excessive sexual contact and masturbation, strong emotional experiences, or social isolation. Finally, magical causes, hexes, brought about by *hechicerosis* (warlocks) and *brujas* (witches) are usually considered to be involved. Severely disturbed individuals are considered dangerous secondary to their unpredictability but they are also pitied because of their lack of contact with reality. They are generally cared for by the entire village. Less severely disturbed categories of mental illness include the *tonto* or *idiota* (idiot) who is grossly deficient in cognitive faculties; *nerviosos* (nervous person); *desorientados* (persons who are abnormally unpredictable or absent minded); *atrabancados* (persons who show a persistent tendency toward impulsiveness and abruptness in their social relationships). It is interesting that these categories do not include any descriptions of overtly depressed individuals.

Karno and Edgerton (1969) used questionnaires and structured interviews (which included the presentation of five distinctive vignettes of psychiatrically disturbed individuals) to ascertain the general concepts of mental illness and thoughts about the potential utility of psychiatrists among Mexican Americans living in East Los Angeles. A total of 444 Mexican Americans and 200 matched Anglo controls were evaluated. They found that a larger majority of Mexican Americans than Anglo controls identified both depressed and schizophrenic patients as individuals who had a mental illness. Furthermore Mexican American subjects, somewhat more than Anglos, believe psychiatry can be helpful, were more optimistic about the curability of mental illness, and believe that the origin of mental disorders begins in childhood. Morales reported (1971b) that 13th and 14th century Aztec Indians had developed concepts of ego formation and psychic structure similar to Freud's later theories, a finding that puts these contemporary Mexican American concepts in greater perspective.

UTILIZATION OF SERVICES

Reports of underutilization of services by Mexican Americans have received considerable attention in the literature. Available data are based either on inpatient or community mental health clinic utilization. Reports on inpatient utilization are actually quite contradictory. Jaco (1959) studied residents in Texas during the 1950s and found that the incidence of the treatment of psychosis was four times greater for Anglos in private hospitals, but equal rates existed for Mexican Americans and Anglo patients treated for psychosis in state institutions. Karno and Edgerton (1969) reported that only 2.2% of admissions to California state hospitals in 1962 and 1963 were Mexican Americans: significantly less than the 9% to 10% of Mexican Americans within the general population. Long et al (1977) also reported a lower percentage of Mexican American inpatients in a Northwest Denver Mental Health catchment area compared to the general population. Bloom (1975) studied the incidence of first admissions to psychiatric inpatient facilities in Pueblo, Colorado, and reported under-representation in 1960 but over-representation in 1970. Finally, Wignall and Koppin (1967) found that admission rates of Mexican Americans were somewhat higher than for Anglos in Colorado State Hospitals in 1967.

Underutilization of traditional community health mental health clinics has been reported by several authors (Karno 1966; Karno and Edgerton 1969; Sue et al 1978). A number of possible reasons for this underutilization have been suggested, but a recent study by Keefe (1978) has shown no correlation between mental health clinic contact and "social economic status, the presence of an integrated extended family, commitment to the folk medical system, attitudes towards mental health services or the reliance on relatives, doctors, clergymen, Mexican American community workers or 'curanderos' for emotional support." In his 1978 review of issues relevant to Mexican American mental health service utilization, Barrera recommended that studies specifically ascertain attitudes of Mexican Americans toward the available mental health facilities. Miranda (1976) notes that many mental health clinics are inaccessible to barrio residents and can be confusing to patients because of their seemingly fragmented and depersonalized process of entry and their lack of immediate response to the patient's problems.

Since 1970 at least five mental health care facilities specifically designed to provide mental health services for Mexican Americans have reported percent utilization of these clinics parallel to the total Mexican American population in the area (Flores 1978; Heiman, Burruel, and Chavez 1975; Heiman and Kahn 1975; Karno and Morales 1971; Long, Horel, and Radinsky 1977; Martinez 1977c; Philippus 1971). The reasons for these clinics' success are that 1) they are centrally located in the barrio, 2) there is a high percentage of Spanish speaking staff with some staff members coming from the immediate area, 3) initial registration is immediate and informal, 4) dropping into the clinics at any time is encouraged, 5) one mental health team member is assigned to each patient throughout treatment, 6) services are initially crisis oriented with immediate social service assistance and/or medical care available, and 7) community boards share in administrative responsibility for the clinics.

The series of papers from East Los Angeles presents a noteworthy progression. Karno et al (1969) reported that Mexican Americans sought help for mental illness from general practitioners because no community mental health clinics were readily available. In 1971 Karno and Morales reported that the very large percentage of Mexican Americans among the first 200 patients attending a new East Los Angeles Mental Health Clinic was representative of the percentage of Mexican Americans in East Los Angeles (70% to 80% of the population). Flores (1978) provides a follow-up report from the same clinic describing the general characteristics of 200 consecutive patients seen between October 1974 and February 1975. Of note is that the clinic had to enlarge to meet a greatly increased demand for direct services, that the percentage of Mexican American clients remained very high (75% with an additional 10% of the patients being of another Hispanic background), that an increasing number of the patients came from outside the catchment area, were monolingual (Spanish speaking only), were native-born Mexicans, and were either self-referred or referred by other patients. It is quite clear from these reports that Mexican Americans will use mental health facilities that are culturally sensitive, receptive, and responsive.

SPECIFIC DIAGNOSTIC AND TREATMENT ISSUES

At this time only very limited information regarding specific diagnostic differences among Mexican Americans exists. Alcohol and drug abuse are considered significant health problems by Mexican Americans in Arizona (almost 200 subjects were surveyed in 1974) but the prevalence of alcohol was reported to be similar to that of Anglo Americans (Biegel, Hunter et al 1974; Beigel, McCabe et al 1974). Alcocer (1977) reported a greater prevalence of alcoholism for Mexican Americans in Los Angeles (1972) but used numbers of arrests and autopsy findings as his data base without consideration of the clear selection bias involved. Stoker and Meadow (1974) reported a higher percentage of Mexican American parents with significant alcohol abuse problems than Anglo parents of the 304 children in two study groups at a child guidance clinic. Long (1977) also found a higher percentage of Mexican Americans with alcohol-related problems at a large community mental health center in Denver. Again Gossett (1971) found less drug abuse in Mexican American adolescents than by Anglo American students in the Dallas Public School system.

The incidence of psychosis is unknown. Contradictory findings of in-patient utilization provide the only available data. Meadow and Stoker (1965) compared the symptoms in 120 Mexican American patients' records from the Arizona State Hospital with 120 matched Anglo controls. Interestingly they found that overall mexican American psychotic patients demonstrated more depressive symptoms as compared to the Anglo patients who were generally found to be more paranoid. Despite this statistically significant finding, however, a larger number of Anglo

Americans had been diagnosed with affective illness while more Mexican Americans were diagnosed as chronic undifferentiated schizophrenics. Fabrega et al (1968) demonstrate the importance of close matching of control groups, noting that when social class, education, estimated IQ, age, sex, and number of previous hospitalizations are controlled for, apparent differences in symptomatology for different ethnic groups are essentially eliminated.

Fabrega et al (1967) also reported a more limited study of 30 Mexican class outpatients in Mexico City in 1967. His findings are significant in that virtually all male patients seeking psychiatric help attributed their difficulties to some somatic cause and verbalized no thoughts about emotional or nervous disorders. In contrast, two-thirds of the women did conceptualize their distress in terms of emotional problems, family difficulties, loneliness, and so on. The remaining one-third of the women also spoke of somatic problems.

Several general aspects of treatment have been described. Burke (1965) reports the contrasting, rapid improvement of minority groups within certain Massachusetts State Hospitals who had tended to have long courses of treatment until staff and group activities were specifically provided to address their issues as ethnic or religious minorities. Normand et al (1974) and C. Martinez (1977b) have reported successful involvement of Mexican American outpatients in group therapy. The group support is supplemented by help with external problems and provides an initial educational process to introduce concepts of psychotherapeutic treatment. Martinez also notes that the patients are quite verbal but do manifest some limitations in expressing their differences with authority figures. Exploration of Mexican American and Anglo American subgroup dynamics have significant value for all patients.

Kline (1969) has emphasized the importance of Anglo mental health workers' being aware that Mexican American patients may initially perceive them as cold, exploitative, and insincere. It is clearly important to allow patients to express such prejudicial apprehensions if a therapeutic alliance is to be established. In contrast to these misgivings Acosta and Sheehan (1976) have actually found that Mexican college students demonstrated a preference for Anglo American therapists over Mexican American therapists of similar educational background. Independent of a therapist's ethnic background, countertransference reactions of overidentification and overcompensation must be monitored (Bradshaw 1978). Morales (1971a) provides two clinical vignettes that illustrate how a narrow clinical approach, seeing the patient's distress as simply a culturally-determined pattern of emotional expression, was ineffective. Eventual exploration of the patient's specific personal history and relationships within the family clarify the reasons for the patient's symptomatology and clinical presentation. Similarly, awareness that a certain percentage of Mexican Americans believe in spirits should not decrease the diagnosis of psychosis when it was clinically indicated. An ongoing assessment of culturally-bound external stresses needs to be balanced with an awareness and gradual exploration of internal limiting conflicts, which may be expressed by culturally-determined patterns of behavior or perceived as external experiences of discrimination.

Finally, the importance of involving the patient's family in both initial evaluation and treatment planning is emphasized (Arce et al 1977; Murillo 1971). As Murillo notes, the degree to which the family is valued by Mexican Americans may prompt a family to "sever all relationships with one of its members if that individual, through his behavior, brings shame or disorder to it." Though severe mental illness is generally seen as a medical problem and not an issue of dishonor, drugs and alcohol are considered to be evidence of little will power and can often stimulate familial rejection, which further complicates treatment efforts.

BILINGUALISM

Unavailability of Spanish speaking staff is clearly a problem for many clinics attempting to serve Mexican American individuals. Lack of confidentiality and loss of the dyadic experience with the therapist are major limiting factors regarding the use of translators for psychiatric evaluation and treatment. The effort of thinking in a second language for patients who have some facility with English but who are experiencing varying degrees of emotional upheaval can make the patient's symptoms seem more severe (Arce et al 1977; Marcos et al 1973). Though truly bilingual patients may be able to enter therapy successfully, a potential for reinforcement of defensive resistance and possible inaccessibility of certain conflicts exists when the second language is used exclusively. As Marcos and Alpert (1976) summarize:

> Psycholinguistic investigators have repeatedly demonstrated empirically that bilingual subjects verbalize different associations in response to semantically identical words, according to the language in which the task is performed. In general, these studies suggest that words referring to concrete, high-imagery objects elicit more similar responses in the bilingual's two languages than do abstract words, which in turn tend to evoke more similar associations than words referring to feelings.

These authors indicate that some of the potential limitations of therapy for bilingual patients interviewed in only one language can be minimized by a therapist's appraising such factors as "the age and developmental stage of the patient when languages were acquired, experiential sorting of language contexts and the nature of the object relations associated with them, and attitudes and values connected with each language." Del Castillo (1970) described the masking of psychotic symptoms by several patients he evaluated during recovery from acute psychotic episodes; the patients were interviewed in their second language as opposed to their primary language. His findings support the proposition that a second language can at times reinforce certain psychological defenses.

CONCLUSION

Mexican Americans are a large minority group that has continued to maintain many aspects of their Mexican heritage while living in the United States. The importance of the Mexican American family bonds and the value given to life experiences, as opposed to the mere acquisition of material belongings, are values that particularly distinguish Mexican Americans from their Anglo American cohorts. Each Mexican American responds differently to the process of assimilation, the pressures of acculturation, the stresses of discriminatory forces, and still for many, the hardships of poverty. Despite their different cultural heritage and traditional folk concepts of disease they do readily seek professional assistance for mental health difficulties, particularly if such services are provided in accessible and culturally-oriented clinics. There is a major need for the development of further treatment facilities as well as the training of more Hispanic and more bilingual mental health professionals so that needed services can be delivered and further clinical studies of mental health problems carried out.

F.H. Martinez (1977) describes the task facing mental health professionals attempting to make the current multifaceted local, state, federal, and private bureaucracies more responsive to Mexican American mental health needs. He also provides a brief history of the National Coalition of Hispanic Mental Health and Human Services Organizations, a Washington, DC, based coalition. Since its establishment in 1974, this organization has been coordinating efforts to further develop research, services, and manpower training activities for all Hispanic Americans. It is a valuable resource for clinicians working with Chicano populations.

The author acknowledges Cervando Martinez, MD, Associate Professor, Department of Psychiatry, The University of Texas, Health Science Center at San Antonio, Texas, for his review and editorial comments.

BIBLIOGRAPHY

Acosta FX, Sheehan JC: Preferences toward Mexican American and Anglo American psychotherapists. *J Consult Clin Psychol* 44:272–279, 1976.

Alcocer AM: Alcoholism among Chicanos, in Padilla AM, Padilla ER (eds): *Improving Mental Health and Human Services for Hispanic Communities.* Washington, DC, The National Coalition of Hispanic Mental Health and Human Services Organizations, 1977.

Alegria D, Guerra E, Martinez C, et al: El hospital invisible. *Arch Gen Psychol* 34:1354–1357, 1977.

Arce AA, Jimenez R, Martinez C: *The Hispanic American* (audio cassette). Smith Kline Corporation, Philadelphia, 1977.

Barrera M: Mexican-American mental health service utilization: A critical examination of some proposed variables. *Community Ment Health J* 14:35–45, 1978.

Beigel A, Hunter EJ, Tamerin JS, et al: Planning for the development of comprehensive community alcoholism services. I. The prevalence survey. *Am J Psychiatry* 131(10):1112–1116, 1974.

Beigel A, McCabe TR, Tamerin JS, et al: Planning for the development of comprehensive community alcoholism services: II. Assessing community awareness and attitudes. *Am J Psychiatry* 131(10):1116–1121, 1974.

Bloom BL: *Changing Patterns of Psychiatric Care.* New York, Human Sciences Press, 1975.

Bradshaw WH: Training psychiatrists for working with Blacks in basic residency programs. *Am J Psychiatry* 135(12):1520–1523, 1978.

Burke JL, LaFave HG, Kurtz GE: Minority group membership as a factor in chronicity. *Psychiatry* 28:234–238, 1965.

Casavantes E: Pride and prejudice: A Mexican American dilemma, in Wagner NN, Haug MJ (eds): *Chicanos: Social and Psychological Perspectives.* St. Louis, Mosby, 1971.

Casper EG, Philippus MM: Fifteen cases of Embrujada combining medication and suggestion in treatment. *Hosp Community Psychiatry* 26(5):271–274, 1975.

Clark M: *Health in the Mexican-American Culture.* Berkeley and Los Angeles, University of California Press, 1959.

Creson DL, McKinley C, Evans R: Folk medicine in the Mexican-American subculture. *Dis Nervous System* 30(4):264–266, 1969.

Del Castillo JC: The influence of language upon symptomatology in foreign born patients. *Am J Psychiatry* 127(2):242–244, 1970.

Diaz-Guerrero R: Neurosis and the Mexican family structure. *Am J Psychiatry* 112(6):411–417, 1955.

Dworkin AG: National origin and ghetto experience as variable in Mexican-American stereotype, in Wagner NN, Haug MD (eds): *Chicanos: Social and Psychological Perspectives.* St. Louis, Mosby, 1971.

Dworkin AG: Stereotypes and self-images held by native-born and foreign-born Mexican Americans. *Sociol Soc Res* 49(2):214–224, 1965.

Edgerton RB, Karno M, Fernandez I: Curanderismo in the metropolis: The diminishing role of folk psychiatry among L.A. Mexican-Americans. *Am J Psychother* 24(1):124–134, 1970.

Fabrega H, Jr, Metzger D: Psychiatric illness in a small Latino community. *Psychiatry* 31(4):339–351, 1968.

Fabrega H, Jr, Rubel AJ, Wallace CA: Working class Mexican psychiatric outpatients. *Arch Gen Psychiatry* 16(6):704–712, 1967.

Fabrega H, Jr, Swartz JD, Wallace CA: Ethnic differences in psychopathology. I. Clinical correlates under varying conditions. *Arch Gen Psychiatry* 19(2):218-226, 1968.

Fabrega H, Jr, Swartz JD, Wallace CA: Ethnic differences in psychopathology. II. Specific differences with emphasis on the Mexican-American group. *J Psychiatr Res* 6(3):221-235, 1968.

Fabrega H, Jr, Wallace CA: Value identification and psychiatric disability: An analysis involving Americans of Mexican descent. *Behav Sci* 13(5):362-371, 1968.

Flores JL: The utilization of a community mental health service by Mexican-Americans. *Int J Soc Psychiatry* 24:271-275, 1978.

Goodman ME, Beman AM: The child's-eye-views of life in an urban barrio, in Wagner NN, Haug MJ (eds): *Chicanos: Social and Psychological Perspectives.* St. Louis, Mosby, 1971.

Gossett JT, Lewis JM, Phillips VA: Extent and prevalence of illicit drug use as reported by 56,745 students. *JAMA* 216:1464-1470, 1971.

Hamburger S: Profile of Curanderos: A study of Mexican folk practitioners. *Int J Soc Psychiatry* 24:19-23, 1978.

Heiman EM, Burruel G, Chavez N: Factors determining effective psychiatric outpatient treatment for Mexican-Americans. *Hosp Community Psychiatry* 16(8):515-517, 1975.

Heiman EM, Kahn MS: Mental health patients in a barrio health center. *Int J Social Psychiatry* 21(3):197-204, 1975.

Jaco EG: *Culture and Mental Health: Cross-Cultural Studies.* New York, Macmillan, 1959.

Karno M: The enigma of ethnicity in a psychiatric clinic. *Arch Gen Psychiatry* 14:516-520, 1966.

Karno M, Edgerton RB: Perception of mental illness in a Mexican-American community. *Arch Gen Psychiatry* 20:233-238, 1969.

Karno M, Morales A: A community mental health service for Mexican-Americans in a metropolis, in Wagner NN, Haug MJ (eds): *Chicanos: Social and Psychological Perspectives.* St. Louis, Mosby, 1971.

Karno M, Ross KN, Caper RS: Mental health roles of physicans in a Mexican-American community. *Community Ment Health J* 5(1):62-69, 1969.

Keefe SE: Why Mexican-Americans underutilize mental health clinics: Fact or fallacy, in Kasas JM, Keefe SE (eds): *Family and Mental Health in the Mexican-American Community.* Los Angeles, Spanish Speaking Mental Health Research Center UCLA, 1978.

Kiev A: *Curanderismo: Mexican-American Folk Psychiatry.* New York, Free Press, 1968.

Kline LY: Some factors in the psychiatric treatment of Spanish-Americans. *Am J Psychiatry* 125(12):1674-1681, 1969.

Kreisman JJ: The Curandero's apprentice: A therapeutic integration of folk and medical healing. *Am J Psychiatry* 132(1):81-83, 1975.

Long EG, Horel R, Radinsky T: *Transcultural Psychiatry: An Hispanic Perspective,* monograph 4. Los Angeles, Spanish Speaking Mental Health Research Center (UCLA), 1977.

Maccoby M: On Mexican national character, in Wagner NN, Haug MJ (eds): *Chicanos: Social and Psychological Perspectives.* St. Louis, Mosby, 1971.

Marcos LR, Alpert M: Strategies and risks in psychotherapy with bilingual patients: The phenomenon of language independence. *Am J Psychiatry* 133(11):1275-1278, 1976.

106

Marcos LR, Urcuyo L, Kesselman M, et al: The language barrier in evaluating Spanish-American patients. *Arch Gen Psychiatry* 29:611–659, 1973.

Martinez C: Community mental health and the Chicano movement. *Am J Orthopsychiatry* 43(4):595–601, 1973.

Martinez C: Curanderos: Clinical aspects. *J Operational Psychiatry* 8(2):35–38, 1977a.

Martinez C: Group process and the Chicano: Clinical issues. *Int J Group Psychother* 27(2):225–231, 1977b.

Martinez C: Psychiatric consultation in a rural Mexican-American clinic. *Psychiatr Ann* 12:74–80, 1977c.

Martinez C, Martin HW: Folk diseases among urban Mexican-Americans. *JAMA* 196:161–164, 1966.

Martinez FH: Chicanos and the "Non-System" for mental health services, in Padilla AM, Padilla ER (eds): *Improving Mental Health and Human Services for Hispanic Communities*. Washington, DC, The National Coalition of Hispanic Mental Health and Human Services Organizations, 1977.

McWilliams C: *North from Mexico: The Spanish Speaking People of the United States*. Westport, Conn, Green Wood Press, 1968.

Meadow A, Stoker D: Symptomatic behavior of hospitalized patients. *Arch Gen Psychiatry* 12(3):267–277, 1965.

Miranda MR, Kitano H: Mental health services in third world communities. *Int J Ment Health* 5(2):39–49, 1976.

Montiel M: The Chicano family: A review of research. *Soc Work* 18(2):22–31, 1973.

Morales A: Distinguishing psychodynamic factors from cultural factors in the treatment of the Spanish-speaking patient, in Wagner NN, Haug MD (eds): *Chicanos: Social and Psychological Perspectives*. St. Louis, Mosby, 1971a.

Morales A: The impact of class discrimination and white racism on the mental health of Mexican-Americans, in Wagner NN, Haug MJ (eds): *Chicanos: Social and Psychological Perspectives*. St. Louis, Mosby, 1971b.

Murillo N: The Mexican-American family, in Wagner NN, Haug MJ (eds): *Chicanos: Social and Psychological Perspectives*. St. Louis, Mosby, 1971.

Normand WC, Iglesias J, Payn S: Brief group therapy to facilitate utilization of mental health services by Spanish-speaking patients. *Am J Orthopsychiatry* 44(1):37–44, 1974.

Padilla AM: Measuring ethnicity among Mexican-Americans: Some questions for Chicanos in mental health, in Padilla AM, Padilla ER (eds): *Improving Mental Health and Human Coalition of Hispanic Communities*. Washington, DC, The National Coalition of Hispanic Mental Health and Human Services Organizations, 1977.

Padilla AM, Carlos ML, Keefe SE: *Psychotherapy with the Spanish Speaking: Issues in Research and Service Delivery* monograph 3, Los Angeles, Spanish Speaking Mental Health Research Center (UCLA), 1976.

Padilla AM, Olmedo EL, Lopez S, et al: *Hispanic Mental Health Bibliography II*. Los Angeles, Spanish Speaking Mental Health Research Center (UCLA),1978.

Philippus MJ: Successful and unsuccessful approaches to mental health services for an urban Hispano-American population. *Am J Public Health* 61(4):820, 1971.

Ramirez M: Identification with Mexican-American values and psychological adjustment in Mexican American adolescents. *Int J Soc Psychiatry* 15(2):151–156, 1969.

Ramirez S, Parres R: Some dynamic patterns in organization of the Mexican family. *Int J Soc Psychiatry* 3(1):18–21, 1957.

Report to the President from the President's Commission on Mental Health. Washington, US Government Printing Office, 1978.

Romano VO: The anthropology and sociology of Mexican-Americans: The distorting of Mexican-American history. *El Grito* 2:13–68, 1960.

Romano VO: The defined and the definers.: A mental health issue. *El Grito* 5:4–11, 1971.

Rubel AJ: Concepts of disease in Mexican-American culture. Am Anthropol 62:795–814, 1960.

Ruiz P: Folk healers as associate therapist, in Masserman JH (ed): *Current Psychiatric Therapies.* New York, Grune & Stratton, 1976.

Ruiz P, Langrod J: Psychiatry and folk health: A dichotomy? *Am J Psychiatry* 133(1):95–97, 1976.

Saunders L: *Patients, Physician and Illness.* New York, Free Press, 1958.

Simmons OG: The mutual images and expectations of Anglo-Americans and Mexican Americans, in Wagner NN, Haug MJ (eds): *Chicanos: Social and Psychological Perspectives.* St. Louis, Mosby, 1971.

Stoker DH, Meadow A: Cultural differences in child guidance clinic patients. *Int J Soc Psychiatry* 20:186–202, 1974.

Sue S, Allen DB, Conaway L: The responsiveness and equality of mental health care to Chicanos and native Americans. *Am J Community Psychol* 6(2):137–146, 1978.

Werner E, Evans MI: Perceptions of prejudice in Mexican-American preschool children, in Wagner NN, Haug MD (eds): *Chicanos: Social and Psychological Perspectives.* St. Louis, Mosby, 1971.

Wignall CM, Koppin LL: Mexican-American usage of state mental hospital facilities. *Community Ment Health J* 3(2):137–148, 1967.

7 Puerto Rican Americans

Angel Gregorio Gómez, MD

The image of the Puerto Rican in "mainland" United States* is not clear to non-Puerto Rican mental health workers—primary physicians, psychiatric trainees, educators on mental health, paraprofessionals, administrators at a policy making level.

Cultural and cross-cultural elements should be considered in psychiatric training as, for example, their relationship with the outcome of mental illness or the promotion and preservation of mental health. Other areas of concern are 1) common denominators between the Puerto Rican and other predominant population segments of the Hispanic American within a cultural and transcultural frame of reference; 2) the Puerto Ricans and culture variables emerging from Puerto Rican pluralism; 3) clinical considerations concerning cultural issues on values and behavior; and 4) problems in communication, transference, and counter-transference, which affect the outcome of prevention and treatment.

---

*For the majority of Puerto Ricans, the "mainland" United States denotes a geographical concept rather than an emotional conviction.

CULTURE AND PSYCHIATRIC TRAINING

In psychiatry — the most sophisticated and integrated offspring of medicine and the behavioral sciences — the study of culture has not yet come into its own according to a very recent statement of Favazza and Oman (1978), even though most social change is accompanied by an intensification of social and cultural sources of psychological conflict (Kiev, 1976). In this regard, Bernal y del Río (1977), who has elaborated on the concepts of ethnophobia and ethnophilia, or the expression of feelings and attitudes for or against certain ethnic groups, has gathered, along with others, pertinent data on the importance of transculturality in psychiatric training (Bernal et al 1977).

In all training programs on behavioral sciences the same basic questions must be answered: who is training whom, and how and what for? Due to issues related to civil rights and the Constitution, federal agencies have recently released specific policy guidelines for federally funded training programs.

The draft "Report of Workgroup on Manpower Training — Research and Development" of the National Institute of Mental Health* clearly states:

> Particular attention in the R and D training efforts should be given to training approaches which would seek to heighten the awareness and sensitivity of the trainees to the life styles, culture, and language of the various ethnic minority groups and their implication for effective service.

Guidelines on training from the National Institute of Drug Abuse (February 21, 1978) advise that

> in order to operate valid training systems, states must be aware of staffing patterns within service delivery programs in order to establish and maintain adequate training support for all workers with special emphasis on the unmet needs of special populations in the state (racial and ethnic minorities as well as women).

The President's Commission on Mental Health (1978)† recommends that the President also direct

> ...The Department of Health, Education, and Welfare to give further priority to (a) minority mental health workers (b) researches from minority groups and (c) persons serving bicultural and bilingual groups.

---

*Research and Development Manpower Initiative for the National Institute of Mental Health. A work group report. December 1976.
†Report of the Task Panel on Special Populations: Minorities, Women, Physically Handicapped. Submitted to the President's Commission on Mental Health, February 15, 1978 (vol. III).

The same Commission points out that in delivering services the priority must be people, not places.

If training is geared to serve minorities in the United States, we must be careful of our definition of *minority groups,* a loose phrase that can mean different things to different people (Heck et al 1973).

For the trainer who looks with optimism to government recommendations, it is important that these will not be just a bureaucratic gimmick, or an expiratory action for "training by guilt." They should be implemented in strict justice. We all know that in the pluralistic United States, culturally alien minorities, which face continuous culture shock or vanish in the melting pot of acculturation due to accelerated social change, show higher vulnerability to wasting away their lives in drug and/or alcohol escapism by seeking "a better life through chemistry." In this regard, there is a continuously increasing bibliography on Mexican-Americans, Puerto Ricans, Cubans, and other Spanish speaking groups.

For training to be relevant, it should serve the needs of the client and not the needs of the caregiver. Therapy is still the key word used to label the emotional transaction between parties. Everyone seems to have a therapeutic (magical?) solution for the treatment of these patients. Today the alternatives range anywhere from drug therapy to folk healing, and from the mysticotranscendent to therapeutic communities, from behavior modification to relationship enhancement programs as culturally transplanted therapies. Whether the new psychotherapies and encounters of the 1970s represent serious progress or fads has already been discussed by Charny (1974) and others.

However, we insist that, whatever the particular therapeutic approach to be employed, ethnic, cultural, and transcultural fac⁺ors should always be present in the mind of the clinician.

On the other hand, in studying cultural differences we must be careful not to fall into the trap of misunderstanding and misapplying knowledge, since there exists the real danger of "transcultural manipulation" through acculturation. According to Meyer (1977), the individual who undergoes a change in the way he values his own heritage and background may enter into conflict with himself, as well as with his family and group.

If culture "consists of patterns, explicit and implicit, of and for behavior acquired and transmitted by symbols, constituting the distinctive achievements of human groups, " and if "the essential core of culture consists of traditional (ie, historically derived and selected) ideas and especially their attached values" (Kroeber and Kluckhohn 1952), we must then conclude that culture in an anthroposocial context is equated to identity, and identity is the essence of life.

For the Spanish speaking or Hispanic-American, preserving at least their historical or ethnocultural identity becomes a matter of survival with dignity. Regardless of their ethnic origin and/or hierarchical position as caregivers, mental health workers should be aware of this, especially since Census Bureau projections indicate that in the 1980s the Spanish speaking population in the United States will reach twenty million, and by the 1990s will constitute the nation's largest minority group. If this conglomerate of people continues to face an adverse social environment as a sort of "culturecide," we will witness an increase in emotional and dependency disorders among them. We agree with Denny (1978) that social environment has recently come to be regarded as one of the most powerful determinants of behavior. This is in turn an emphasis on Gelb's (1972) previous statement: "Mental health is not an individual's state of mind but, rather, the quality of his human activity. And, if all human activity depends upon and takes place in a social matrix, one must, therefore, have healthy social experience in order to remain healthy." Preserving and enhancing one's cultural identity in pluralistic America to enrich interpersonal relationships or group interaction constitutes a healthy social experience indeed.

THE PUERTO RICANS: AN OVERVIEW

In our book entitled *A Guide to Mental Health Services* (Heck et al 1973) we emphasized that every culture has developed a complex set of standards for making a distinction between normal and abnormal functioning, and that these standards must be considered in any judgment about the "normality" or "abnormality" of a particular person's mental functioning. Therefore, when we talk about the mental health of Puerto Ricans or any other ethnic group we cannot avoid dealing with the essential core of their culture.

Concerning culture and mental illness among Puerto Ricans in Puerto Rico, Fitzpatrick et al (1971) agreed with others that certain causes of mental illness appear to be associated with the culture of the Spanish speaking in their native cultural environment. Particular culture traits function in the native environment but appear to become dysfunctional in the new cultural environment. New York City is a good example. Culture traits that are normal in a Spanish speaking background may be diagnosed as abnormal by psychiatrists in the United States. Particular kinds of treatment are culturally more suitable to the members of one culture than to members of another.

The case of Puerto Ricans in the United States, particularly along the Northeastern seaboard and in Chicago, has transcended the academic interest of urban anthropologists and social researchers. As an important segment of the 19 million United States Hispanics "awakening minority," they are increasing in political power and therefore becoming important people, notwithstanding that "the Puerto Rican experience today is all too often one of blighted hopes," and that "for them, life is mostly a grinding struggle for survival" (*Time,* Oct. 15, 1978, p 17).

The Sociocultural Dimension

Anyone engaged in the delivery of mental health care, human services, or primary care to Puerto Ricans in the United States should keep in mind the decisive force created by social and cultural variables. The sociocultural force in its interaction toward a biopsychosocial adaptation includes minority group problems involving prejudice and inadequate facilities for health, education, and welfare (Freedman et al 1976). The Puerto Rican immigrant who on the mainland becomes a manifold minority because of his ethnicity, skin color, language, belief system, place of living, and other variables. For the older person, culture shock is overtly manifested by a sudden and massive reduction of social skills by the stress of new environmental contingencies.

Lack of social skills has been called the essential behavioral deficit owing to conflict of a person with the environment (Phillips 1978). In his review of the 1974–1976 literature on social and cultural influences in psychopathology, King (1978) concluded, based on the collected data, that indeed there is a relationship between social and cultural forces in the emergence of mental illness.

In pointing out sociocultural influences, the Report of the Research Task Force of the National Institute of Mental Health (1975) emphasizes the relationship between societal stratification and psychological functioning. The report states:

> Over the last several decades, evidence has accumulated to the effect that the individual's location in the (society) stratification system bears strongly on his thoughts, dealings, and behavior....one promising hypothesis holds that the constricted conditions of life experienced by people of lower social class position may foster conceptions of social reality so limited and so rigid as to impair people's ability to deal resourcefully with the problematic and stressful.

Mental Health, Mental Illness, and Life-Styles in Puerto Rico

The study of Rogler and Hollingshead (1965), indicated that 14 years ago there was "a rate of 435 psychotics per 100,000 population in Puerto Rico." Since then, diagnostic labeling and statistical methods in the definition and categorization of mental illness have changed because research methods and case reporting have also changed. Yet, it remains painfully true that in Puerto Rico, as in any other country of the world going through sometimes paradoxical, economic, social, and cultural changes, the discrepancy between the achieved and the expected standards of living creates tensions contributing to family disorganization and vulnerability to mental illness.

While the life span for the American white in the United States is 2 years less than for the Puerto Rican living on the island, the quality of life in the United States is obviously more detrimental to the latter. (We suffer more not because we live more, but because we suffer more.) Puerto Ricans are more exposed to stressful existential situations than their American counterparts who are not forced to struggle with a problem of national identity in terms of political ambivalence or confusion, or with rampant poverty and its side effects of high unemployment, inadequate housing, crowding, insufficient school and health facilities, intoxicating ecology and the like.

Such stressful living conditions are externally oppressive, unavoidable elements pushing the Puerto Rican to seek for an anxiolytic, autoplastic change as a sort of coping mechanism even if the change is self-defeating or self-destructive, as in the case of alcohol or drug addiction, and addiction related crime.

Applying the Hunt Formula, the Puerto Rico Department of Addiction Services (DAS) estimates that, among three million Puerto Ricans residing on the island, there are approximately 1600 (estimated) addicts to "hard drugs" for every 100,000 inhabitants. On the other hand one can count by the thousands those who show psychological dependence on other controlled substances, particularly marihuana and pills of all types.

Alcoholism is considered the principal addictive disorder in Puerto Rico, where there are about 250,000 alcoholics or alcohol abusers. Puerto Rico ranks third in the world in the consumption of hard liquor per capita, after Russia and Poland, followed by France and the United States.

The so-called dual addiction is now an incipient and growing phenomenon among young Puerto Ricans. Drug and alcohol related crimes are the concern of all islanders because of their impact on domestic tranquility.

The government of Puerto Rico has been dealing with problems related to lack of mental health and/or presence of negative life-styles. For example, over the last few years, Dr. J. Rivera-Dueño, Secretary of Health, Commonwealth of Puerto Rico, has been publicly stating in all kinds of forums that factors concerning the general life-styles of the Puerto Rican make the lack of mental health the number one health problem in Puerto Rico. Rivera-Dueño, a dynamic pediatrician and health administrator, who once worked for the federal government in New York, has embarked on an ambitious island-wide program of health education, to be followed by the reorganization of the prevention, primary care, and treatment aspects in the health service delivery system. This approach aims to promote and maintain mental health and to alleviate burdens of mental illness or emotional daily problems of living.

Also, the DAS, under the enterprising and enthusiastic directorship of Mrs. Sila Nazario de Ferrer—who came to her executive position after several years of work in the social research field, and lately after 8 years as senator in the Puerto Rico Legislature—is doing its share of work. Since its creation 6 years ago, DAS has been delivering pertinent services at all levels of prevention and treatment through the best scientific approaches known for the addictive disorders and through singular, avant-garde programs for addicted offenders at both the criminal and the juvenile justice systems. At DAS the well-being of the family ranks with the priorities of prevention and treatment of alcoholism and drug addiction.

The accelerated social changes of the past decade have produced a significant shift in the traditional life-styles of the Puerto Rican. Without even leaving the island (something done very often), the Puerto Rican is becoming more and more a person influenced by the fast changes taking place all over the world. Constant traveling, better education, and the daily impact of mass media information and advertisement account for our trends to become "people for all seasons," *gente del mundo,* or people of the world, or in subtle terms, one might say subliminal acculturation. Without giving away our cultural heritage and historical background, without resigning our traditional values we are becoming not only more Americanized, but also, in some ways, more Europeanized or Africanized. We include more English words, phrases, or jargon in our daily Spanish vocabulary; we enjoy more exotic dances and music; we drink more wine, whiskey, vodka, or gin; we play more football, golf, and tennis; we smoke more pot; and we bend or defy more moral rules than ever in our individual and collective life history. Subliminal acculturation affects all socioeconomic classes in Puerto Rico but seems less evident in the poor, particularly when the Puerto Rican poor need to reinforce their identity (as at the special clusters or barrios in the United States).

On the other hand, it appears that Puerto Ricans, like Cubans, often show verbal and nonverbal behavior focusing attention on themselves as a need to assert their presence. Such activity could be a compensation for our internalized sense of smallness in our everyday comparison with the perceived hugeness of American objects. In that context, our "noisy behavior," our loud pitch of voice, our exaggerated gesticulation, and reaction with "national pride" whenever we celebrate an outstanding achievement by a Puerto Rican in sports, arts, and science all over the world, are understandable modes of expression.

The Puerto Rican-ness of the new Puerto Rican is getting diluted throughout cross-cultural pathways, as it happens, for example, with the

Italian-ness of the new Italian, the Black-ness of the new Black, the Cuban-ness of the new Cuban, the Mexican-ness of the new Mexican American, the Irish-ness of the new Irish or the Jewish-ness of the new Jew in pluralistic America.

Yet, when a Puerto Rican needs to "put on" an identifiable appearance, he goes back to his historic ethnocultural root within the anthroposocial trunk of the Taíno Indian, Spaniard, and African ethnic triad. Each of us resorts to one or more of these ethnic roots, and symbolically we wear the ethnic clothes suitable for the occasion. It seems we will retain the Puerto Rican affect regardless of any psychological fragmentation or intellectual confusion.

That is the essence of the Puerto Rican culture in its dynamic dimension. It holds the capacity or potentiality for Puerto Ricans to move freely across cultural situations without becoming amorphous molecules within any kind of melting pot. My personal experience is that at the top of El Yunque Rainforest, a few minutes away from my home, I feel the Taíno, the Spaniard, and the African streams merging and running in my veins. In Mexico City, particularly at the Museum of Anthropology and Natural History, I am the Continental Man. If it happens I am visiting Italy, in any historic place of Rome I become the Universal Man. In terms of culture, it could be wise to consider a Puerto Rican, even if he is illiterate, in that transgeographical dimension.

Culture Variables and Pluralism

Those interested in learning about key aspects of Puerto Rican culture should read Hilda Hidalgo's (1971) concise, sharp, bright, and practical document written 8 years ago for the National Rehabilitation Association. This compact document gives clear guidance on the Puerto Rican sense of dignity, language, religion, diet, music, entertainment, race, family structure, sex roles, values closely related to Puerto Rican culture, and more. Also, in the past decade literature concerning Puerto Ricans has increased. Pertinent bibliography may be obtained in the United States from the National Institute of Mental Health Clearinghouse. Perhaps more specifically from the Hispanic Research Center, Fordham University, and at the Center for Puerto Rico Studies, John Jay College of Criminal Justice, New York. Therefore, I should not repeat in this chapter what already has been so clearly printed. However, some clarifications are necessary.

What kind of Puerto Ricans are we talking about? Most of the literature available to mental health trainees in the United States makes reference to Puerto Ricans who, in a given historic moment resided on the mainland, as if they were the main interesting population. This group represents only one part of the picture and has been so misunderstood that often human services programs seem geared to deal with a caricature of Puerto Ricans.

For a pragmatic and fair understanding, Puerto Ricans should be grossly divided according to place of birth/place of living, educational (knowledge/skills), and socioeconomic variables.

The geographic variable seems to be decisive; when referring to place of living one must add "at a given time"; for we are a highly mobile people going through a constant "domestic migration" within the island's scarce territory, which implies moving from the rural to the urban or from the less urban to the more metropolitan setting, and also going through the "outside migration" from the island to the mainland, and vice-versa, as part of our fringe benefits and privileges as United States citizens.

Within the geographic context the mental health worker could possibly deal with classes as follows:

1. Those Puerto Ricans who reside or give indications of permanent residence in Puerto Rico could be referred to as "Islanders." Occasionally they travel to the United States for business or entertainment, to seek specialized education or health services, or seemingly to visit relatives and friends. This group enjoys relatively good (satisfactory to high) educational and socioeconomic living standards, but they do not necessarily constitute an elite. They get public or private mental health services in Puerto Rico and sometimes, depending on what they can afford, they will get private psychiatric hospitalization in the United States or Europe, particularly in Spain.

2. The Puerto Rican "newcomers" are those who have been forced to migrate or to settle on the mainland for prolonged periods (from a few months to many years). The reasons for their emigration are varied: a real need of a job or a better job (socioeconomic factor), and/or the hope to enjoy the well-advertised American dream (emotional-political factor). This group is naturally caught in the trap of poverty or deprived urban areas of Puerto Rico. Frequently they are less educated and less skilled than those who remain on the island. Sometimes the mental health worker meets them isolated in places such as correctional settings or state hospitals.

3. The Puerto Rican "merry-go-rounders" group consists of those who, with relative frequency, commute back and forth between the island and the mainland in a migratory revolving door. Among these air commuters are to be included seasonal farm workers, people lacking emotional and economic stability, or Puerto Ricans who are looking for a "national identity" in terms of historical and ethnocultural perceived, interpreted, and internalized roots.

4. An interesting group, from the anthroposocial viewpoint, is formed by those persons who were born on the mainland of Puerto Rican

parents, or those who during their infancy or early childhood settled in the United States with their parents or their extended or surrogate families. These are the "Mainlandricans." By reason of birth or settlement during an early age they consider themselves a part of their natural or foster home places or belonging there. They have been labeled as the "Niuroricans" or "Neoricans" from New York or New Jersey, the "Chicagoricans" from Chicago, "Bostonricans" from Boston, and "Philliricans" from Philadelphia. They also have been subjected to great prejudice and considered aliens in both the mainland and Puerto Rico. Nevertheless, throughout the last decade, and because of the phenomenon of reverse migration they have been able to integrate in the mainstream cultural life of the island, where now they feel they are welcome and accepted. While living in the United States, in geographical terms, their sense of belonging was imprinted on a map of a given state or city district. Concerning ethnic identity some of them, tired and frustrated of repetitive rejection by other predominant ethnic groups, resorted to their own parental roots and rediscovered themselves within a buoyant frame of ethnic pride. Generally speaking, they encounter no major difficulties in adjustment or readaptation to life on the island through common cultural denominators, or in the Puerto Rican clusters or barrios in the United States.

However, a fistful of them seem to be striving for a non-Puerto Rican identification and tend to think of themselves as different Puerto Ricans, as if they were a light year away from the islanders. They resort to self-denial as a main coping mechanism. They will never adequately adapt to a (possible) living opportunity on the island; they are full of resentment and sometimes they overly voice hatred against their ethnic origin, doing their best to stay away from the Puerto Ricans. They speak shyly of their origin and feel ashamed if it is discovered. They try to feel and think as "full-blooded Americans." In psychodynamic terms this could be viewed as an imitation of the perceived ideal or as an identification with the aggressor. To this regard, Mizio (1974) states:

> The Puerto Rican who, by placing himself into the proverbial melting pot, is able to metamorphose as white with an Anglicized name and life-style, makes it finally possible to provide for his family an American standard of living. The price he must pay is denial of self and heritage and a sacrifice of personal integrity. Whether society permits him a self-definition of white or black he is faced with an identity problem...

5. A special group consists of a combination formed by some of the Puerto Rican "merry-go-rounders" and some of the "Mainlandricans." They like to think they belong to some place, either Puerto Rico or the mainland, but at the same time they feel uncomfortable in both. In terms of mental illness or emotional disorders this is a highly vulnerable group.

One of them told me that the place where he feels most at home was in the airplane whenever he travels from the island to mainland and vice versa. This group in which anomie is pervasive seems to be always in the middle of nowhere. These are the "Unsettledricans." For them, nomadism seems to be an egosyntonic behavior even within the context of social hyperkinesis.

Labels for the five above mentioned Puerto Rican groups are not intended to be pejorative but descriptive of what are unavoidable sociocultural phenomena impacting the Puerto Ricans. Not included in those groups are, of course, those who move to the United States mainland simply because they like it better than the island; they may be married or not to non-Puerto Rican spouses; they enjoy their work and do not care too much about ethnic pride or national identity. They belong to the place where they can hang their hats. Maybe they are not too happy, but because of their flexible, adaptive, sociosyntonic, psychological resources, they say they are satisfied.

The educated person in Puerto Rico, as in other parts of the world, does not necessarily have a good socioeconomic status, but undoubtedly he enjoys a better quality of life. If for one reason or another he lives on the mainland he will survive, in Darwinian terms, in the American urban jungle of the ghetto, and eventually he is likely to become an agent for social change if he remains on the mainland. In the mental health arena he is sometimes found on the other side of the fence, in a role of a caregiver rather than a caretaker.

Quite often within the geographical, educational and socioeconomic variables, another type of Puerto Rican shows up, the political dissident from the middle left to the extreme left. This group includes all kinds of people, from hard laborers to sophisticated academicians, pointing out that the political relationship of the United States with Puerto Rico is colonial and Fanon (1973) emphasizes that colonialism is a cause of maladaptive behavior.

CLINICAL CONSIDERATIONS CONCERNING
CULTURAL INFLUENCES ON VALUES AND BEHAVIOR

Concerning the mental health of the Puerto Rican, especially the young generation, one cannot avoid the influence of the universal technological revolutions of our society; they impinge on and affect the dynamic aspect of culture. Puerto Rican society—as American society—can be divided in three "before and after" periods: before and after the man on the moon, before and after the contraceptive pill, and before and after the Beatles. These three events are symbolic of main universal shifts in technology, mores, and tradition from which the Puerto Ricans and many other people around the world cannot escape. Therefore, clinicians should look at Puerto Rican culture not as a static process, of course, but rather as a dynamic process constantly changing under the influence of a technological world and a revolutionary society bridging gaps between geographically distant and ethnoculturally different groups.

Just a decade ago some of the "findings" and statements of social researchers on Puerto Rican issues made sense. Not any more. Ten or 15 years ago readers of Puerto Rican literature could swallow statements like, "...the cultural requirement for dependence and submissiveness in the female results in frustration which, in turn, give rise to fantasies of romantic life especially in adolescent girls...," or, "...due to the constant presence of others, all components of behavior become overly-socialized including sexual behavior...," or, "the attitude of fatalism cushions the shock of failure, the person can always attribute his failing to God's will...."

Statements of that sort, which at one time would seem part valid to some Puerto Ricans in given historical situations, have permeated the scientific literature and have unintentionally contributed to reinforcing the Puerto Rican cultural myth. The clinician may be caught unaware in a countertransference process detrimental both to him and the Puerto Rican patient or client.

Clinicians in the United States treating or intervening with Puerto Ricans must 1) make a careful assessment of the person he is treating within the context of Puerto Rican pluralism, and 2) recognize his capacity or limitation to communicate directly or indirectly with his patient, on both linguistic and cultural terms. Besides an assessment of the so-called Puerto Rican culture the clinician should weigh the levels of acculturation and resistance. In this regard he should take into consideration issues related to patterns of migration and adaptation to new environments, communication, expressions of mental illness as perceived by the non-Puerto Rican, sex roles as conflicting among generations and affecting traditional family life-styles, belief system, and the impact of family roles on aspects of both mental health and mental illness to name just a few.

Migration, Adaptation, Acculturation, and Resistance

As I mentioned elsewhere (Gómez 1976), once in the United States, Puerto Ricans tend to congregate in visible population clusters, for economic, social, and political reasons rather than because of a "natural preference to associate with their 'own kind' due to strong kinship of friendship ties" as indicated in an article (*Boston Sunday Globe,*

December 20, 1970, p A-3); when pushed to low-income urban districts, Puerto Ricans organize neighborhoods, or barrios, where they share and maintain cultural values. On the other hand, Puerto Ricans develop a psychological stance that allows them to escape when it becomes intolerable because of the ease with which they can return to their island (Cohen 1970), where—just a few hours later—they find themselves being not a minority or a majority, but plain human beings.

Confronted with the "love it or leave it" dilemma, Puerto Ricans arriving in the United States generally go through a crisis of adaptation that can be transitory or long-term in nature.

Canino and Canino-Stolberg (1978) describe how the Puerto Rican traditional family, in terms of structure and interaction, is required to change its patterns of transactions when the family migrates to the United States. The authors point out how the level of stress, together with the flexibility of the family system to adjust to new patterns, will determine whether the family adapts or becomes dysfunctional, and they emphasize the intergenerational conflict of Puerto Ricans in the United States.

On the other hand, in pointing out home–school conflict and the Puerto Rican child in the United States, Montalvo (1974) states that despite good intentions and special projects, education is critically affected by lack of knowledge and appreciation of different cultural patterns.

In dealing with levels of acculturation, Arce and Torres-Matrullo (1978) call attention to values, expectations, stresses, presenting problems and treatment behaviors of newly migrated Hispanic groups (particularly Puerto Ricans) and contrast them with clients who are considered to have achieved a greater level of acculturation.

Issues on Communication

The basis for any emotional transaction and interpersonal relationship is communication, verbal and nonverbal. Good examples would be the crying spells, and gestures, and the restful quietness of the newborn as expressions of anxiety or tranquility.

Language is acquired through a cultural filter and the acquisition of the symbolic world of nonverbal expression. Eisenberg (1972) states that "one trait common to man everywhere is language; in the sense that only the human species displays it, the capacity to acquire language must be genetic."

With regard to verbal communication, as in the case of the Spanish speaking, bilingualism and its relation to psychopathology have received little attention in the general research and clinical literature (Laski and Talesporos 1977). Ruiz's warning (1975) concerning that subject is pertinent:

> Even in the use of the same language, the meaning of words varies from person to person and from place to place. The exchange of ideas is influenced by unconscious and conscious material being mixed in an indiscriminate way, which creates conflict in people relating to each other. The conflict is intensified when two languages are being used, as for instance, Spanish and English. As a person switches his language, he also shows a change in his behavior, as if he were two people operating under different consortships. Often, unconscious material comes out more easily in the original language.

Judith Nine-Curt (1976), a Puerto Rican educator, calls attention to the fact that "by the time we are seven and we are ready to enter school for the first time, every single one of us is already a cultural and linguistic entity; in other words, we are already Puerto Ricans, or Chinese, or Americans...". For her, every single person is the heir of an unimaginably vast cultural wealth. According to American anthropologist Ray L. Birdwhistell, communication is at most 35% language, and Nine-Curt indicates that "the remaining 65% of communication which is mostly made up of nonverbal activities, is still functioning among the American Puerto Ricans in New York City and Chicago and other large cities of the United States as it functions in Puerto Rico. Their NVC (non-verbal communication) systems are Puerto Rican, their ethnicity — that is, their racial make-up — is Puerto Rican. Only their language has changed, for most of them speak English." Concerning the Puerto Ricans in the United States, she points out that they look and behave very much like those on the island with one exception: they speak English; however, most of their nonverbal ways of communicating among themselves are Puerto Rican, even in second or third generations in the States."

According to Torrey (1973), therapists generally tend to relate better to patients or clients who speak the same language, share a common world view and/or common thoughts on causation. Therapists and clients have, in Torrey's words, "cognitive congruence." Communication problems create serious difficulties in developing empathy toward the patient (Ruiz and Langrod, 1976).

As Rogers (1961) pointed out, communication and empathic understanding, or "understanding *with* a person, not *about* him," are clues to successful therapy, and can bring about major changes in personality. Rogers states:

> Although the tendency to make evaluations is common in all interchange of language, it is very much heightened in those situations where feelings and emotions are deeply involved. So the stronger the feelings the more likely it is that there will be no mutual element in the communications.

There will be just two ideas, two feelings, two judgments, missing each other in psychological space. Real communication occurs and this evaluative tendency is avoided, when we listen with understanding. What does this mean? It means to see the expressed idea and attitude from the other person's point of view, to sense how it feels to him, to achieve his frame of reference in regard to the thing he is talking about.

Expressions of "Psychopathology"

I agree with the clinical experience reported by Abad et al (1977) who call our attention to common physical complaints of Puerto Rican patients (headaches, dizziness, muscular aches, chest pain, and palpitations, "brain ache" or *dolor de cerebro* located in the occipital and upper cervical areas), which are often of psychosomatic nature. These authors indicate that, in a clinical setting in the United States, the approach to somatization found most useful to clinicians "is one that accepts and seeks to relieve the bodily complaint of the patient and, in that process joins the confidence of the patient which allows exploration of underlying problems," and that "seen almost as frequently as patients with somatic complaints are patients who are nonpsychotic yet describe hallucinatory experiences (pseudohallucinations).

Compared with hallucinations of a psychotic patient, pseudohallucinations generally tend to be less dramatic and often occur just prior to falling asleep at night. In general they are less disturbing psychologically and more culturally syntonic than hallucinations of the psychotic. Their onset is frequently precipitated by situational stress of transitory nature and typically includes visual imaginings or auditory sensations of hearing one's name being called, knocking at the door, or strange noises about the house. Voices or visions of people recently deceased are not uncommon.

Some authors, who are quite aware of how language and prejudice have clearly influenced the labeling of psychopathologic illness and service delivery to Puerto Ricans, are also concerned about both overestimation and underestimation of disease by Anglo psychiatrists and other clinicians who cannot communicate directly with the Puerto Rican patient in the United States.

As examples of misinterpretations of cultural traits of Spanish speaking patients seeking medical help from Anglo psychiatrists, and of the eventual translation of such traits to diagnostic entities, I remember a few cases in which my consultation as a Spanish-speaking psychiatrist was required. It happened in the case of three Mexican Americans, one Cuban, one Chilean and nine Puerto Ricans all with the diagnosis of schizophrenia or manic-depressive illness when they were just going through acute personal and familial crises.

On the other hand, an Anglo psychiatrist in Puerto Rico diagnosed a depressive neurosis, severe in an 11-year-old girl who, through a quick urinalysis was found to be suffering a kidney condition. In another instance, an Anglo psychiatric trainee under my supervision, very eager to understand cultural issues pertaining to Puerto Rican patients, insisted that a young man "was going through a cultural-situational crisis under the influence of witchcraft" when in reality the patient was overtly psychotic.

Another clinical challenge for the non-Puerto Rican therapist could be what is already known as the "Puerto Rican syndrome." Maldonado-Sierra et al (1960) in their studies on mental disease among Puerto Ricans, contributed to the psychiatric literature pointing out this peculiar syndrome, which had been well conceptualized in its dynamics and cultural determinants by Fernández-Marina (1961). The syndrome, named *el ataque* (the attack) consists of bizarre seizure patterns, usually considered psychogenic in nature and identifiable as uniquely Puerto Rican; it can function as a basic ego defense against psychotic breaks, or as a limit to extreme regression or total disorganization of the ego. A good clinical warning (Abad et al 1977) is that "often misdiagnosed, the *ataque* is a hyperkinetic episode, including a display of histrionics or aggression on the part of the patient, and sometimes culminating in stupor. It is critical for clinicians to be able to differentiate an *ataque* from an epileptic seizure or other pathology."

A variant of the *ataque* can be observed during funeral rites as an expression of grief, from immediate relatives and close (or even distant) friends of the deceased. In dynamic terms, the funeral just offers the opportunity for a physical release of accumulated repressed anger, or discomfort, through a socially acceptable fit.

Sex Roles

In Puerto Rico, young girls are not prevented any more from freely seeking a compatible mate for marriage because of the family's cloistering her in their anxiety to protect her virginity until marriage. Chaperoning is a laugh-provoking cultural residue. Yet, virginity still is highly valued, as it is for millions of non-Hispanic Americans.

Machismo, conceptualized or functional, seems to be a dirty word or an obscene trait within the cultural mythology of the island. *Machismo* has been defined as "the quality that exemplifies man's superiority over women, the value of demonstrating by acts considered virile such as fathering children, seducing women, being waited upon by them, avoiding tasks that are considered "women's tasks," that the man is *macho completo* (all man)" (Hidalgo 1971).

A favorite, popular joke among Puerto Rican goes as follows: A man from Central America, with a big moustache and using strong gestures was bragging that in his country "all of them were *machos*..." A smiling Puerto Rican who was listening replied: "In Puerto Rico we are half *machos* and half *hembras* (rough females), and we enjoy it a lot." That joke should not be taken lightly as a popular expression that in Puerto Rico sex roles are clearly defined for it alerts one to something else. Nowadays, when a Puerto Rican man publicly voices his *machismo,* he exposes himself to find his statement is detrimental for his own masculinity. On the other hand, Puerto Rican *machismo,* is less tyrannical in comparison with American *machismo*, which is portrayed by an increasing number of wife beaters, an expression of physical abuse that is vanishing in Puerto Rico.

When a family migrates from the island to the mainland, traditional values and structures are challenged, particularly the relationship between husband and wife. In this regard Tomasulo (personal communication 1975) states that as the woman often finds employment more quickly and easily than the man, "the...[demoralizing]...situation threatens the man's concept of his manliness, while at the same time forces the woman to question her subordinate role in light of her new economic power and resulting emerging autonomy." This phenomenon is common among working class couples in the island, where *hembrismo* (*machismo's* counterpart) is an emerging expression of a sociocultural phenomenon (Gómez 1977).

Hembrismo — in terms of woman's emancipation — has been looked upon as a female revenge (Habach 1972). According to my clinical experience as well as observations on the street, I have concluded that in Puerto Rico *hembrismo* is a form of assertiveness of the woman who, through a frustrated intent to imitate a male *(macho),* becomes a primitive female or rough woman *(hembra). Hembrismo* is not a search for an (unreachable) identification psychosexually with the man; it is rather an imitation taking place in a sociosexual spectrum of idealized roles; and it is the natural outcome of an evolutional social process, a normal reaction, within a historical context. It should not be confused with the American women's liberation movement, although it shares some common elements concerning social (and maybe political) goals.

In Puerto Rico I have advised therapists to avoid countertransference problems, for *hembrismo,* like *machismo,* has certain personal healthy adaptive values and properties; both become noxious if they are institutionalized or systematized.

Also, in regard to cultural aspects of countertransference while dealing with sex roles in Puerto Rican patients, Torres-Matrullo (1978) alerts clinicians in the United States to be careful "not to aggravate those conflicts/stresses impinging on the family unit, by, eg, encouraging a woman to assert herself without regard to the negative consequences which may result on the part of the male partner whose position within the home is already being undermined." That author goes on in her caution against expecting all Puerto Rican women to fall within the traditional cultural stereotype for there are real differences among Puerto Rican men and women according to the level of acculturation and education.

Belief System

Subjugation of nature and surrendering to fate's contrivances are part and parcel of cultural values among Spanish speaking populations. Because of his Taíno-Spanish-African cultural heritage, the Puerto Rican often exhibits, and clings to, a peculiar belief system. Most Puerto Ricans are Catholics only in a traditional way, and they are experiencing a growing influence from the Protestant church. Regardless of religious regulations or parochial prohibitions, Puerto Ricans of all social strata are inclined to seek other supernatural interpretations, or explanations, about the cause and effect of the good and the evil in their behavior. That usually happens in the absence of strong (church) religious values, and also when one is experiencing a loss, real or symbolic, of a family member or a beloved person, or of a job, or health, or of just good luck.

Often, in the midst of a stressful situation with moral implications, when the person feels threatened by God's immediate and unavoidable punishment, the Puerto Rican prays or looks for assistance from his church, asks for forgiveness and works through his emotional crisis by means of church devices (ie, penitence or personal *sacrificio* which implies not to seek pleasure or gratification during a given period of time). This reparative, compensatory good behavior, sometimes is channeled through *promesas* (promises for inhibitory, unpleasurable, behavior); and it is not rare to see Puerto Rican women making public announcement of their *promesas* by wearing humble clothes of a given color, according to the saint or patron in whom their faith relies. All this has to be seen in a religious-cultural context.

If a very personal, individual, inner feeling of an emotional crisis persists, clinically expressed by either anxiety or depression, or both, and personally interpreted as bad luck, *brujería o mal de ojo* (witchcraft or evil eye), the Puerto Rican like any other person from the Caribbean, might seek help from a source who could give an "acceptable," concrete explanation according to his belief system based on traditional, cultural, and religious constructs. In those instances he may resort to the spiritual healer or *espiritista* who undoubtedly could play an important role. But you may rest assured that before going to the *espiritista*, the Puerto Rican will have searched for the help of formal caregivers (physicians, people of the church, professionals of all sorts) or informal caregivers (bartenders, beauticians, relatives, the friend around the corner) as a first step or as a primary care source.

A sizeable body of literature is available concerning the role of *espiritismo* (or "spiritualism") as a tradition among Puerto Ricans. In this regard the contributions of Vivian Garrison (1977) and of Koss (1979) are well known. As a result of a study of a Puerto Rican community mental health resource, Harwood (1977) summarizes what has been written on the subject up to a few years ago.

Espiritismo has been considered a form of "folk psychiatry," or "psychotherapy." It is debatable if its function is to prevent the labeling of the participant as crazy, since the spiritualist session has created a permissive group setting wherein all abnormal behavior is given meaning and is made acceptable. It is debatable and sometimes social researchers and sophisticated onlookers of a given culture tend to forget that tradition is both an egosyntonic and a sociosyntonic process; and that "abnormal behavior" is sometimes a biased perception of the evaluator's being alienated from the cultural life experience of the group being observed. In that context, a pseudohallucination suggesting a link to religious beliefs and the supernatural, for example, is a normal expression of behavior.

Not all Puerto Ricans resort to *espiritismo* as a healing art or science; it is not dogma even for most of those to whom *espiritismo* is an appealable source of help, for they regularly attend their churches. For them, *espiritismo* is clinging to a cultural, acceptable process of socialization in which a secondary gain is to feel safe in a no-man's land of beliefs. In this regard, Puerto Ricans tend to think and to act in a hopeful, though ambivalent way, showing a protective shield in which the wise motto "Por Si Acaso" (just in case) is built.

In some predominant Puerto Rican milieu on the mainland it is, of course, understandable to pay attention to the cultural value of *centros espiritistas,* or clinical set-ups. I agree that when feasible, the psychiatric or mental health establishment—from medical schools to neighborhood centers—should collaborate with *espiritistas,* for it is evident they are a cultural, practical, and most valuable outreach source. That could also be the case of *curanderos* or those who practice *curanderismo,* which Kiev (1968) has labeled as Mexican-American folk psychiatry.

In his summary of a panel discussion, "Voodoo, Spiritualism and Psychiatry." Ralph (1977) indicated:

> There was a consensus among participants that a mental health professional must know more about an individual's cultural background if he or she is to be effective. The point is obvious when one considers a person from a society which has institutionalized the belief of good and evil spirits and the practice of witchcraft, but it is just as true when dealing with persons in the United States who are significantly, though not as

obviously, culturally different. Mental health professionals must accord respect to all belief systems which link individuals to socially validated world views and which provide meaning to their own, very human, experience.

On the other hand, other authors (Abad et al 1977) state that decisions whether to involve *espiritistas* in mental health programs depend on the prevailing climate of the individual Hispanic community and the psychiatric setting, for the degree of receptivity may vary between communities. They based their reservations on the ambivalent attitudes of some Puerto Ricans toward *espiritismo,* and they express concern "that individuals strongly involved in a religious faith may feel offended by an official endorsement of *espiritismo;* and the preference of many patients attending *centros* to keep their visits a private matter." Like Harwood (1977) they feel that "research is needed to clarify those circumstances where folk healers might be most effective and where they would be less so, or even contraindicated."

Harwood's indication is that:

> Provided ethical problems could be overcome (and these are many and weighty), a controlled experiment comparing cure rates of Puerto Rican spiritist patients who had been matched and assigned to spiritist and psychiatric forms of therapy would yield important evidence pertinent to the general question of the relative effectiveness of indigenous and psychiatric therapies.

Family Roles

The emerging issue on the evolution of sex roles of the Puerto Ricans tends to give a blurred image of what is known as the traditional family structure. I agree with Hidalgo that the patriarchal extended family is still the predominant family structure, and that the nuclear family is becoming more and more prevalent, especially among the growing middle class.

However, a clear definition of the Puerto Rican family in the 1970s has been an uphill task for social researchers and human behavior theoreticians. I can remember more than a dozen occasions when bright people with significant expertise and from the most ample and diverse educational backgrounds had to adjourn endless meetings without arriving at a consensus of an agreeable, acceptable definition (for them) of what is the Puerto Rican family nowadays. Puerto Rican islanders as Fernández-Marina (1960, 1968) who elaborated on the psychological functions of Puerto Rican families, and Vales (1978) who defined the concept of *familismo* (familism) as a system of values have made important contributions. I believe that this difficulty also occurs when a definition of family is put under the microscope of such variables as history and culture, socioeconomic and sociopolitical factors, migratory patterns, and the structural versus the functional-dynamic role.

Macroscopically, the Puerto Rican family can be viewed as a cohesive group linked by blood ties, psychological interests, or community common denominators. In a given historical situation (a social party, a voyage, a civic or political meeting, or in an unexpected encounter) a distant relative or a person from one's home town automatically will be welcome as "a brother" or a "sister."

Cohesiveness is deeply ingrained in the Puerto Rican's traditional, ethnocultural homogeneity without exception of classes and regardless of socioeconomic status. Cohesiveness is shown in friendly nonverbal communication (a smile, a handshake, a tap on the shoulder or other affectionate expressions of touch), and in the genuine readiness to give a hand, to help someone who is in disgrace. This proves true regardless of exceptional instances in which the Puerto Rican remains indifferent through dehumanized inhibitions, such as a negative imitation of the perceived, stereotyped, American way of living as "mind your own business."

The cohesive element in the Puerto Rican family is the cue to understand why, in some instances a given family is inclined to reinforce or perpetuate a disorder that seems to be pathological or detrimental for an outsider. In such instances, disequilibrium or imbalance means equilibrium. For in the (conflictual) intrafamilial structure and psychodynamics a strange homeostasis takes place in order to accept, understand, and maintain self-defeating or self-destructive behavior of any of the family. In given moments that sort of selective blindness or denial serves as a coping mechanism. That does not mean that mental illness or deviant behavior represent a "normal" or acceptable way of effecting intrafamilial transactions; however, the lack of a stigmatizing label for a given family at a given time appears to lessen the traumatic effect of negative behavior, or negative collective life-style in that family.

When a diagnostic label is used to describe a patient's problem, it is commonly said that that person *is* neurotic or psychotic or compulsive or whatever. As if by magic, the label stretches integrally over the patient. The patient *is* as opposed to what the patient *does*. Instead of being a functional description of a specific mental impairment, the diagnostic label serves as an ambiguous and pejorative statement about the patient's whole personality (Heck et al 1973). The same criterion could be applied whenever we refer to a family unit (ie, "the González or the Pérez families") who probably have been already playing a scapegoat role at a community level.

The same person who would not admit that a close family member is showing deviant behavior (for example: mother-daughter, wife-husband, or father-son relationship), later on would admit it with sorrow and desire to help. This would happen in those instances when other systems would intervene to affect the "deviant" person, such as mental health, criminal justice, or the juvenile justice systems.

Needless to say, the cohesive element — the glue that preserves Puerto Rican-ness — is best used in the promotion and preservation of mental health. In this regard, within a cultural frame — tradition and folklore holding hands — the psychiatric or mental health establishment could invest useful energy in the planning, implementation, and development of preventive programs. This could be channeled through mass media education, neighborhood groups, and primary care projects, to name a few. In dealing with strategies, people from all walks of life should be involved, of course.

Grossly defined, the Puerto Rican family is, and will continue to be in the foreseeable future, a helping institution. Good advice to the Anglo psychiatric establishment: when dealing with Puerto Rican families for the understanding of a mental health condition or a social health situation, or when recruiting the family efforts for the prevention, promotion, or preservation of mental and social health, the best way to do it is through a culturally oriented helping-the-helper-to-help-himself type of program. A clinical vignette is pertinent at this point.

One chilly morning in December, 1970, I was in Boston visiting the Office of Employment (a Massachusetts State agency) at Cardinal Cushing Center. At that time I was a Fellow at the Harvard Laboratory of Community Psychiatry and had a liaison and field placement with a mental health service sponsored by Boston University Medical School. At the time I was not only one of the two available Spanish speaking psychiatrists in the whole Boston Metropolitan Area where approximately forty thousand Spanish speaking people were living, but also I was considered "an expert on Puerto Rican affairs," a title designed to cover up my token role. Part of my self-assigned duties consisted of rambling around the South End, Roxbury, and North Dorchester areas, where myriads of Puerto Ricans resided, to get an idea and a feeling of the interaction among the Boston academic establishments, federal, state, and city agencies, and Puerto Rican community-based self-help groups.

When I talked to Mr. V, Director of the Office of Employment, he informed me that Puerto Ricans were having problems getting a job because of language barrier, cultural adjustment, low level of education and high index of illiteracy in English, plus a lack of motivation to study, and, low job market. While there, I witnessed an incident I should describe, for it will give an idea of the feelings of a Puerto Rican going through a life crisis ordeal in Boston:

> The small office was crowded with applicants looking for jobs. A 33-year-old, male Puerto Rican entered the office and gave a piece of paper to Mr. V — angrily voicing his complaint "that for the third time he

was refused a job in spite of being referred by Mr. V's office." The man sat down talking (in Spanish) to other applicants. Then he said: "One of these days I am going to kill someone, at least in prison one does not pay rent." He was showing free-floating anxiety and went on with his homicidal ruminations until I asked him whom he was going to kill and how. The man stared at me and somewhat confused said: "I...don't know...." I told him that was part of the problem, not knowing whom he was going to kill, but that I believed him and I was taking his words very seriously because there was no question that he was quite desperate, that he was building up a lot of tension and that, given the situation and condition to blow up, he might kill someone. As I talked to him he calmed down a bit and gave me a condensed personal history. About a year previously he had been admitted to a local (Boston) hospital "because he was going out of his mind." At the hospital, "they found something wrong with his blood." After 5 months of hospitalization he left the institution against medical advice. He went to Patterson, New Jersey, "looking for a job" while his wife and children remained on welfare in Boston. The man's argument was that he did not want his family to be on welfare since he was the man of the house and he wanted to work as he always had; he did not want his family "living on charity." The man recognized "he was reaching the bottom of the hole" and that when he said he was going to kill someone he was not joking at all. That kind of thought was something that bothered him once in a while "especially when he feels he is being rejected" as for instance, when he is refused a job. The man realized he was in need of (social, medical, and psychiatric) help because he was feeling "physically and mentally wasted." On my advice he agreed to get in contact with his doctor at the hospital where he was a former patient, "that same afternoon." I told him I was also in the helping professions and that I wanted to contact his family to see what could be done. When he said goodbye, his handshake was strong and warm.

Next day, a follow-up on that Puerto Rican's problem resulted in a family crisis intervention which proved to be the most beneficial for all concerned. The wife and other close relatives shared responsibilities to alleviate the man's burden as head of the family, in that case a "troubled head." That Puerto Rican was seeing himself reflected in the mirror of his family. Every day he was feeling more inadequate; he was very preoccupied about the value judgment of others concerning the way he was responding to his family needs and demands. When the family, in its helping role, expanded from nuclear to an extended structure and became a source of gratification and of moral support, the man's intrapsychic world turned to be less conflicted and threatening.

The influence of parents and their neuroses on the developing child has long been recognized, and the importance of unconscious conflicts in the parents as a cause of conflicts in the child is gaining more acceptance (Cavenar and Butts 1979). This must be kept in mind by Anglo psychiatrists who, in dealing with Puerto Rican families on the mainland should make an assessment of the younger generation within a family context, for the Puerto Rican child in the mainland is caught in the middle of two main cultural influences and all kinds of cross-cultural impacts, sometimes making his cultural identity crisis a permanent one.

A Final Note to Anglo or Non-Puerto Rican Psychiatrists

Clinicians should be aware of cultural value clashes while engaging in individual, group, or family therapy. The therapist who accepts cultural stereotypes without question runs the risk of misinterpreting symptoms and response to treatment, as Raquel Cohen maintains (1974). I agree with Chediak (1971) that, in the effort to understand another's behavior, the therapist should possess empathy, intuition, and a set of theoretical constructs as his three basic professional tools. We also agree that attitudes in understanding another's behavior are based on the negative stereotyping of the other's culture and ethnic background (Weiss and Perry 1977).

In his approach to the mind, the psychiatrist depends on his educational formation in terms of specific training, on his ethnocultural life experience, and on his own rigidity or open-mindedness. Whether his approach to another mind is physical, intrapsychic, interpersonal, existential, naturalistic, or supernatural, he must be aware of the role that basic values of culture play in human behavior. In order to understand the psychodynamics of the individual we must first understand his cultural status (MacKinnon and Michels 1971).

The basic value of Puerto Rican culture is a form of individualism that focuses on the inner importance of the person (Fitzpatrick 1971). On the mainland, individualism is seen by judging a person for what he *does* and what he *has* rather than what he is (Tomasulo, personal communication, 1975). To this regard, Maurice Nicholl's words (1973) are more important than ever: "A man is his understanding. If you wish to see what a man *is* and not what he is *like,* look at the level of his understanding."

On no less importance at this point is the advice given by Bluestone and Purdy (1977):

> Perhaps the "American" clinician who can best treat Puerto Rican patients is the one who finally realizes that the Puerto Rican culture is different—it is not "American"—and that it not only confounds him at times, but frustrates him in his practice and may even cause him to err in his diagnosis. If he can recognize that *he* has to learn, and wants to, then he will find that his skills can be more appropriately applied. We would add that a clinical service itself must go through this process so that it can provide the clinician with the opportunity and the impetus to learn.

Aware of such reality, Victor Bernal and others at the Puerto Rico Institute of Psychiatry embarked on a training effort, a Don Quixote dream difficult for non-Puerto Ricans to analyze and interpret. Bernal, who developed his Ethnic Self-Awareness Inventory (1973) as a practical tool that came out of his remarkable transcultural observations (1971), has been trying to implement two avant-garde training projects at his institute. One of the projects, entitled The Laboratory of Socio-Cultural Detoxification, was intended "for the detoxification of cultural prejudices and racial misunderstanding." The trainees were intended to be highly placed professionals from the mainland—who have within their aegis the delivery of services to the minorities. Highly placed professionals in Puerto Rico were prepared to form the "trainer group." The other project, entitled The Selective Recruitment Program, was aimed at developing special training on "bicultural psychiatry." In that program, trainees from mainland "sister institutions" were chosen each year for 3 years, to become psychiatric residents at the Puerto Rico Institute of Psychiatry, which serves as "the mother institution." The goal was that at the end of a fully approved residency program in Puerto Rico, the psychiatrist, besides getting good clinical training, would have profited from a unique set of clinical skills on bicultural psychiatry; then, he would go back to the mainland to engage in the training, development, and supervision of mental health teams who would serve the best interests of Spanish speaking populations (Bernal et al 1977). Elsewhere I have stressed this need for special consideration in structuring mental health and human services for the Spanish speaking in the United States (Gómez 1975, 1976; Gómez and Silva 1977).

At this point I cannot help quoting Judith Nine-Curt, for her indications are relevant to the practice of any non-Puerto Rican clinician or mental health worker:

> We cannot continue to live our lives among others, particularly among people from other ethnic backgrounds, always worried about being hurt and hurting others, always in a resentful and rejecting mood. We must try hard to learn to switch cultural channels at the same time we retain our cultural styles among our own. We may finally come to feel that we are not living among "strangers" but among people just like ourselves.

At the San Juan International Airport, as one walks across to the United States Immigration Service, an English-speaking officer asks the same routine question: "Where were you born?" The laconic answers of passengers reflect their place of origin: Puerto Rico, Wisconsin, New York. Very few people are aware that Mrs. Culture and her family travel in the same airplane, wearing universal clothes.

BIBLIOGRAPHY

Abad V, Ramos J, Boyce E: Clinical issues in the psychiatric treatment of Puerto Ricans. *Transcultural Psychiatry: An Hispanic Perspective,* monograph 4. Los Angeles, Spanish Speaking Mental Health Research Center (UCLA), 1977.

Arce AA, Torres-Matrullo C: *Acculturation: Its Impact on Treatment Strategies.* Read at Special Session "The Hispanic-American Family: Stresses and Strengths." American Psychiatric Association Annual Meeting, Atlanta, May 1978.

Bernal y del Río V: *Imitation, Identification and Identity (Remarks on transcultural observations).* The Herman Goldman International Lecture Series, New York Medical College, May 14, 1971.

Bernal y del Río V: *The Ethnic Self-Awareness Inventory.* San Juan, The Puerto Rico Institute of Psychiatry, 1973.

Bernal y del Río V: *Ethnophobia and Socio-Cultural Detoxification.* Special lecture delivered at Harvard Medical School, Boston, March 1977.

Bernal y del Río V, Gómez AG, Martineau B: *Transculturality in Psychiatric Training: The Puerto Rico Experience.* Read at the Annual Meeting of the American Psychiatric Association, Toronto, May 1977.

Bluestone H, Purdy B: Psychiatric services to Puerto Rican patients in the Bronx. *Transcultural Psychiatry: An Hispanic Perspective,* monograph 4. Los Angeles, Spanish Speaking Mental Health Research Center (UCLA), 1977.

Canino IA, Canino-Stolberg GJ: *Impact of Stress on the Puerto Rican Family: Treatment Considerations.* Read at Special Session "The Hispanic-American Family: Stresses and Strengths." American Psychiatric Association Annual Meeting, Atlanta, May 1978.

Cavenar JO, Butts NT: Unconscious communication between father and son. *Am J Psychiatry* 136(3):344-345, 1979.

Charny I: The new psychotherapies and encounters of the seventies: Progress or fads? *Reflections* 10(2):1-13, 1974.

Chediak C: Discussion on G.R. Ticho's cultural aspects of transference and countertransference. *Bull Menninger Clin* 35(5):326-330, 1971.

Cohen R: *Preventive Mental Health Programs for Ethnic Minority Populations: A Case in Point.* Speech delivered before the XXXIX Congreso Internacional de Americanistas, Lima, Peru. (Available from the Laboratory of Community Psychiatry, Harvard Medical School), August 1970.

Denny NR: Social environment as a therapeutic agent. *Psychiatr Ann* 8(2):75-79, 1978.

Eisenberg L: The human nature of human nature. *Science* 176:123-128, 1972.

Fanon F: *Los Condenados de la Tierra.* Fondo de Cultura Económica, Mexico, 1963.

Favazza AR, Oman M: Overview: Foundations of cultural psychiatry. *Am J Psychiatry* 135(3):293-303, 1978.

Fernández-Marina R: Cultural stress and schizophrenogenesis in the mothering one in Puerto Rico. *Ann NY Acad Sci* 84:864-877, 1960.

Fernández-Marina R: The Puerto Rican syndrome: Its dynamic and cultural determinants. *Psychiatry* 24:79-82, 1961.

Fernández-Marina R: The psychological functions of Puerto Rican families. *Proceedings of The Family in the Caribbean,* Institute of Caribbean Studies of the University of Puerto Rico, March, 1968, pp 21-23.

Fitzpatrick JP: *Puerto Rican Americans: The Meaning of Migration to the Mainland.* Englewood Cliffs, NJ, Prentice-Hall, 1971.

Freedman AM, Kaplan HI, Sadock BJ: *Modern Synopsis of Comprehensive Textbook of Psychiatry/II*. Baltimore, Williams & Wilkins, 1976.

Garrison V: The "Puerto Rican syndrome" in psychiatry and espiritismo, in Crapanzano V, Garrison V (eds): *Case Studies in Spirit Possession*. New York, Wiley, 1977a.

Garrison V: Doctor, espiritista or psychiatrist?: Health-seeking behavior in a Puerto Rican neighborhood of New York City. *Med Anthropol* 1(2):65–180, 1977b.

Gelb LA: Mental health in a corrupt society, in Ruitenback H (ed): *Going Crazy: The Radical Therapy of R.D. Laing and Others*. New York, Bantam, 1972.

Gómez AG: *Service Delivery in the Spanish-Speaking Community*. Read at Session VIII, Forum on "Delivery of Services to Minority Groups," Annual Meeting of the American Psychiatric Association, Anaheim, Calif, May 1975.

Gómez AG: Some considerations in structuring human services for the Spanish-speaking population of the United States. *Int J Ment Health* 5(2):60–68, 1976.

Gómez AG: *Hembrismo: Expresión de un Fenómeno Socio-Cultural del Puerto Rico Actual*. Read at the Annual Meeting, Section of Psychiatry, Neurology and Neurosurgery, Puerto Rico Medical Association, San Juan, October 1977.

Gómez AG, Silva JT: *Mental Health Services to Addict Offenders in Puerto Rico*. Read at Session II, Annual Meeting of the American Psychiatric Association, Toronto, May 1977.

Habach E: Ni machismo, ni hembrismo. *Colección: Protesta*. Caracas, Publicaciones EPLA, 1972.

Harwood A: *Rx: Spiritist as Needed. A Study of a Puerto Rican Community Mental Health Resource*. New York, Wiley, 1977.

Heck ET, Gómez AG, Adams GL: *A Guide to Mental Health Service*. Pittsburgh, University of Pittsburgh Press, 1973.

Hidalgo H: *The Puerto Rican. Ethnic Differences Influencing the Delivery of Rehabilitation Services*, series 3. Washington, DC, National Rehabilitation Association, 1971.

Kiev A: *Curanderismo. Mexican-American Folk Psychiatry*. New York, Free Press, 1968.

Kiev A: Cultural perspectives on the range of normal behavior, in Masserman JH (ed): *Social Psychiatry, vol 2. The Range of Normal in Human Behavior*. New York, Grune & Stratton, 1976, pp 37–41.

King LM: Social and cultural influences on psychopathology. *Ann Rev Psychol* 29:405–433, 1978.

Koss J: *Therapist-Spiritist Project in Puerto Rico*. Read at Symposium 33: Minorities and Transcultural Psychiatry, 132nd American Psychiatric Association, Annual Meeting, Chicago, May 1979.

Kroeber A, Kluckhohn C: *Culture*. Cambridge, Mass. Papers of the Peabody Museum 47(1), 1952.

Laski E, Talesporos E: Anticholinergic psychosis in a bilingual: A case study. 134(9):1038–1040, 1977.

Maldonado-Sierra ED, Trent RD, Fernández-Marina R, et al: Cultural factors in the group psychotherapeutic process for Puerto Rican schizophrenics. *Int J Group Psychother* 10:373–382, 1960.

MacKinnon RA, Michels R: The psychologically unsophisticated patient—the Spanish speaking lower class patient. *The Psychiatric Interview in Clinical Practice*. Philadelphia, Saunders, 1971, pp 394–396.

136

Meyer GG: The professional in the Chicano community. *Psychiatr Ann* 7(12):9–19, 1977.

Mizio E: Impact of external systems on the Puerto Rican family. *Soc Casework* 55(2):76–83, 1974.

Montalvo B: Home-school conflict and the Puerto Rican child. *Soc Casework* 55(2):101–110, 1974.

Nicoll M: *The New Man, Part II.* Baltimore, Penguin, 1973.

Nine-Curt CJ: *Non-Verbal Communication in Puerto Rico.* Fall River, Mass, National Assessment and Dissemination Center for Bilingual Education, 1976, p 57.

Phillips EL: *The Social Skills Basis of Psychopathology. Alternatives to Abnormal Psychology and Psychiatry.* New York, Grune & Stratton, 1978.

Ralph J: Transcultural psychiatry: An Hispanic perspective (panel discussion). Los Angeles, (UCLA), Spanish Speaking Mental Health Center, monograph 4, 1977.

Rogers CR: *On Becoming a Person—A Therapist's View of Psychotherapy.* Boston, Houghton Mifflin, 1961, pp 331–332.

Rogler L, Hollingshead A: *Trapped: Families and Schizophrenia.* New York, Wiley, 1965.

Ruiz EJ: Influence of bilingualism on communication in groups. *Int J Group Psychother* 25(4):391–395, 1975.

Ruiz P, Langrod J: The role of folk healers in community mental health services. *Community Ment Health J* 12:392–398, 1976.

Research in the Service of Mental Health. Report of the Research Task Force of the NIMH. Washington, DC, Dept HEW Pub No (ADM) 75-237, 1975.

Torres-Matrullo C: *The Impact of Cultural Sex Role Differences and Change on Treatment of Puerto Ricans.* Read at the COSSMHO National Conference on the Hispanic Family, Houston, Tex, October 1978.

Torrey EF: *The Mind Game—Witchdoctors and Psychiatrists.* New York, Bantam, 1973.

Vales P: *Values of Familism: An Interactional Effect Across Social Classes in Puerto Rico.* Presented at the COSSMHO National Conference on the Hispanic Family, Houston, Tex, October 1978.

Weiss JMA, Perry ME: Transcultural attitudes towards antisocial behavior: Opinions of mental health professionals. *Am J Psychiatry* 134(9):1036–1038, 1977.

8 Discussion: Cultural Aspects of Mental Health Care for Hispanic Americans

A. Anthony Arce, MD

Among the most important results of the social upheavals of the past two decades have been the resurgence of ethnic consciousness and the emergence of the ethnic group as a new social form. The myth of the melting pot has heretofore obscured the degree to which Americans have historically retained an ethnocultural identity through the preservation of ancestral traditions and values and through myriads of subnational affiliations. This increasing fragmentation of our social fabric along ethnic lines is emphasized by the more recent demands for recognition by white ethnics of diverse European national origins; for example, the Institute of Cultural Pluralism of the American Jewish Committee, which has been spearheading this effort. Concern over the official minorities (eg, American Indians, Asian Americans, Blacks and Hispanics) has extended to include white ethnics and other newly arrived immigrant groups.

Ethnic identity provides an individual with a sense of historical continuity to life, a continuity based on a preconscious recognition of traditionally held patterns of thinking, feeling, and behaving that is the cornerstone of a sense of belonging. The reassertion of ethnic identity and the increasing awareness of the culturally pluralistic nature of American society has far-reaching implications for psychiatric practice, an area of endeavor where feelings, attitudes, and behavior are the prime targets for intervention.

The traditional foundations of modern psychiatry, ie, neurosciences and psychology, focused attention on the dysfunctions of individual organisms. The emergence of sophisticated social science theory and methods has contributed to our understanding of the interactions between sociocultural factors and individual and group behavior, and their contributions to the genesis of psychologic dysfunction. Transcultural and epidemiologic studies have shown that the stresses contributing to the onset, development, and course of behavior disorders, the tolerance for social deviance, and the methods of response to such deviance tend to be functions of sociocultural factors such as family structure, economic systems, political organization, and religious beliefs and practices.

However, despite a rapidly blossoming body of literature on the cultural aspects of psychiatry, the addition of a cultural dimension to psychiatric training lags far behind. As Grinker (1975) has said, psychiatric training has not kept pace with the "vertigo-inducing problems" of dealing with a pluralistic society "divided into social, ethnic, and economic groups, each of which has different problems in coping with the strains of the mythical whole...The similarity of training programs produces a stereotyped result because curricula are almost identical everywhere in the country." And he goes on to say,

> All of this means that psychiatry is necessarily a part of the process of social change...We can no longer afford the luxury of making public generalizations for narcissistic purposes. Those who treat should treat adequately the problems of difficult lives...If we plan to educate therapists...we need to redefine our system of a biopsychosocial conglomerate in order to educate wisely for the future.

To be sure, efforts in this direction are beginning. Bernal y del Río's development of a Laboratory for Sociocultural Detoxification and a Selective Recruitment Program, both at the Puerto Rican Institute of Psychiatry, have been alluded to by Gómez in his paper. The American Psychiatric Association has also recently established a Task Force on Cultural and Ethnic Factors in Psychiatry, chaired by John Spiegel. Among its goals are to: 1) heighten understanding of APA members of specific cultural, national, or ethnic backgrounds called for by the cultural diversity and pluralistic nature of our society; 2) inventory the curricula of residency training programs to see if this subject matter is included; 3) develop model courses and bibliographies for use in training programs; 4) emphasize specifics of culturally differentiated diagnostic and treatment techniques for various ethnic groups and propagate these insights through publications; and 5) generalize and correlate a multiethnic and culturally appropriate mental health approach with other medical specialties.

I found the contributions of Drs. Gómez, Ruiz and Wilkeson exceedingly interesting, timely, relevant, scholarly and thoughtful. All address issues common to all Hispanic subgroups when exposed to a different value system: culture shock, erosion of traditional family structure, changing sex roles, problems in communication, and so on, and contain enough novel ideas to generate lively debate.

The papers highlight first of all the cultural diversity among Hispanics. It is common practice to lump together all Spanish speaking peoples as if they constituted one huge homogeneous mass, while glossing over the multiple differences among and within Hispanic subgroups. All share a common language and Spanish heritage, as well as a set of cultural values which are based on cooperation and mutual aid; on the strengths and supports provided by the family and the community; on the status and prestige ascribed to the person because of what he/she is rather than what he/she has achieved; on the recognition of a person's dignity and respect regardless of station in life; and on the interpersonal sharing of emotional aspects of life. However, beyond these parameters, the similarities diminish. Each group has maintained its autonomy and is clearly distinguishable from the others. It is very easy for us Hispanics to pick up the peculiar sing-song of the various groups as they speak Spanish, to pick up various idiosyncratic linguistic patterns and idioms. Each of these groups has its own life-style; its own social context; its own idiosyncratic patterns of thinking, feeling, and behaving; its own linguistic forms; its particular strengths and weaknesses. While all groups face basically similar problems in American society and have a limited number of choices among alternatives, each arrives at different culturally determined solutions. As Gómez has said, in spite of a possible cultural dilution through exposure to American society, the Puerto Rican-ness of the Puerto Rican, the Cuban-ness of the Cuban and the Mexican-ness of the Mexican American continue to be visible in both verbal and nonverbal behavior. The same observation is of course applicable to other groups. We have heard, for example, from the Asian-Americans who represent an equally heterogeneous and complex group with diverse religions, cultures, languages, and histories.

Ruiz begins his analysis with a brief exposition of the historical antecedents to the Cuban presence in this country, which certainly predates the Castro regime, because of the geographic proximity of Cuba to the United States. Following the Castro ascendancy, between 1959 and 1966, the vast majority of Cuban émigrés were of the upper and middle social class, but since then there has been an increasing influx of lower socioeconomic groups. Patterns of mental health and service delivery in Cuba are then related by Ruiz to social class status and reference is made to the persistence of socioculturally determined patterns of service-seeking behavior in the new setting.

His mention of the mutualist clinics, which offer not only health and mental health services but also social and recreational services aroused my curiosity. Mutual assistance organizations are probably not unknown to most of us. They certainly flourished among early Jewish, Irish, and Italian immigrants to New York and elsewhere, during the early part of this century and, as a matter of fact, continue to function in many ways in those settings. In Puerto Rico, the Sociedad Espanola de Auxilio Mutuo y Beneficencia (Spanish Society for Mutual Help and Welfare) established a hospital which to this day is one of the most prestigious medical institutions on the island. What was arresting about the Cuban mutualist clinics is the integration of social and recreational services into a health and mental health (Health Maintenance Organization) type of provider. We agree that social and recreational activities play a significant part in promoting mental health and in the treatment of the emotionally disabled. Yet our tradition-bound service system pays too little attention to this aspect of care. Ruiz states that this model of service delivery is currently flourishing in Miami and that it serves to reinforce and preserve cultural identification. In our search for more relevant and accessible patterns of health care delivery, the mutualist clinic deserves further exploration.

In a more clinical vein, Ruiz then acknowledges the universality of psychiatric syndromes and attempts to describe specific characteristics that are culturally determined. He also suggests some general intervention approaches and warns of possible pitfalls in attempting to overdiagnose and overtreat. Unfortunately, I found this section less enlightening than I had hoped. Reactions of anxiety, depression, and intrafamilial conflict are common to all human beings who are faced with sudden dislocations in their lives and permanent severance of social, political, and economic ties with their homeland. Ruiz fails to demonstrate the distinctively Cuban coloration of these symptomatic manifestations, other than their relationship to the reality of migration and the political situation in Cuba. In other words, it is not as dramatic as the Chinese *koro,* my first experience of hearing about a syndrome that I could say is culturally bound (because I do not think that even the Puerto Rican *ataque* fits that kind of bill).

Anyway, these observations are not to minimize the importance of these manifestations; that is, anxiety, depression and so on, from a clinician's point of view, but to underscore their universality. It is important to recognize their possible transitory nature and to avoid both *misdiagnosis,* by attributing to them a greater pathologic significance than they actually possess, and *overtreatment,* through psychopharmacologic or psychoanalytic modalities. Ruiz suggests short-term supportive interventions, perhaps in group formats, utilizing the extended family network systems.

In our own work at Hahnemann, we have found this approach to be exceedingly useful with recent Puerto Rican arrivals. In fact, a special partial hospitalization type of program with a behavioral, problem-centered approach was set up utilizing bilingual, bicultural staff. Male and female cotherapy teams were chosen to colead the groups, which were same-sexed groups (in contrast to Anglo partial hospitalization programs). Separate male and female groups were necessary because culturally the sexes are segregated and also because we found differences between the sexes in the nature of their problems and degree of severity. Women were less severely depressed, and their problems revolved around marital conflicts and childrearing issues. Men were more severely depressed and often had serious drinking problems. The groups became an extended system of support for these newly migrated families and provided an opportunity for learning survival skills. They also provided an opportunity for training our residents in the management of these cases.

I think an understanding of the Cuban immigrant, as distinguished from the Puerto Rican or the Mexican, must take into consideration the forced quality and the likely permanence of their migration. There is something yet to be said about the effect on the individual of having burned one's bridges behind one, especially when it is done involuntarily. Certainly the effect must be of a different order of magnitude, both qualitatively and quantitatively, than when migration is voluntary and when there is always the possibility of returning to the familiar homeland.

However, even when undertaken voluntarily, migration affects the individual's perception of his/her self-worth. Wilkeson alludes to the gradual erosion of the positive self-image of Mexican Americans born in Mexico when exposed to discrimination in this country. On the other hand, the option to return to the familiar homeland is not altogether without problems by way of reverse discrimination as experienced by Puerto Rican Americans and Mexican Americans born in this country who visit their respective homelands.

As if to underscore this point, Gómez develops a typology of Puerto Ricans based on migratory patterns and theorizes briefly as to their possible psychodynamic implications. This fringe benefit of moving freely from island to mainland and vice versa may very well represent a facet of that "identity safe-conduct" by means of which Puerto Ricans rewind themselves and recharge their ethnocultural identity. It also may provide, as Gómez suggests, a dynamic dimension to Puerto Rican culture as a result of which the Puerto Rican is gradually becoming a person of the world. The implications of Gómez's typology, though not clearly spelled out, are that these five groups face differential stresses in their encounters with the alien society, requiring different types of intervention.

Now, in terms of the various syndromes that Ruiz discussed, let us briefly focus on transitory paranoid states. Among the three predominant Hispanic groups in this country, the Cubans are the most politically oriented and the most entrepreneurial. Witness the Cubanization of Miami. Given that 1) a major segment of migrants came from the powerful upper and middle classes, individuals who obviously had a vested interest in the political future status of Cuba; 2) Castro agents have been known to dispose of former enemies in the United States; and 3) United States and Cuban foreign relations are unpredictable at best, one would have little problem in anticipating the emergence of transient paranoid states based on more than a mere grain of reality. The question, of course, is can an Anglo therapist approach the person with sufficient understanding of the reality, the requisite degree of empathy, and the necessary communication skills to help?

The final segment of Ruiz's paper describes in relatively broad strokes the origin and development of *santeria,* the Cuban variant of a belief system widespread among Hispanics, especially, though by no means limited to, those of the poorer classes. Gómez discusses the Puerto Rican variant, *espiritismo,* and Wilkeson the Mexican variant *curanderismo.* As all three authors point out, the prevalence of these folk belief systems is based on the Hispanic's cultural orientation toward a fatalistic view of the world in which man's behavior is controlled by natural and supernatural forces. There are differences between *santeria, espiritismo* and *curanderismo* if one thinks of them as being somewhat culturally determined. *Santeria* obviously, as Ruiz described, has much more of an African influence; *espiritismo* is based on the writings of Kardec, and *curanderismo* resembles in many ways the medicine man of the American Indians. There is also another difference: the word *santero* in Cuba is obviously a folk healer who follows practices of *santeria.* In Puerto Rico, a *santero* is a man who carves figures of saints for sale but with no relationship to the cult of the Cuban *santeria.*

This particular belief system, the folk belief system, is perhaps the aspect of Hispanic culture that is most misunderstood, even in the face of a growing body of literature on the subject. For instance, the underutilization of mental health services by Hispanics has been explained on the basis of preference for folk healers and practices because of their cultural relevance. However, both Torrey and Garrison have demonstrated that psychiatric clinics and folk healing operations serve nearly the same segment of the Hispanic population. Torrey has concluded that Mexican Americans will avail themselves of mental health services in preference to folk healers when such services are psychologically accessible through the presence of bilingual, bicultural staffs. And Gómez points out that an appeal to the *espiritisa* follows a futile search for help from physicians, clergymen, and informal care givers in the community, such as relatives and friends. The futility of that search is in all likelihood due to the failure of others to provide an acceptable explanation for the behavior and an ego syntonic process for solution, rather than to any irrational holding on to a superstitious belief.

Another feature that Ruiz points out, and points it out so rapidly that I think it ought to be emphasized, is that folk healers view symptoms in general as a sign of positive strength as well as an expression of unusual qualities possessed by the patient. That is, the folk healer believes that the patient may, in fact, be an embryonic folk healer herself or himself. The folk healer thus approaches the symptom from the point of view of its restorative functions, rather than as a sign of dysfunction, a diametrically opposite view from that taken by Anglo therapists. I am reminded of the dictum that symptoms are an attempt at restoration, albeit painful and maladaptive, an observation that we often overlook at our mad rush to cure. Vivian Garrison's (1977) brilliant analysis of *espiritismo* concludes that:

> The spiritist system of treatment capitalizes on this natural restitutive process....the two types of healers (the folk and the professional) interpret the same feelings and behaviors in similar ways, have similar treatment goals and to some extent similar treatment techniques, but they talk about what they see and do within very different systems of conceptualization of the self and the world...It is a great oversimplification and ethnocentrism to consider one system (the spiritist medium cult) "magical" and the other (modern Western psychoanalytically-oriented psychotherapy) "scientific." It is also a great oversimplification to equate possession beliefs and behaviors with any one or two categories from the psychiatric nomenclature.

Kreisman (1975) has pointed out that a major problem in dealing with folk illness is recognizing it as a significant factor in the malady. It is unusual for a Hispanic to volunteer this information; that is, the belief of possession, so the therapist must be alert to the subtle signs that indicate that a patient's cultural concept of illness is interfering with a traditional therapeutic program. Kreisman (1975) suggests that two of these signs may be 1) the achievement of a plateau stage with failure to progress beyond initial improvement, and 2) the reaction of the family—demanding discharge, threatening to take the patient to a private physician, and criticizing the hospital, the physician, and the treatment process. He suggests four alternatives for the therapist: 1) ignore the belief system; 2) acknowledge it but compete against it; 3) cooperate benignly with it; and 4) integrate it into his therapeutic endeavors. This is of special interest in terms of how we are going to include the integration of this folk belief system into the training programs for psychiatric residents.

Gómez and Wilkeson have ably condensed the many aspects of their respective cultures that are relevant to a culturally syntonic treatment approach and thus of importance in the training of psychiatrists. Gómez highlights the concept of *hembrismo,* reflecting the changing pattern of male and female relationships on the island.

At several points all three authors refer to the process of acculturation with what I perceive to be negative connotations. In fact, Gómez implies that it is "culturecide." For the long-time residents on the mainland, acculturation is a reality that must be recognized because of its relationship to clinical configurations and treatment strategies. Insufficient attention has been paid to this variable even though we perceive its effects in, for example, the experiences of "reverse migrants," Puerto Ricans who return to the island after long-term residence on the mainland. A recent study by the University of Puerto Rico is at variance with some of the statements made by Gómez. The study describes some of the problems that the reverse migrants encounter when confronted with a "new culture." They think, act, and talk differently and often find their language ridiculed and their cultural habits scorned. Most feel like outsiders and report that it takes an inordinately long time, 10 years in one case, to adjust to the island's life-style. Their neighbors resent the greater degree of personal independence and assertiveness displayed by these new arrivals, which contrasts sharply with the traditional cultural values of conformity and the repression of aggression. *The New York Times Magazine* also carried an article on some of the problems these reverse migrants face when coming back to the island. To be sure, not all of them experience these problems, but I believe that the vast majority of them do. The degree to which they become acculturated to the new setting and the rapidity with which this is accomplished are of course matters that should be studied more.

There is an issue which I would like to touch upon: the seeming equation of acculturation with assimilation. At times, the two terms seem to be used synonymously. I think we ought to clarify that they are not synonymous and that, as a result, we have to think of the process of acculturation for Hispanics in this country as being of special significance for our training program, as well as for psychiatrists, both Hispanic and non-Hispanic, who treat these patients.

Gordon has defined assimilation as the process or processes by which people of diverse racial origins and different cultural heritage occupy a common territory and achieve a cultural solidarity sufficient at least to sustain a national existence. Assimilation has not taken place until the immigrant is able to function in the host community without encountering prejudice or discrimination. So, assimilation is essentially the melting pot, which we know now is a mythical concept. Although they are United States citizens and have been migrating in substantial numbers to the mainland since World War II, Puerto Ricans in this country are still the victims of prejudice and discrimination and continue to be a visibly different cultural minority, so they have not achieved assimilation. The same is true of Mexican Americans born in this country.

On the other hand, Redfield et al (1936) point out that acculturation involves those phenomena that result when groups of individuals having different cultures come into continuous first-hand contact, with subsequent changes in the original cultural patterns of either or both groups. While ideally the process of acculturation should enhance the cultural repertoire of both groups through the incorporation of what is best in each, in the real world, the prevailing patterns of the majority group are expected to be absorbed by the minority group. As a result, there are many psychodynamic and behavioral adjustments required of individuals undergoing acculturation, if they are going to acquire competence in adapting to the new environment. Acculturated individuals develop new life-styles that are reflected in changes in the quality of interpersonal relationships and in the utilization of coping mechanisms. I do not believe that becoming acculturated while, at the same time, maintaining one's ethnic identity and pride in one's roots has to pose necessarily an irreconcilable conflict. Acculturation does not imply a total repudiation of traditionally held values as Wilkeson states. In fact, acculturated individuals may enjoy a decided advantage through the more flexible utilization of the broader range of adaptive mechanisms available to them.

The behavioral changes induced by the acculturation process can be predictably reflected in contrasts between acculturated and unacculturated individuals along several dimensions, such as presenting problems, expectations of mental health services, and responses to treatment.

Our community mental health center serves a large Puerto Rican population, one of the largest Puerto Rican populations in Philadelphia, as well as a large Black population, so that most of our clients are either Blacks or Puerto Ricans. The residency training program at Hahnemann is an integral part of the community mental health center's activities so that the residents spend a lion's share of their outpatient experience in the community clinics dealing with Black and Hispanic patients.

Among the Puerto Ricans, we have found that there are significant differences between acculturated and unacculturated patients in the kinds of clinical configurations that they present and the kinds of treatment modalities that they can become engaged in for any length of time. By that I mean that they simply come back, that they are engaged in the treatment process without there being any value judgment as to outcome.

The clinical picture for nonacculturated subjects; that is, the new immigrants, is dominated by an affective state of depression in a setting of family conflict as a result of the disruption of the traditional marital roles. We consider the nonacculturated subjects to be those who have lived on the mainland fewer than 10 years. The degree of overall pathologic disorders exhibited by the males in this group points to a more rigid, culturally-restricted coping repertoire. Among recently arrived migrants the women bring sewing and other marketable skills from the island, while the men, primarily from agrarian backgrounds, lack the skills sought in this highly industralized society. Because of their employability, women are compelled to assume the role of family provider, which changes the traditional character of male and female relationships. Both marital partners respond with a loss of self-esteem. For the husband, this loss stems from the considerable reduction in male authority; for the wife, from conflicting feelings of helplessness at dealing with unaccustomed assertiveness, while at the same time being expected to remain docilely subservient to the male.

Puerto Ricans as a group have difficulty dealing with aggressive feelings and anger. The culture places great value of the individual's ability to maintain outward calm for the sake of *las apariencias;* that is, so as not to appear to be out of control and bring about public humiliation and shame on oneself and one's family. In that respect, they are similar to the Chinese. When such feelings are openly expressed, they are followed by intense feelings of guilt over the violation of a highly valued cultural standard. The suppression and repression of anger, together with the guilt induced by these feelings, sets the stage for the emergence of depression as the most predominant affective state among new arrivals. Depression is further enhanced by the process of demoralization that is part of being poor, uneducated, and culturally different in this country, and by the effects of social dislocation.

The newly arrived woman appears to cope much more effectively with depression than her male counterpart. This may be due in part to her assumption of responsibility for insuring the social and biological survival of the family unit. But it may also be that certain coping mechanisms, such as somatization, are more readily available to her as culturally sanctioned means of release. Physical symptoms referrent to the vegetative system are considered to be typical female problems and therefore a sign of weakness. Men are expected to be strong and to show contempt for anything that smacks of femininity, in spite of the kind of changing conceptions of sex roles that Gómez points out.

The severity of the everyday problems in survival, the limitations in psychological awareness, and the need to develop adaptive coping styles quickly make behavioral and support-oriented psychotherapy both in individual and group formats the approach of choice with nonacculturated patients. The aims of such an approach are to provide ongoing orientation to available social services, to increase interpersonal problem-solving capacities, and to promote the development of survival skills essential for successful adaptation to the new environment.

In contrast, acculturated patients have succeeded in acquiring skills that enable them to respond more adaptively to everyday stresses. After the family has achieved some baseline of personal adaptation to the prevailing culture, the clinical picture is dominated by the presence of free-floating anxiety in a setting of family conflict characterized by both marital and intergenerational strife. It is they and their children who will subsequently experience culture shock if they become new arrivals in Puerto Rico.

Although family income may still lie below the poverty level, both partners are likely to be sharing the responsibility for family support and mere biological survival is not their chief concern. A sense of accomplishment restores a modicum of self-esteem with an overall reduction in the intensity of depressive symptoms. Women, however, appear to experience a greater degree of discomfort because of increasing dissatisfaction with marital and family relationships. They resist attempts by the husband to restore his former position of total authority while bearing the brunt of the intergenerational conflict because they continue to be the core of the family and home functioning.

The lives of acculturated individuals, as contrasted with the new arrivals, are less suffused with the emergency of survival. Having established a foothold in this setting, the conflicts they experience resemble to varying degrees those of the general population. Exposure to the media and the cross-cultural traffic tend to heighten their level of personal awareness about the nature of these conflicts. Such awareness requires greater reliance on conscious control as a defensive maneuver which, in turn, generates free-floating anxiety.

Dynamically-oriented psychotherapy, either group or individual, which aims at increasing insight and the consideration of personal behavioral options, appears to be more suited to the needs of the acculturated group. However, even under these circumstances, interventions must take into account deeply ingrained cultural attitudes and values. The availability of bilingual, bicultural staff continues to be a critical feature of service delivery, though less so than for services aimed at the unacculturated group.

These observations are of importance because in our eagerness to emphasize cultural differences, we must not ignore the very real presence of the process of acculturation. As people become acculturated, the problems manifested in their clinical configurations resemble more and more those of the poorer classes of the total mass of America, whether they are Blacks, whites, or whatever, but with distinctive culturally-determined colorations.

148

BIBLIOGRAPHY

Garrison V: The "Puerto Rican syndrome" in psychiatry and *espiritismo,* in Crapanzano V, Garrison V (eds): *Case Studies in Spirit Possession.* New York: John Wiley and Sons, 1977, pp 383–449.

Gordon M: *Assimilation in American Life: The Role of Race, Religion and National Origins.* New York, Oxford University Press, 1964.

Grinker RL: The future educational needs of psychiatrists. *Am J Psychiatry* 132:259–262, 1975.

Kreisman JJ: The "curandero's" apprentice: A therapeutic integration of folk and medical healing. *Am J Psychiatry* 132:81–83, 1975.

Redfield R, Linton R, Herskovits, M: Memorandum on the study of acculturation. *Am Anthropol* 38:149–152, 1936.

Cultural Aspects of Mental Health Care
for Native Americans

9 Native Americans

Johanna Clevenger, MD

The *Encyclopedia Britannica* says these are the characteristics that American Indians have in common: medium skin pigmentation; straight, coarse hair; high frequency of shovel-shaped incisors; sparse body hair, a very low incidence of male pattern balding; and the absence of blood type B and Rh negative type blood. I would add, diversity. The diversity of our groups or tribes, dialects, social patterns, and economic enterprise is striking. There are some 800,000 of us living within the boundaries of the United States, composing more than 200 tribes or bands, and speaking one or more of over 200 living language groups. We reside on large reservations, such as my reservation, the Navajo, which extends from northern New Mexico into a large portion of Arizona and parts of Utah. The Navajo Reservation is far larger, for example, than the state of Connecticut. Some reservations are quite small. The Tewa tribe lives on a small portion of land completely surrounded by the city of El Paso, Texas. Some tribes are recognized by the federal government. Others, such as the Alabama-Conchiti who live near Houston, Texas, are not federally recognized. Some of us live in rural circumstances, such as the Jicarilla Apaches. Perhaps 50% of us, however, are now living in urban centers, such as Dallas, Los Angeles, and Seattle.

THE AMERICAN INDIAN
DOES NOT HAVE A WRITTEN LANGUAGE

Our nonwritten communication is very powerful and follows a type quite foreign to Anglo observers. White physician-administrators in the Indian Health Service, attempting to take up some health matter at the local Chapter meeting in a community on the Navajo Reservation, might listen for hours before being allowed to address the group.

I personally feel that television is a very Indian medium. It is visual,verbal, circumstantial, repetitive, and the late night news recoups the business of the day.

THE AMERICAN INDIAN IS A SURVIVOR OF CHANGE

The drastic changes that we as a dominant society are experiencing — such as the scarcity of gasoline, which threatens our livelihood, our entertainments, and maybe even our identity— are identical to what has been going on in my family history for 100 years. My grandfather was one of the 8000 Navajos taken from their homes and put into a concentration camp at Fort Sumter in 1876. There they stayed for 4 or 5 years before being allowed to return to our present reservation. And, I assure you, it was not for any humanitarian reason that the United States government gave up on my grandfather and his cohorts and let them go back. It had cost the taxpayers some five million dollars for our stay away from our reservation. In the treaty that the Navajos signed promising to end their raiding, the government promised schools. And it was at one of these schools at Tohatchie, New Mexico, that my mother learned English and began the studies that led to her being a teacher. She would no longer be the sheepherder her mother was. And my brother and I were born at the segregated Indian hospital in Albuquerque where I was later to do my rotating internship (as it had by then been "integrated" into the county hospital district). From those few survivors of Fort Sumter the Navajos have prospered and increased 20- or 30-fold. This surely has been because of adaptability to change.

THE AMERICAN INDIAN
HAS A SPECIAL SENSE OF AUTONOMY

In my opinion this sense of individual autonomy is key to the group cohesiveness and lack of competition characteristic of Indian school children.

I would like to emphasize that I am speaking as a Navajo woman who has a census number and who is officially ⅛ Navajo, but I am speaking for myself only. This is characteristic of an American Indian as I know him. He speaks for himself. During my stay as a general practitioner in the employ of the Indian Health Service, at Shiprock, New Mexico, in the mid-1960s, it was not unusual for an Anglo physician to recommend hospitalization or perhaps surgery for a youngster, only to have the parents turn to the child and say, in very soft Navajo terms, some communications. The parents would then turn back to the physician and say, "No, we won't do that. He won't stay." The physician would almost invariably be perplexed and say, "But why?" And the parents would say, "Because he doesn't want to." And he would not. And they would politely and graciously leave. Of course, as middle-class professionals, we would want our children to have thoughtful, intelligent, and age-appropriate orientation to decisions made in their behalf, but to leave the decision to them is a foreign idea.

I am speaking for myself and I will be speaking about things I know about myself and my clan. It was common, in taking a collaborative history from a family that a psychiatrist might ask, for example, "How does your husband feel about the death of his father?" The Indian wife would respond, "I don't know." As clinicians we would find this hard to accept, but if we were to press her further, asking if his work habits had changed, perhaps, or if he seemed depressed, or if there were other changes noted, she might say that her husband had lost his job soon afterwards and went back to the reservation. Then we would interpret that the death of his father was an important loss to him, and she would respond, "I don't know—he didn't say." As an Indian, she would not presume to speak on behalf of anyone else, even someone as intimate as a spouse, and as an Indian, I hope to keep this clear perspective.

THE AMERICAN INDIAN EXISTS
IN A COMPLEX SOCIAL STRUCTURE

I will quote a statement of Chief Luther Standing Bear (1933), made a century ago:

> We did not think of the great open plains, the beautiful rolling hills and winding streams with tangled growth as wild. Only to the white man was

nature a wilderness, and only to him was the land infested with wild animals and savage people. To us it was tame. Earth was bountiful and we were surrounded with the blessing of the great mystery. Not until the hurried man from the East came, and with brutal frenzy, heaped injustices upon us and the families we loved, was it wild for us. When the very animals of the forest began fleeing from his approach, then it was that for us the Wild West began.

I do not wish to extend this statement in a noble savage perspective, but to underline for you as future psychiatrists and clinicians that the person you evaluate or have in psychotherapy who is Indian, is a person who is part of a complex social structure. We are neither primitive nor are we simple. If you are told that your next patient is a Navajo woman and your mind clicks off a few peculiarities of Navajos— for example, that they shake hands with everybody in a very gentle manner upon greeting— you would be right. But if that is all you know, you would be ill-equipped to understand her familial clan or tribal status. I am Navajo; my mother was full-blood and was born in the reservation near Crown Port, New Mexico. We belong to the Toadalheeni Clan, or Bitterwater Clan, and it is one of five beginning, or major clans. My maternal grandmother and her younger sister were both married to my maternal grandfather and in nearby camps the women raised their children—20 or 22 between the two of them. A previous marriage and later marriage of my grandfather were not as long-lived, and those children are not included in my kinship. Polygamy was banned long before my grandfather's death in 1933, but undoubtedly still exists. Marriage within the clan is forbidden. A man joins the clan of the woman he marries and goes to live with her people. Their children are members of her clan. And all clan members are brothers and sisters. The clan to which a person belongs describes a large family unit which has its own mythology, history, and political power. My clan's history and special myths are not well known to me, because I have not yet earned the privilege of being told. At age 42, I am still a youngster to my elders.

THE AMERICAN INDIAN
HAS A COMPLEX SPIRITUAL REALITY

Art, music, and poetry are very much a part of the Navajo's day-to-day life. The art forms of weaving, painting, and jewelry making are probably what are most identifiable to outsiders about us, but beyond these ordinary and surface symbols, there exists a lively healing system that combines medicine with drama and art in ceremonies that make family psychotherapy sessions I conduct in Dallas, for example, seem pallid. As Navajos we see misfortune, accident, and illness as caused by disharmony within the universe, and I suspect that this is a universal theme. The cause might be something we did, such as eating fish, or coming in contact with a bear, or it might be something done to us, such as witching by someone who is offended by us.

During my first years as a clinician treating members of my own tribe, I had my first glimpse of the cultural differences surrounding issues of health and disease. The young white medical officers were confronted again and again with the Navajo mother, her infant on a cradle board. The physician would ask, by means of an interpreter, what was wrong with the baby. The mother would reply, by means of an interpreter, that the baby had been crying. Inquiries about fever, cough, vomiting, and diarrhea, were often fruitless. The issue remained: the infant was crying. By this time the physician would generally be conceptualizing "hysterical mother" and feeling his time was being wasted. What he was not understanding was the significance of this complaint, the conception of illness by the Navajo mother. From birth, the baby had been swaddled, safely bound on his cradle board, and carried everywhere with the mother. He had been nursed and rocked whenever he was restless. If he cried, he was immediately attended to and comforted. Their bond was immediately in harmony. If he continued to cry, despite all his mother's efforts, something was indeed not right. He was sick. The white physician was used to the concept of an infection causing fever and cough as illness; the Navajo mother used the concept of disharmonious relationships as illness.

Suppose I were living in Shiprock, New Mexico, and something was wrong. How would I go about attending to this? First, I would consult a diagnostician. This person would, by several means, such as hand trembling, star gazing, and talking to me, establish what was not right in my world. Once I had the diagnosis, I would then consult a medicine man medicine man who specialized in the ceremony which fit my disorder. In Shiprock, we would often hear visiting medicine men who came from other tribes in Oklahoma and Colorado to conduct their particular specialities. Once a healer was called, my family would come to help prepare the accommodations, the food, and to participate with me in the ceremony. The prescribed ceremony might be a 1-, 5-, or 9-day sing. And believe me, the 9-day sings are very costly enterprises. Robert Bergman, in his 1973 paper entitled "School for Medicine Men," describes this process:

> Important sings or important ceremonies last 5 or 9 nights and are difficult and elaborate to a degree approached among physicians, I think, only by open heart surgery. The proper performance of a major sing requires the presence of the entire extended family and many other connections to the patient. The immediate family must feed all these people for days. Many of the people present have imporant roles in the performance, such as chanting, public speaking, dancing in costume, leading group discussions, and many other prescribed activities of more or less

ritualized nature. For the singer, himself, the performance requires a letter-perfect performance of 50 to 100 hours of ritual chant, something that approaches the recitation of the New Testament from memory, the production of several beautiful and ornate sand paintings, the recitation of the myth connected with the ceremony and the management of a very large and difficult group process.

From a training aspect, Bergman goes on to make an important distinction between the training of medicine men and the training of psychiatrists:

In their training, ritual is the main focus. What is unvaryingly their practice from one case to another, is at the center of their thought. Informal interaction with the patient and his family is considered more important in an informal sort of way. This kind of interaction is not one that is taught explicitly, but only what is taught, by-the-by. For us in psychiatry, the emphasis is exactly the opposite.

Our ritual, and I agree with Bergman, is equally elaborate, is not taught as the central explicit ritual, and it is ritual that is being taught by-the-by. He goes on,

In any event, the singers do manage an intricate family interaction that I think has several important effects. The patient is assured that his family cares for him, by the tremendous effort being made. Two, the prolonged and intense contact makes it inevitable that conflicts are revealed, and if things are handled skillfully, resolved; and, three, a time of moratorium and turning point are established.

I do not feel as negative about witchcraft as Dr. Leighton does (see Chapter 14), and this was brought to me very vividly when I was living up in Shiprock. I lived in government housing which had an indoor toilet that was properly maintained, running water, and a washing machine. I owned a very well-running car. I used to go up and down a dirt road that ran by the river, in and out of Shiprock, where the post office and trading post were located, and I would sometimes take my babysitter out to where she lived, some five miles down the way. One time she pointed out to me as we were buzzing along this dirt road, "Oh, yes, there's a witch," and there was a very ordinary Navajo lady sitting out in the sun. It seemed as I talked with my housekeeper, the main offense this lady had committed to offend people was that she was too wealthy. At a later date, I was going down the same road with a clan sister, Gail, who lived only about three miles away and I told her of my interchange with my housekeeper. I told Gail that every time I went down that road I would stop and pick up somebody, either coming or going, feeling that because I was well paid, well nourished, and had a good car, I should share this in a Christian way with those less fortunate than I, who were walking along the road. Gail laughed at this point and said, "You know, our cousin Ed does the same thing." What Ed was operating under, though, was the effect of witchcraft. His behavior was exactly the same as mine; he would stop along the way, and, pick up people going and coming into Shiprock; but he was afraid that if he did not, one of them would be a witch, and put a spell on him, then he would be sick.

THE AMERICAN INDIAN HAS A LONG AND UNIQUE HISTORY OF DEALING WITH THE UNITED STATES GOVERNMENT

In the 1960s, when I was a psychiatry resident, I was one of a group of residents who challenged the IRS ruling that our psychiatry stipends from the medical school were not fellowship awards and therefore were taxable as income. Each of us had been called in for an audit, and we met with a series of increasingly important bureaucrats. Their desks got bigger and their nonthinking became more obvious. Each seemed to take particular delight, I felt, in our discomfort. Somewhere along the way we were interviewed by a quiet young attorney, who was obviously sincere (which won us over), and who encouraged us to pursue our hopeless cases into tax court. I have since reaffirmed that I will henceforth be suspicious of sincere young helpers. So, as a group, we had our day in court, and we each testified, outlining the differences between what we did in the hospital, for which the hospital paid us, and what we did at the medical school, for which we were getting fellowship stipends from the medical school. We enumerated our duties and the time spent. It was all folly, and it was a pretty naive process. Our fate, of course, was to pay the taxes. And I proposed that any eight year old Sioux boy in South Dakota would have been far more experienced than we in dealing with the United States government, and he would have already been far better able to cope than we with our disappointment.

If you do treat American Indians, there are at least three bureaucracies that you should know about. The first is the Bureau of Indian Affairs, then the Indian Health Service, and finally, the National Institute of Mental Health.

The Bureau of Indian Affairs was formerly under the Department of War, when Indian tribes were seen as nations and seen as entities to be dealt with on a treaty level. Over the years since, a couple of things have happened that I think are significant: 1) until recently, we were not considered nations, but wards, and there was a very paternalistic attitude toward us, as people; and 2) we are no longer in the Department of War, but in the Department of Interior. The Bureau of Indian Affairs has wide-reaching enterprises on reservations, such as boarding schools, irrigation, housing, census office, and relocations projects, which take Indian families from reservation areas into such populous places as Dallas and Chicago.

In 1955, the Indian Héalth Service was taken away from the Bureau of Indian Affairs and eventually became a service of the Department of HEW. In the 20 some years that they have been in charge of a comprehensive health plan, I think their record has been impressive. Infant mortality rates are markedly down; tuberculosis is disappearing, and in the last 10 years or so, they have addressed such mental health issues as alcoholism and drug abuse.

The National Institute of Mental Health (NIMH) has been on the scene and has had important participation with us. For example, there is a grant from the NIMH that funds the Navajo medicine man school in Rough Rock, Arizona, which is a fine institution for training medicine men.

However, despite some obvious pluses in each of these three bureaucracies, I would like to quote from an article by Dr. Robert Leon, which was in the August 1968 issue of *American Journal for Psychiatry,* entitled, "Some Implications for a Preventive Program for American Indians." He says,

> The unfortunate fact is that the Battle of Wounded Knee has been re-enacted at a psychological level over and over again, often with the first shot being fired by a frustrated Bureau official who misunderstands the behavior of an Indian or perhaps correctly perceives the unconscious hostility of the Indian and reacts with his own unconscious hostility. To correct this, we must take a dynamic view of the process of intervention and finally begin to deal with the covert messages which the government and the Indians have been exchanging for over 100 years, but rarely if ever openly acknowledging.

> Unfortunately the federal government is not geared toward working in this way. This does not mean that many officials of the Bureau of Indian Affairs cannot understand this way of working, but they too are caught in their own system. Congress appropriates money for programs; new schools are built or housing programs are developed. Once the money is appropriated the Bureau is under pressure to show results: if the program is to build bathrooms with inside toilets and running water for Indians, the Bureau must be able to report to Congress how many bathrooms were built and how many families still do not have them. It is difficult for such programs to take into account whether or not inside toilets are the major concern for a particular family and whether or not the family can utilize and maintain the new facilities to their own advantage.

THE AMERICAN INDIAN: A BRIEF CLINICAL CASE

Bernice R, who appeared in my office in November 1978, was 42 years old. She was an Indian woman from Oklahoma but had lived for the past 10 years or so in Dallas. She worked for the post office and therefore could afford my very high fees. She was the mother of four sons, one of whom was still living at home, and she consulted me because of compulsive eating. She said,

> It's my eating. I eat everything. I can't control it and it is getting worse all the time. I just can't cope with it. I've tried everything; staples in the ear, weight watchers, liquid protein—they all work. I lose pretty good. Sometimes as much as 20 pounds and then I just blow it, and before you know it, I've gained back 30. It's really scary. There's really no excuse for that. It's just a matter of self-discipline. And I can't discipline myself. I'm miserable with myself and with everybody else.

Then she went on to describe problems in her relationship with her best friend at work, with her boss, and her mother. Clinically, she appeared as an industrious, family-oriented woman, whose good humor showed briefly from time to time. But she was now depressed. Near the end of our first session she acknowledged, "You know the main problem is my mother. When I was five, she put us all in boarding schools." She explained to me, not knowing that I was Navajo, that boarding schools are Indian orphanages. She said,

> I always thought it was something she had to do and I never resented it. It was a good school and I liked it. She later remarried and her husband was white and resented us kids. But you know, all the time I was in boarding schools, I thought that some day she would come and get us if she only could. During all those years I was never with her for more than 2 weeks at a time.

In our therapy together during the next 10 weeks, she allowed herself the resentment so long repressed toward her mother and she acknowledged at last that her mother had abandoned her and that her serious self-criticism grew out of her wish to suppress this concept. She grieved again for that and again for the loss of her third son, who had been killed in an accident some eight years before, which had marked the onset of her clinical symptoms.

I present Bernice for two reasons. First, she did not consult me because I am Indian. She came to my office as she might come to yours—because my office happened to be near the post office where she worked, and because I am a woman. I also present her because the problems she exposed for me to understand and help her with were really not that difficult. I did not have to be an Indian to understand each of the points she had to make. She could have explained her family system for me. I do think that because I was Indian and knew about boarding schools and knew about the concepts she was mentioning, it was a faster process, but I think she would have done well with any good connection.

RESOURCES

The research and development center for American Indians is the White Cloud Center at the University of Oregon in Portland, which is run by an Indian psychologist, Bob Ryan (White Cloud Center, Gaines Hall, 840 Southwest Gaines Road, Portland, Oregon 97201). The White Cloud Center is named for one of the early Chippewa physicians, Thomas Whitecloud, who was there with a group of us only eight years ago when the Association of American Physicians was founded in Oklahoma City. He is now deceased but his son, Tom, who is an orthopedic surgeon, remains a member of our group. From the White Cloud Center, there will be research projects and also information available to each of us who needs specific and special information about American Indians.

The White Cloud Center is the keeper of the annotated bibliography: *American Indian Annotated Bibliography of Mental Health,* volume 1, edited by Dr. Carolyn Attneave. She has very faithfully included a number of interesting articles and also given some commentaries which I have found, in my work, most helpful. Diane Kelso remains with the project at the White Cloud Center and has also been helpful to me in researching some matters.

Lastly I would like to include as a resource the *White Cloud Journal,* which is a forum for the publication of articles about mental health issues of American Indians and Alaskan Natives.

BIBLIOGRAPHY

Bergman RL: A school for medicine men. *Am J Psychiatry* 30(6):663–666, 1973.

Leon R: Some implications for a preventive program for American Indians. *Am J Psychiatry* 125(2):232–236, 1968.

Land of the Spotted Eagle Boston Houghton Mifflin p.xix, 1933.

10 Discussion: Cultural Aspects of Mental Health Care for Native Americans

Marlene EchoHawk, PhD

Dr. Clevenger has presented some very good information regarding the diversity of American Indian tribes, her personal experiences as a member of the Navajo nation, and the main agencies that affect the lives of Indian people.

I am going to emphasize and expand on the topic of diversity. American Indians are represented in almost every state of the Union. The increase in the Indian population, combined with a newly awakened sense of pride in their cultures and languages, adds to the importance of learning about American Indian tribes.

Too narrow a focus on cultural differences between Indian and non-Indian cultures may tend to obscure other important differences that exist between Indian tribes. For instance, there are over 250 different Indian languages. Customs, including pattern of child rearing, attitudes toward health and illness, family structure and roles, vary widely from tribal group to tribal group. This is true even for tribes within the same geographic region, such as Oklahoma, which has 38 different tribes and the second largest Indian population within the United States. Varying levels of acculturation, urban versus rural setting, and interracial marriages are some factors contributing to diversity. Some background information is necessary in order to understand and appreciate the present-day diversity of Indian tribes.

The history of American Indians has included a variety of intrusions on the life-style of Indian society. Some of the Anglo systems that have influenced traditional patterns of Indian tribes are the educational, legal, and religious systems.

The term *education,* as used here, refers to the Anglo educational system, but it must be recognized that American Indian tribes also have educational systems. Stated another way, education is not an invention of the Anglos.

The school on the reservation was not a neutral agent where knowledge would be transmitted. It was the arena of an intense social drama, the place where not only the long-term aims of federal policy were to be achieved, but more particularly where the Indian children were to be remolded and equipped to be satisfactory American citizens. The children were the prime targets, and one of the acknowledged goals of the school was to break the parental influence. Indians were forced to surrender any effective control over the formal education of their children. Concentration on a specific goal, the "civilization" of the Indian, brought with it a disregard for the process by which this was to be achieved. Only the final result was important. Controlled, financed, and organized by the Bureau of Indian Affairs, the Indian concept of education assumes a sinister character. While present intentions in BIA boarding schools are quite different, including attempts to respect cultural background, there are still problems. One crucial factor is that large numbers of present-day Indian parents and grandparents grew up in boarding schools and in so doing lost the kind of exposure to family and community that would help them maintain cultural ties and prepare for parenthood.

The confusion resulting from the educational system led to a serious problem involving the legal system. Because of the kinds of social disarray that existed, breakup of traditional communities and family structure, rampant depression, alcoholism as well as lack of parenting experiences, a particularly distressing phenomenon was created as a side effect of the jurisdictional issues involving Indian tribes: namely, Indian children in proportions far greater than non-Indians are placed outside of their families and often in non-Indian homes.

The valiant struggle of the American Indians to retain their land is a well-documented and familiar story in United States history. The less familiar part of American Indian history relates individual tribal negotiations of treaties with the federal government and in some instances with states. Treaties recognizing tribal sovereignty have not always been honored, leading to a jurisdictional dilemma for the American Indian population.

The tribes, relying on the validity of treaties with the federal government, value their sovereignty. However, certain states have enacted laws that do not recognize tribal governments. Other states recognize tribal governments in a limited number of legal matters, but not in all matters.

The gray area revolving around jurisdictional issues has created one of the main obstacles for agencies providing services to American Indian tribes. The insidious nature of the jurisdictional problem becomes more acute when young Indian children and their parents are concerned.

There are vigorous attempts to provide more suitable alternatives as well as to prevent any need for placement. Tribal groups throughout the country are more and more aware of the problem and are themselves attempting to engage in remedial action. A recently enacted bit of federal legislation, The Indian Child Welfare Act of 1978 (PL 95-608) establishes nationwide procedures for the handling of Indian child placements.

If there were ever an area that Indians had in common it might be said to have been the area of religion and spirituality. A deep reverence for nature and a belief in a supreme force were tenets held by all tribes. Their deeply held beliefs made them vulnerable to the confusion of many denominations professing Christianity. Many of today's Indians claim membership in most of the major Protestant and Catholic denominations. However, many of the traditional religions still exist. The point to be made here is that there is now diversity in the area of religion among Indian tribes.

The significance of traditional religious practices and the spirituality of Indian people is frequently lost in a scholarly interpretation; therefore, I have chosen not to dwell on the topic of Indian religions.

Given these outside influences contributing to the diversity of American Indian tribes, it is easier to understand the challenge to psychiatrists in determining where, on the continuum of acculturation, an Indian patient may be and how to use that knowledge in developing a treatment plan. We do not have empirical data to indicate which treatment approaches work best with Indian people. Until such data become available, we have only personal experiences and professional training to guide us.

Cultural Aspects of Mental Health Care for Black Americans

11 Black Americans

Jeanne Spurlock, MD

It is essential that one aspect of psychiatric training should be directed toward a better understanding of the Black population in the United States and of the transference–countertransference patterns that make an impact on the kind of services given. A curriculum that is culturally relevant for Black trainees and Black patients should be considered relevant for all trainees and all patients and should be integrated into general psychiatric residency training programs. The following objectives of psychiatry residency training are suggested: 1) teaching sufficient theory and technique, including adequately supervised clinical experiences, to assist trainees in the development of skills for the competent practice of psychiatry; and 2) assisting the trainee in developing an understanding that differences are not necessarily deviances and in developing the self-awareness to permit the effective handling of transference and countertransference phenomena.

Some training directors have actively sought to modify their respective programs to better meet the needs of minority group populations — both psychiatry residents and patient (actual and potential) groups. The interest in developing a model curriculum, with particular reference to Black Americans, has surfaced in several groups in a relatively short time. The topic was addressed at a Solomon Fuller Roundtable Conference (Sharpley 1977), "Treatment Issues: FMGs and Black Patient Populations." The topic was also discussed at a special session at the 1977 Annual Meeting of the American Psychiatric Association. The Black Psychiatrists of America conducted a "training conference for Black psychiatry residents and postresidency psychiatrists" in March, 1980.

THE NEED FOR CULTURALLY RELEVANT CURRICULA

Previous efforts at developing a model curriculum for culturally relevant training have been both indirect and direct. Jones et al (1970) pointed to a number of deficiencies in training programs. They reported that most of their supervisors tended to minimize, or disregard, the impact of social factors on personality development. They viewed themselves as subjected to "whitening." Jones and his collaborators expressed particular concern about the patronizing attitudes of supervisors. This reference and others point to the need for a training experience for supervisors. Kramer et al (1973) underscored a number of important omissions in psychiatry texts prior to 1970:

> A recent compendium on community mental health (Bindman and Spiegel 1969) contains fifty-five articles, none of which deals frontally with the questions of Blacks and mental health. Nor, again, are entries found in the subject index.

In offering an explanation for these kinds of oversights, Kramer et al suggested, "Psychiatry and other mental health disciplines are no less immune to the pervasive influence of racism and prejudice then other intellectual and service institutions of this country." Pierce (1976) points to the "ubiquitous effects of racism, a contagious lethal mental and *public health disease*" (italics added). In another reference, Pierce (1974) discusses the delusional aspects of racism. "The tragic result of this delusion, afflicting virtually the entire population of this country, has had unsettling effects not only for us in this day but for the entire world now and for some time in the projected future." Pierce's references to the effects of racist practices in the areas of mass communication and formal education are of significance to psychiatric educators in view of the psychiatric consultations sought and provided to school systems and in the film and television industries. A *Time* (magazine) Essay (Morrow 1978) summarized the situations which negatively depict Black Americans. The series, "Hey, Baby I'm Back," is illustrative. The Black father is presented as handsome, conniving, immature, and irresponsible. The Sapphire image of the Black woman is provided by the character enacted by the grandmother in the series. The script writers of "Good Times" and "The Jeffersons" reinforce the negative stereotype of Black men in the characters of J.J. (in "Good Times") and George Jefferson. News reporters also reinforce the negative image. Yette (1976) recalled the following broadcast:

> On December 5, 1975, when the NBC "Today" show's bicentennial focus was on the State of Illinois, reporter Bob Jamison narrated, as the camera panned the Chicago North Shore, the skyline off Lake Michigan, and the commercial opulence of Michigan Avenue. Then, to close his narration, to sum up his report on the city whose name has become synonymous with gangsterism and big city wheeling-dealing, reporter Jamison said: "But there is a poor side, a corrupt side of Chicago..."
> And, as he said "corrupt," the camera moved in from the richness of the North Shore, and focused solely on the face of a small Black child, standing beside a fence that looked like it could have been taken from the set of either the "Sanford and Son" junkyard or the "Good Times" tenement.

The foregoing accounts of psychological assaults daily mar the mental health of Black people. Some will "weather the storm." Some will break down. The psychiatrists to whom these patients are referred (whether in a private practice or an institutional setting) must have knowledge of their patients' background in order to understand the psychopathologic problem and effectively treat it.

MYTHS: ADVANCED AND CORRECTED

Scores of accounts of misconceptions about Black people have been published in professional literature. No doubt, some of these misconceptions have been incorporated into clinical procedures. For example, Bender (1939) wrote:

> There has appeared to be a special pattern in behavior disorders of Negro children that displays itself in several ways. This is related to the question of motility and impulse. Two features which almost anyone will concede as characteristic of the race are: 1) the special capacity for laziness, and 2) the special capacity to dance. The capacity for laziness is the ability to sleep for long periods of time, when it fits the needs of the situation. The dancing represents special motility patterns and tendencies.

The adage, "the more things change, the more they remain the same," is pertinent to the subject of the perpetuation of misconceptions in the field of psychiatry. McDonald (1970), taking off from a discussion of Spitz's account of the effects of early maternal deprivation on later development, writes:

> The serious and permanent intrapsychic defects caused by such deprivation have been well documented and this research is having its influence upon social programs aimed at improving the lot of the poverty-striken victims of racial prejudice. Negro children, raised in a distorted family setting and deprived of adequate mothering have been forced, through early environmental influence, to develop into inferior adults.

Prudhomme and Musto (1973) have summarized a literature search in a pithy account of the integration of racist myths in theoretical concepts throughout the history of psychiatry. Some of the issues have been addressed by a number of others, including Bernard (1953), Davis and Coleman (1975), Hill (1971), Meers (1970, 1978), Kramer (1973), Pasamanick (1963), Pinderhughes (1973),Spurlock (1973), Thomas and Comer (1973), Thomas and Sillen (1972), and Wilkinson (1970). Wilkinson traces the historical path of the myth describing the alleged inferiority of Blacks. "...(E)arly American myths...held that Black persons were inherently inferior to whites. In present day America, the genetic basis for inferiority is being replaced with a sociopathological basis caused by the oppressiveness of slavery and the failure to rectify the ills that followed this subjugation."

Bradshaw (1978) emphasizes the need to dispel the still-existing myths during the course of psychiatric training. He implies that several misconceptions, which can be classified under two headings, warrant particular attention: 1) misconceptions about the structure and functioning of the Black family, and 2) the nature of the Black American's response to stress. Efforts to rectify these misconceptions are visible in a number of mental health professional journals and other volumes, but whether these references are used in psychiatric training programs is questioned. In addition to the references already identified, others include Billingsley (1968), Staples (1970), and Herskovits (1958). Haley's *Roots: The Saga of an American Family* (1976), popularized by two television productions, vividly illustrates the stability of many Black American families. Guttman's *The Black Family in Slavery and Freedom, 1750–1925* (1978) is another classic example.

Only a modest number of pertinent references have been cited here; others of particular significance are listed at the end of the chapter. It is essential that a representative sample be included in literature seminars or in other pertinent components of the psychiatric training program (ie, normal growth and development, family development and dynamics).

CULTURAL ASPECTS OF PSYCHOPATHOLOGY

Thomas and Comer (1973) write of "direct linkages between the quality and level of mental health in individuals and groups and the opportunities and limits that exist within the society." King (1978) reports, from an "analysis of the 1974–76 literature on social and cultural influences in psychopathology," that the "data suggests *[sic]* ...a relationship between social and cultural forces in the emergence of mental illness." In studying such relationships, King points out the need to assess three factors: 1) perception of the diagnostician in the context of his model, medical or otherwise; 2) perception of the individual or community in its context; 3) objective manifestations of signs and symptoms in the person being diagnosed."

Class-related factors cannot be overlooked in a study of cultural aspects of psychopathology or mental health. Herzog and Lewis (1970, 1971) address this issue in a reference to studies of fatherless families: "They suffer too, as does so much research, from inadequate controls for socio-economic status and — especially in studies of children in poverty — from confusing socio-economic differences with color differences." Staples (1978) also calls attention to the matter: "...data indicate a close correlation between female-headed households and socio-economic status." In a reference to out-of-wedlock or unwanted pregnancies, Staples writes, "The options exercised by the middle class are not as easily available to women of the underclass."

Characteristics of a cultural grouping are shaped, in part, in response to the broader environment. The following excerpt from Myrdal's *An American Dilemma* (1944) is illustrative:

> The good humor that is associated with the Negro's emotionalism is the outcome, not only of the attempt to enjoy life to its fullest, but of stark fear of the white man. Much of the humor that the Negro displays before the white man in the South is akin to that manufactured satisfaction with their miserable lot which the conquered people of Europe are now forced to display before their German conquerors. The loud high-pitched cackle that is commonly considered as the "Negro laugh" was evolved in slavery times as a means of appeasing the master by debasing oneself before him and making him think that one was contented. Negroes still "put it on" before whites in the South for a similar purpose...

Justice (personal communication 1979) suggests that characteristics and problems of Black Americans are highly related to experiences of exclusion. Significant differences often play a lesser role.

Perception of the Diagnostician

The premise advanced by Bender (1939) is illustrative of the "diagnostic blindness" in part by cultural influences. Another example is found in a review (Prudhomme and Musto 1973) of early American psychiatric literature. "The supposed low insanity rate of the Black was often interpreted during the nineteenth century as a result of the comforts of slavery or the dull strength of the uncivilized." Thomas and Sillen (1972) make reference to early accounts of the very low incidence of clinical depression among Black Americans and attributed these observations to reflect the stereotypic view of Blacks as "happy-go-lucky." Obviously, such misperceptions yield a faulty diagnosis.

Wadeson, in a personal communication, reported an internship experience that is pertinent to this issue. A staff physician had sharply criticized him for diagnosing a gastric ulcer in a Black patient. The attending physician's reasoning was that the happy-go-lucky personality pattern of Black people does not lend itself to the diagnostic picture of gastric ulcer. Davis and Jones (1973) have noted that a significantly greater proportion of Black patients are diagnosed as schizophrenic, while a significantly greater proportion of Caucasians are diagnosed as alcoholic or depressed. Cannon and Locke (1967) reported similar findings; they suggest "diagnostic differences found between Blacks and whites could be a reflection of the diagnostic habits of psychiatrists or could be due to differences in the quality of communication between Negro patients and a white psychiatrist as compared to white patients and a white psychiatrist."

Undue Emphasis on Environmental Factors?

Parallel to the recent emphasis on racism's generating social ills and impaired health, there appears to be a pattern, in some clinical settings, of diagnosing the disturbed or disturbing behavior of many Black children and adolescents as "adjustment reaction." In many such instances, clinicians minimize or overlook, perhaps for complex reasons, intrapsychic factors and fail to recognize the diversity among Black people; that there is no one response of Black people to the stresses generated by racism. Parenthetically, the role of bias in patient assessment, whether of Black and other minority persons, or those from the dominant group, cannot be overemphasized. Implicit is the need to recognize the importance and effect of culture on the individual, and simultaneously, the need to perceive the patient as an individual having developed (with illness and health) within the culture. Recognition of these manifestations must become an integral aspect of psychiatric residency training.

Impact of Specific "Cultural" Factors

Spurlock (1975) made reference to the frequently encountered experiences, of a racist coloring of Black Americans, that are reflected in psychiatric illness. "Where the incidence of deprivation, great stress, traumatic relationships, and inadequate or unavailable treatment is greater for persons of one color than another, one may find a higher incidence of certain stress-related illnesses and more severe cases of these illnesses." Davis (1968) addressed the subject of the special ways in which being Black in America may affect the manner and degree to which the individual achieves personal identity and identity as a member of society.

> The chances for successful negotiation are significantly decreased for the child of any family at the lowest end of the socio-economic scale, but there will be a larger proportion of dark-skinned children emerging from infancy with specific vulnerabilities to later damaging experience since their families occupy a disproportionately large segment of the population at that end of the scale.

Spurlock and Lawrence (1979) noted a number of circumstances that lend to the development of potential hazards for the Black child in utero. "The high incidence of hypertension and toxemia in Black pregnant women put the lives of the mother and infant in jeopardy. The extreme youthfulness of a great many Black mothers, their malnutrition and inadequate prenatal care often produce premature births and low birth weight." (The same ills can, and do, befall the young mother of any ethnic identity. However, the incidence of adolescent pregnancy has been reported to be higher in Black girls.) Lythcott et al (1975) cite data to support the validity of this premise in New York City. "Sickle cell disease can be life threatening....Even the newborn is a victim of the widespread use of substance abuse in many Black communities."

Meers (1973) views the "chronic external conflict and distress" that is readily observable in most Black urban ghettos and as a source of "a flood of unpredictable stimuli"—a constant threat. This being so, he cautions that clinicians who are called on to make an assessment of the mental health of children who live in ghetto settings must "distinguish between 1) symptoms and regressive, adaptive behaviors that are situationally reactive to external conflicts, and 2) those symptoms that derive from internalized conflicts." He further suggests the importance of noting that neurotic conflicts may be masked by "situational traumas of everyday life."

Davis and Coleman (1975) discuss the hazards of ego development in the "modern ghetto." However, they stress that there is evidence of "resilient strengths which serve to establish effective means of autonomous function in relation to vital task requirements," as well as defective ego development.

Characteristics of some Black family units that have been viewed as indicative of pathologic disorders are perceived as a cultural norm by a sizeable percentage of the population within the particular culture. Ladner (1972) addresses this topic as related to sex codes.

> The low-income Black community has always been stereotyped as having "loose morals" and "promiscuous behavior" in the area of sex....What is not taken into consideration in these assertions is that a different set of moral codes regulates the sexual behavior of Black people....Premarital sex is not regarded by the majority of low-income Black people as an immoral act.

However, Ladner acknowledges that there are differences within the community. It follows, then, that this pattern of sexual behavior is not viewed as expected behavior for all residents of low-income Black communities, and/or all such communities. It should be noted that what was considered a cultural norm at one point in the history of a group may become, at a later time in history, a feature of a pathologic problem. The discussion of sexuality by Staples (1978) is illustrative:

> ...the inclination of Blacks toward natural responses to sexual stimuli has become somewhat dysfunctional in the urban setting....In the rural South a new birth was an asset since the child could easily be accommodated into the family. But in the urban environment, the unexpected birth of children to teenage mothers more often means an increase in high school dropout, inadequate parenting, a risky early marriage, or welfare dependency...

Herzog and Lewis (1970, 1971) write "It is, unfortunately, no myth that the proportion of fatherless families is very high in our inner cities. Even though the majority of inner-city children are in two-parent homes at any given time, a smaller proportion remain in the same two-parent home throughout their first 18 years." The question, raised by these authors, of the validity of research in this area was previously referred to in this communication. In a study designed to test the hypothesis that "Black boys from homes having no adult male figures would have significantly poorer self-attitudes than girls from this type of home, and boys and girls from homes with adult males and females," Rubin (1974) determined there to be no significant difference. Rubin's conclusions parallel those of Herzog and Lewis: "father absence is only one among an interacting complex of factors which mediate and condition its impact on a growing child;...even if eventually a significant association can be demonstrated between father absence and one of the adverse effects attributed to it, that impact is dwarfed by other factors of the interacting complex." It should also be noted that fathering is often provided by a male relative or the mother's "significant other."

A review of a record of the diagnostic study of a Black male child is of significance here. The child had been referred to a child psychiatry facility, which had earned a national reputation as a superior training institution. Ellis (a fictitious name) was 8 years of age at the time of the referral, which was initiated by the schoolteacher because of academic slowness and withdrawn behavior. It was written that Ellis was a product of a common-law union. According to the record, the mother had reported that the child's father was a frequent visitor and regularly made financial contributions for the support of Ellis and his sister, 2 years his senior. In outlining the formulation of the case, the diagnostician had recorded that there was no father in the home and that Ellis apparently lacked a stable male figure with whom to identify. It was obvious that the diagnostician reacted to a set frame of reference and could not attend to the information that had been provided—that this child did have an ongoing relationship with his father, who apparently was not as unstable as depicted in the record.

Patterns of Behavior

In addressing the consequences of racism for the Black child, Spurlock (1973) calls attention to some "specific patterns of behavior" that are often generated "through the Black child's efforts to find ways to cope with the conflicts triggered by discriminatory experiences," both overt and covert. Aggressive behavior and explosive anger (which probably most often receive the diagnostic label of "unsocialized aggressive reaction of childhood") was observed to be that pattern considered of greatest significance by the larger community. Too often, a diagnostician fails to see the underlying depression and the healthy, defensive use of the anger or hostile, aggressive behavior. Grier and Cobbs (1978) addressed this in *Black Rage*. Toni Morrison (1970) in her novel, *The Bluest Eye,* poignantly describes the anger of a Black girl reacting to an encounter with a grocer. To the grocer, the child is apparently invisible, for she notes

> the total absence of human recognition—the glazed separateness....Yet this vacuum is not new to her...She has seen it lurking in the eyes of all white people. So. The distaste must be for her, her blackness. All things in her are flux and anticipation. But her blackness is static and dread. And it is the blackness that accounts for, that creates, the vacuum edged with distaste in white eyes.

The child finds a way to be rid of the despair, at least temporarily.

Anger stirs and wakes in her; it opens its mouth, and like a hot-mouthed puppy, laps up the dredges of her shame.

Anger is better. There is a sense of being in anger. A reality and presence. An awareness of worth. It is a lovely surging.

No doubt, similar encounters and responses have been experienced by other children who are not visibly different from the dominant group. This, too, evidences the need to make culturally relevant training an integral part of general psychiatric training.

Rainwater (1966) identifies three kinds of "survival strategies" utilized, at least by the lower class Black population: 1) expressive life-style (directing efforts to make oneself attractive so as to better manipulate others and to receive immediate gratification); 2) violent strategy; 3) depressive strategy ("goals restricted to the bare necessities for survival"). Meers (1970) suggests "intellectual or academic retardation as a possible 'symptom choice' that might be specific to the cultural milieu of the modern ghetto."

Responses to Mental Illness

A cursory review of the literature reveals relatively little about the "cultural patterns" in the responses of Black families to mental illness. However, my own clinical experiences (which involved ongoing contact with the families of identified patients), have uncovered a variety of responses, most of which are not dissimilar from those of families of other ethnic groups. The widespread use of denial, at least for a limited period of time, is an example. The 35-year-old wife of a plasterer attributed his paranoid ideations and explosive behavior to "the way he's always been, except he's just gotten more evil; he's got the devil in him." The parents of a 15-year-old boy insisted that their son's lethargy and withdrawn behavior stemmed from his growing laziness. It was painfully difficult for them even to consider the possibility of a "nervous breakdown," and they repeatedly wondered about the need for "another test" to determine the possibility of drug addiction. Black families who hold voodoo medicine beliefs are likely to react with apprehension and grave concern about the "hexing." Obviously, the believers are less likely to accept psychiatric intervention, if at all.

Bland acceptance and tolerance or distancing and abandonment are other responses; the appearance of the specific response appears to be related to the manifestations and severity of the illness. Should the patient quietly and safely reveal her or his symptoms, it is likely that the family will be tolerant. When mental illness strikes the family's primary breadwinner, responses of concern and anxiety may escalate to panic and despair, if not family disorganization.

Black Folk Medicine

Through interviews with "Afro-American healers" Stewart (1971) collected data that illustrated the diversity of the diagnostic techniques utilized by these practitioners. Listed were 1) use of Biblical phrases and/or material from an "old folk medical book"; 2) observations; and 3) entering the spirit of the client. Therapeutic measures included the use of herbs and various rituals (ie, reading of bones). The wearing of special garments and/or accessories is also used in therapeutic intervention. Reassurance has also been described by the healers as an effective treatment measure. Jordan (1973) writes of the three principal characters in Black folk medicine:

> ...(1) the "Old Lady" ("granny" or Ms. Markus"), well versed in herbs, who functions as the local consultant for common ailments; (2) the Spiritualist, the predominating and most heterogeneous character today; (3) the oldest character, and in many ways the most powerful, the Voodoo Priest, or Hougan.

Most of the clients of a "granny" are "young mothers who seek help with infant raising or in treating the illnesses of young children." She does not dispense medications, but provides advice and instruction. Spiritualists are "called" to their practice, unlike Hougans, who are formally trained — "learning the philosophy of elders, as well as the techniques of dealing with people and their problems." Jordan describes many of the clients of the spiritualists as fearful and phobic; the spiritualist "helping them to cope better with their everyday life." It was noted that many spiritualists practice by mail; "frequently, complete psychotherapy is conducted by mail." The Hougan (or voodoo priest) is trained for broader responsibilities. According to Jordan, their responsibilities "combine aspects of many professions, including judicial, medical and legal...The new Prist must be well oriented in the skills of dealing with family and personal problems, and in interpreting signs as good or bad omens."

The voodoo Priest must be well acquainted with the habits of animals, for he bases his diagnostic abilities and proper treatment measures on knowledge of sickness in animals and their selection of herbs for healing. The symbolic characterization of animal life is an important factor in diagnosis and treatment. For example, the spirit of evil is represented by the snake; "the chicken symbolizes man's ability to overcome his weakness." Therefore, "drinking the blood of a freshly killed chicken imparts an awareness of oneself, a feeling of being in control of one's own destiny."

EFFECTIVE PSYCHIATRIC TECHNIQUES: TRADITIONAL AND MODIFIED

The efficacy of the use of traditional psychotherapeutic techniques in treating Black patients has been emphasized by a number of clinicians. Meers (1970), in a report of the analysis of two Black latency-age children, wrote that he found no need to "introduce something new into the treatment of disadvantaged Black patients" who show "a constancy of purpose, a tolerance of my ignorance, and have used their treatment much as most other children I have seen." Spurlock and Cohen (1969) called attention to individual treatment as a preferred and successful psychotherapeutic modality for some Black patients, who are also among the lower socioeconomic group. The diversity of their patient population was noted. Effective treatment was more likely with those families in which there "was a social unit and intactness" regardless of the family composition.

Pinderhughes (1973) discussed common resistances that were observed in Black patients who were in individual treatment before the late 1960s. Some (such as denial, transient paranoid feelings, distrust) were noted to "reflect a sense of victimization"; others (such as silences, lateness, missed appointments) were viewed as representative of "indirect expressions of hostile aggression on the part of persons in whom more direct expression has been inhibited." In such instances successful treatment is more likely when the therapist's thrust is to stimulate and encourage the use of those ego functions that support the drive for self-assertion. When this approach is not used, the probable results will be a reinforcement of resistances. The concept of multiracial mindedness (Pinderhughes 1966, 1973) warrants attention in the treatment process.

> Every Black person has a "White mind" and a "Black mind"...and every White person has a "White mind" and a "Black mind." The White mind constitutes the elements which are uniting and not disruptive to one's groups and are therefore socially acceptable. The Black mind constitutes those elements which are disruptive to one's groups and therefore excluded from society....In our racist society the "white part" of both Black and White persons is projected upon Whites, who are aggrandized, while the "Black part" of both Black and White people is projected upon Blacks.

More than 30 years ago therapists were cautioned about ascribing all problems of Black patients to conflicts specifically related to racial identity

(Adams 1950). Bernard (1953) cited a possible danger in the development of "a new form of racial stereotype...ie, the Negro personality whose frustrated hostility toward whites must always automatically constitute his central conflict and the core of his personality organization." The cautions addressed by Adams and Bernard continue to warrant attention.

Although the preceding comments have been directed to individual psychotherapy and psychoanalysis, they also apply to family and group therapies, and to some extent, behavior modification and the organic and adjunctive therapies. In each of these approaches, particular attention should be given to the transferences and countertransferences.

Social Therapy-Community Psychiatry

Sabshin et al (1970) emphasized the need for environmental therapy. Correction of deficiencies in the environment necessitates social action, which depends, to a great extent, on community organization. In many community mental health centers, the work of an advisory council is an integral part of the program. Often, the focus of the activities of this group is on social action (Spurlock 1973). Thomas and Comer (1973) have suggested an "advocacy approach which involves a dialog between the consumer and the technical source responsible for providing mental health services." However, social action alone is not necessarily enough. "Innovative social therapy" must be coupled with "conventional medical therapies" (Pinderhughes 1973) for adequate treatment of the majority of Black people in need of psychiatric intervention.

SUMMATION

There are many cultural influences on the mental health and illness of Black Americans. To modify the "traditional" psychiatric training programs, culturally relevant training should extend to continuing education in psychiatry, not just as an adjunct, but integral to a general program. In the development of such a program, a number of essentials warrant attention: 1) recognition of the hazards of the "deficit model" and attention to the possible norms in differences; 2) a representative sample of Black-related references in assigned reading for literature seminars or other pertinent components of the training program; 3) clinical experiences with patients from different cultural backgrounds than the trainees; supervisors should have had a similar experience.

Because some experiences of Black Americans are class-related and shared by people from other cultural backgrounds, and in view of recent and potential changes in the practice of medicine (ie, health maintenance organizations, national health insurance), the benefits of culturally relevant psychiatry training should be widespread.

The author expresses appreciation to Ledro R. Justice, MD, for his assistance in the preparation of this chapter.

BIBLIOGRAPHY

Adams WA: The Negro patient in psychiatric treatment. *Am J Orthopsychiatry* 20(2):305–310, 1950.

Bender L: Behavior problems in Negro children. *Psychiatry* 2:213–228, 1939.

Bernard VW: Psychoanalysis and minority groups. *J Psychoanal Assoc* 1:256–267, 1953.

Billingsley A: *Black Families in White America.* Englewood Cliffs, NJ, Prentice-Hall, 1968.

Bradshaw WH, Jr: Training psychiatrists for working with Blacks in basic residency programs. *Am J Psychiatry* 135(12):1520–1524, 1978.

Cannon M, Locke BZ: Being black is detrimental to one's mental health: Myth or reality? *Phylon* 38(4):408–428, 1967.

Davis EB: The American Negro: Family membership to personal and social identity. *J Natl Med Assoc* 60:92–99, 1968.

Davis EB, Coleman JV: Interaction between community psychiatry and psychoanalysis in the understanding of ego development, in Wadeson RW (reporter): Psychoanalysis in community psychiatry: Reflections on some theoretical implications. *J Am Psychoanal Assoc* 23(1):177–189, 1975.

Davis WE, Jones MH: Race-related variations in psychiatric diagnosis. *Newsletter Res Men Health Behav Sci* 15(4):31–32, 1973.

Grier WH, Cobbs PM: *Black Rage.* New York, Basic Books, 1968.

Guttman HG: *The Black Family in Slavery and Freedom 1750–1925.* New York, Random House, 1978.

Haley A: *Roots: The Saga of an American Family.* Garden City, NY, Doubleday, 1976.

Herskovits MS: *The Myth of the Negro Past.* Boston, Beacon, 1958.

Hill RB: *The Strengths of Black Families.* New York, Independent Publishers' Group, 1971.

Herzog E, Lewis H: Children in poor families. *Am J Orthopsychiatry* 40:375–387, 1970; also in Chess S, Thomas A: *Annual Progress in Child Psychiatry and Child Development.* New York, Brunner/Mazel, 1971, pp 307–322.

Jones B, et al: Problems of Black psychiatric residents in white training institutions. *Am J Psychiatry* 127(6):798–803, 1970.

Jordan WC: Voodoo medicine, in Willaims RA (ed): *Textbook of Black-Related Diseases.* New York, McGraw-Hill, 1975.

King LM: Social and cultural influences on psychopathology. *Ann Rev Psychol* 29:405–433, 1978.

Kramer BM: Racism and mental health as a field of thought and action, in Willie CV, Kramer BM, Brown, BS (eds): *Racism and Mental Health.* Pittsburgh, University of Pittsburgh Press, 1973, pp 3–23.

Ladner JA: *Tomorrow's Tomorrow: The Black Woman.* New York, Anchor, 1972.

Lehman HE: Unusual psychiatric disorders and atypical psychosis, in Freedman AM, Kaplan HI, Sadock BJ (eds): *Comprehensive Textbook of Psychiatry II.* Baltimore, Williams & Wilkins, 1975, pp 1732-1733.

Lythcott GI, et al: Pediatrics, in Williams R (ed): *Textbook of Black-Related Diseases.* New York, McGraw-Hill, 1975, pp 130-197.

McDonald M: *Not by the Color of Their Skin.* New York, International Universities Press, 1970, p 220.

Meers DR: Contributions of a ghetto culture to symptom formation: Psychoanalytic studies of ego anomalies in childhood. *Psychoanal Study Child* 25:209-230, 1970.

Meers DR: Psychoanalytic research and intellectual functioning of ghetto-reared black children. *Psychoanal Study Child* 28:395-417, 1973.

Morrison T: *The Bluest Eye.* New York, Pocket, 1970, p 42.

Morrow L: Blacks on TV: A disturbing image. *Time,* March 27, 1978, pp 101-102.

Myrdal G: *An American Dilemma.* New York, Harper & Row, 1944, pp 960-961.

Pasamanick B: Myths regarding prevalence of mental disease in the American Negro. *J Natl Med Assoc* 56(1):6-17, 1964.

Pierce CM: Psychiatric problems of the black minority, in Arieti S (ed): *American Handbook of Psychiatry,* vol 2. New York, Basic, 1974, pp 512-523.

Pierce CM: Teaching cross-racial therapy, in Busse EW, et al (eds): *The Working Papers of the 1975 Conference on Education of Psychiatrists.* Washington, American Psychiatric Association, 1976, pp 224-227.

Pinderhughes CA: Pathogenic social structure: A prime target for preventive psychiatric intervention. *J Natl Med Assoc* 58(6):424-435, 1966.

Pinderhughes CA: Racism and psychotherapy, in Willie CV, Kramer BM, Brown BS (eds): *Racism and Mental Health.* Pittsburgh: University of Pittsburgh Press, 1973, pp 61-121.

Prudhomme C, Musto DF: Historical perspectives on mental health and racism in the United States, in Willie CV, Kramer BM, Brown BS (eds): *Racism and Mental Health.* Pittsburgh, University of Pittsburgh Press, 1973, pp 25-57.

Rainwater L: Crucible of identity: The Negro lower-class family. *Daedalus* 95(1):172-216, 1966.

Rosenthal AH: *Psychiatric Education: Prologue to the 1980's.* Washington, American Psychiatric Association, 1976.

Rubin R: Adult male absence and the self-attitudes of Black children. *Child Study J* 4:33-45, 1974.

Sabshin M, Diesenhaus H, Wilkerson R: Dimensions of institutional racism in psychiatry. *Am J Psychiatry* 127(6):787-793, 1970.

Sharpley RH: *Treatment Issues: Foreign Medical Graduates and Black Patient Populations.* Cambridge, Mass, The Solomon Fuller Institute, 1977.

Spurlock J: Some consequences of racism for children, in Willie CV, Kramer BM, Brown BS (eds): *Racism and Mental Health.* Pittsburgh, University of Pittsburgh Press, 1973, pp 147-163.

Spurlock J: Psychiatric states, in Williams RA (ed): *Textbook of Black-Related Diseases.* New York, McGraw-Hill, 1975.

Spurlock J, Cohen RS: Should the poor get none? *J Am Acad Child Psychiatry* 8(1):16-35, 1969.

Spurlock J, Lawrence LE: The Black child, in Noshpitz JD, et al (eds): *Basic Handbook of Child Psychiatry.* New York, Basic, 1979.

Staples R: The myth of the Black matriarchy. *Black Scholar* 1:8–16, 1970.

Staples R: Black family life and development, in Gary LE (ed): *Mental Health: A Challenge to the Black Community.* Philadelphia, Dorrance, 1978, pp 73–94.

Stewart H: Kindling of hope in the disadvantaged: A study of the Afro-American healer. *Mental Hyg* 55:96–100, 1971.

Thomas A, Sillen T: *Racism and Psychiatry.* New York, Brunner/Mazel, 1972.

Thomas C, Comer JP: Racism and mental health services, in Willie CU, Kramer BM, Brown BS (eds): *Racism and Mental Health.* Pittsburgh, University of Pittsburgh Press, 1973, pp 165–181.

Wilkinson CB: The destructiveness of myths. *Am J Psychiatry* 126(28):1087–1092, 1970.

Yette SF: The mass media and the Black mind: Creating the behavior statistics. Presented at the National Minority Conference on Human Experimentation, Sheraton Conference Center, Reston, Virginia, January 6–8, 1976.

12 Discussion: Cultural Aspects of Mental Health Care for Black Americans

Robert L. Bragg, MD, MPH

My interest in the cultural issues attending mental health care to different ethnic groups, particularly Blacks, has been intensified as a result of my holding bimonthly clinical case presentations with the staffs of various clinics of our Community Mental Health Program, Division of Mental Health Services, University of Miami/Jackson Memorial Medical Center.

In Miami we had many different ethnic groups to consider in setting up our Community Mental Health Center.* Several different clinics were organized and established based on the ethnic groups in the different geographic sections of our catchment area; namely, clinics for 1) Blacks, 2) Haitians, 3) Cubans, 4) Puerto Ricans, 5) Bahamians, and in addition, two geriatric clinics — one for Blacks and the other for non-Black ethnic groups. A client or patient does not have to go to the clinic in his geographic area but may attend any one of them.

---

*The organization of mental health and psychiatric services to the individuals and families of the catchment area was based upon the findings of Weidman and collaborators in the Health Ecology Project (Weidman 1978).

At the case presentation conferences, the staff members of the various ethnic clinics present cases to me. Very often, the cultural impact on the mental health of the client/patient, or family is discussed with a great deal of enthusiasm. The staffs of these clinics, professional and paraprofessional, are almost wholly of matching ethnicity to the populations served. These clinics emphasize a social psychiatry that focuses on external stressors on adaptive strengths in the respective communities and the intrapsychic processes of the clients/patients and/or families.

Research at this Community Mental Health Program is directed at looking into some of the cultural issues that affect the skills and techniques to be used by the therapists in order to deliver effective mental health services.

Dr. Spurlock directly addresses herself to the topic. I think that one statement in her introduction summarized beautifully the issue: "...a curriculum that is culturally relevant for all trainees and all patients and should be integrated in general psychiatry training programs."

I feel quite strongly that supervisors, as a group, and faculties of departments of psychiatry will have to have training relative to the significance of cultural issues attending mental health care to Black Americans so that they may be more effective as supervisors and have greater impact on their students.

We are all aware of the potential and actual significance of role models, and certainly, ideally, supervisors should serve as positive role models for their residents-in-training. Supervisors, then, certainly cannot bring into the supervisory sessions culturally relevant issues related to mental health services for Black Americans if they are not aware of these cultural, relevant issues. This, I think, suggests the need for training in this area for all supervisors of residents in psychiatry.

Do these culturally relevant issues have different degrees of significance in some of the different modalities of treatment; for example, crisis intervention, short-term psychotherapy, long-term psychotherapy, and psychoanalysis? I think of Franz Alexander's discussion of sector analysis when he raised the issue of matching the therapist with the patient relative to some selected variables, with the thought in mind that, if the therapist and the patient had some experiences or personality traits in common, the speed of the psychotherapeutic process would be enhanced. Spurlock mentioned this when she stated in her introduction the transference-countertransference patterns that make an impact on the kinds of services given.

Spurlock mentioned in her introduction that the interest in developing a curriculum with particular reference to Black Americans has surfaced in several groups in a relatively short time. I wonder if some of the variables involved in this surfacing of such a need have been related to the dropping out of Black Americans, (as well as other ethnic groups), from psychiatric evaluation, crisis intervention, and various forms of psycho-therapy because the patient was aware that the intervener or therapist did not understand where the patient was at and coming from at the time.

Too often the answer given by the intervener and therapist is that the dropout of patients is related to the patient's lack of motivation for help. This, in many instances, was and is a rationalization used by the intervener or therapist. I discussed this question with Harriett Lefley, Director of Research at our Community Mental Health Center (personal communication, 1979). I shall quote her:

> The need for involving more Black staff and, certainly, for training more Black professionals is evident. It is not only that we believe that cultural expertise aids in diagnosis and treatment — which it most certainly does. Also involved are avoidance of confounding transference/counter-transference issues with ethnocentrism, ease of psycholinguistic com-munications, mutual understanding of cultural referents, and perhaps a long-range positive role-modeling effect. Further, statistics indicate that Black people tend to underutilize predominantly white facilities; they drop out, fail to keep appointments, or do not come at all. This pattern would also lend itself to another racist myth were it not for the fact that in our Community Mental Health Center facilities, run by Black service providers, utilization rates are highly concordant with the distribution of Black people in the general population. In fact, there is almost perfect match (approximately 52% of our caseload and 52% of the catchment area are Black).

Dr. Lefley continued:

> Minority utilization, including Hispanics, reflects 80% of our case load, representing many individuals who would not normally seek help in a clinical setting. Our no-show rates are also revealing. With no-show rates ranging from 40% to 56% reported by most Community Mental Health Centers, particularly for Black and Hispanic clients, we have a current no-show rate of 11%. It has never gone above 14% since we have been tabulating it. Our dropout rate is under 5%, buttressed by a high degree of consumer satisfaction as reported by patients. Our therapeutic out-come studies similarly show a high degree of goal attainment and a low recidivism rate (4% to 5%) for previously hospitalized patients. All of this suggests that Black people will utilize and can benefit from high quality, culturally appropriate mental health services.

Lefley's communication on cultural aspects of psychopathology stresses that Blacks have been excluded, to a great extent, from the decision-making groups; this element is an important variable in the establishment of programs relevant to the problems of the Blacks. We are all aware of, but do not understand, the problems of those for whom they make decisions. Paternalism and other factors are involved.

The diagnostic differences found between Blacks and whites certainly reflect the kinds of experiences and understanding of cultural factors of various ethnic groups that the diagnostician brings to the interaction between himself/herself and the Black patient.

I also asked Lefley to react to the diagnostic differences between Blacks and whites as reported by many different health-providing agencies. She stated: "I submit that the differential is inflated by misdiagnosis—particularly by the documented tendency of white psychiatrists to see schizophrenia and not see depression in Black patients." Spurlock also stated this in her chapter.

Dr. Lefley continued:

> Over the years, studies have shown that Black Americans are over-represented for schizophrenia, which more often requires hospitalization, and underrepresented for depressive neurosis, which typically results in another type of case disposition. Comparisons for rates for affective disorders, primarily depression, indicate a rate for Black people ranging from one-quarter (Malzberg 1963) to one-seventh (Jaco 1960) the rate for whites. In contrast, Black people's rate for schizophrenia ranges from 65% (Taube 1971) to 300% (Wilson and Lantz 1957) higher than that of whites.

Spurlock mentioned the "happy-go-lucky" myth as one explanation of low depression incidence, and that there is no one response of Black people to the stresses generated by racism, and would extend this to responses to any type of stress. Too often all Blacks are perceived as being alike. Too often the defenses of the Blacks are misinterpreted in many different kinds of situations: the schools, industries, social and working situations. Too often these misinterpretations are to the disadvantage of Black or other minorities. I must add that many (non-Black teachers, non-Black diagnosticians, etc) are unaware that their indifference toward the Black is a hostile, discouraging experience.

I thought that the quote of Davis and Coleman (1975) by Spurlock relative to the hazards of ego development in the "modern ghetto" was of particular importance and will repeat a part of it: "They stressed that there is evidence of resilient strengths which serve to establish effective means of autonomous function in relation to vital task requirements, as well as defective ego development." It appears to me that we are dealing with a vital need for survival and therefore have the responsibility for the establishment of the kind of environment that will enhance survival. This, of course, means development of ego strengths to include defense mechanisms that will permit survival and at the same time healthy means of dealing with various kinds of stresses.

Lefley emphasized the need for adopting a community stance—which should apply to all patients, but is particularly needed when one is

Black and poor. While intrapsychic conflict and family dynamics may follow the same pattern across cultures, probably there is simply more environmental stress on a patient's coping capability when the person does not have the insight to deal with the reality problems that impinge daily on his/her mental health.

In a recent study, soon to be published in *Hospital and Community Psychiatry,* Lefley and her staff investigated the effects of environmental interventions and therapeutic outcome—specifically on whether succss in alleviating external stressors would predict more functional, insightful behavior in patients. The relationship was statistically significant at the p = 0.001 level. Their data suggest that psychotherapy is enhanced by supportive interventions attending to the reality problems of the patient, and in fact may not be optimally effective unless this is done.

One cannot lump all Blacks together in terms of values, attitudes, or needs. This includes attitudes toward sex as well as other issues.

Spurlock stated that Meers (1970) suggested "intellectual or academic retardation as a possible 'symptom choice' that might be specific to the cultural milieu of the modern ghetto." The question that occurs to me is: Is it actual intellectual or academic retardation, or is it *interpreted* as intellectual or academic retardation? I raise this question for there are so many instances in which Blacks are placed in predominantly white environments in schools, tend to withdraw, do not speak when they have something to say, know the answers to questions, feel that they are not a part of the group, and respond to the daily stresses in which they are misinterpreted as being of low intelligence.

Spurlock mentioned that in her addressing the consequences of racism for the Black child, there are some specific patterns of behavior. Later, she quoted Morrison (1970) who described a Black girl as apparently invisible to a white grocer. I would like to mention that, in my opinion, this does extend to the older age group as well. The invisibility of the Black to the majority in many different instances engenders anger, a sense of not belonging, as well as other feelings that sometimes influence in a negative way the performance of the Black in these situations.

Lefley suggests that, given the multiplicity and magnitude of stressors in the daily experience of most Black people, it is astonishing that the rate differential of mental disorders is not higher than it is. There may indeed by *fewer,* rather than more, pathogenic factors in the early life experience of Black children. The strengths in this experience should be emphasized; among them, the extended kinship network and community support systems that insure an availability of loving caretakers for infants and minimize isolation of the mother. Also, Spurlock's mention of male role models even in "father absent" families is well taken. Far from being deprived of adult male companionship, the ghetto child probably has greater access to older males than the child of the affluent or suburban father. It is another sad commentary on our pervasive racism that sociological commentary focuses on absent or negative role models, rather than attempting to research effects of *positive* role modeling on development of Black children.

In Chapter 11 of this text on Effective Psychiatric Techniques: Traditional and Modified, it seems to me that the real issue here is that one must consider the individual or specific family and use the appropriate psychiatric techniques, traditional or modified as indicated. Socioeconomic status and ethnicity alone must not be the determining factors for the technique(s) used. I might add that we must also take into consideration what is going on in the environment. I have in mind the attitudes that many had toward psychiatric treatment in the late 1960s — perceived of by many as a form of brainwashing. At earlier times, for some at least, it was popular to state to one's friends: "I must see my shrink today."

Insofar as environmental therapy is concerned, consumers must be included in the advisory councils of the community mental health centers. Such a council is only a part of what must be included in providing appropriate and relevant treatment for the consumers. Spurlock stated this and I mention it for reinforcement.

Spurlock has well documented the need for psychiatric training directed toward a better understanding of culturally relevant issues related to mental health services for Black Americans, for residents, supervisors, and others involved in the delivery of mental health services to Blacks.

More research should be undertaken to delineate more clearly the significance of cultural factors in the delivery of mental health services to various ethnic groups.

I would like to conclude my discussion with a quote from Landy in 1977:

> A society's medicine consists in those cultural practices, methods, techniques, and substances, embedded in a matrix of values, traditions, beliefs, and patterns of ecological adaptation, that provide the means for maintaining health and preventing or ameliorating disease and injury in its members.
>
> A society's medical system is the total organization of its social structures, technologies, and personnel that enable it to practice and maintain its medicine (as defined), and to change its medicine in response to varying intracultural and extracultural challenges.
>
> Thus, a society's medicine and medical system are interrelated—in fact, are part of—its culture and social system.

BIBLIOGRAPHY

Jaco EG: *The Social Epidemiology of Mental Disorders — A Psychiatric Survey of Texas.* New York, Russel Sage Foundation, 1960.

Landy D (ed): *Culture, Disease, and Healing.* New York, Macmillan, 1977, p 131.

Malzberg B: Mental disorders in the U.S., in Deutsch A, Fishman H (eds): *Encyclopedia of Mental Health,* vol 3. New York, Franklin Watts, 1963, pp 105–166.

Taube C: Admission rates to state and county mental hospitals by age, sex, and color in the United States 1969. US Dept HEW, NIMH Biometry Branch, statistical note 41, 1971, pp 1–7.

Weidman and Collaborators: Miami Health Ecology Project Report: Vols 1 and 2. University of Miami, Offprint. Miami, 1978.

Wilson DC, Lantz EN: The effect of culture change on the negro race in Virginia as indicated by a study of state hospitals mentioned. *Am J Psychiatry* 114:26–32, 1957.

13 Discussion: Cultural Aspects of Mental Health Care For Black Americans: Cultural Aspects of Psychiatric Training

Richard I. Shader, MD

I think that Dr. Spurlock and Dr. Bragg covered the material in the previous chapters in a very comprehensive and thorough way. In trying to think of a vantage point I could contribute to offer something unique, I examined some of the roles that I fulfill in life to see what perspective they might offer. There are really two areas in which I have done considerable work that were not touched on so far. I have worked for many years, through the American Psychiatric Association and as a residency training program director, in manpower recruitment and development. I thought I first would say a bit about my view of the issues of minority recruitment. Then, relating to Spurlock's comment that perhaps there has been too much of an emphasis on environment and not enough emphasis on the intrapsychic, my view is from another perspective: there has not been any emphasis on the biologic aspects of culture and ethnicity as they relate to psychiatric training.

RECRUITING AND TRAINING

My own training in psychiatry is somewhat confusing in regard to cultural psychiatry. Among the many excellent teachers that I had, two had a particularly strong influence on me. One was the late Elvin Semrad, who said that we did not have to concern ourselves with racial or ethnic or cultural issues, because people at heart are very much the same—they need to be loved, to be able to love, to feel mastery, security, and success, or else they can walk through life feeling frightened or defeated or hurt; they need to be able to express their sexual feelings as a part of their love or in some other way. Semrad felt that if we paid attention to those dimensions that were alike in people, then cultural differences would not be so important. That is true, up to a point. Unfortunately, some of the major problems in communication that can stand in the way of seeing similarities among people do not get addressed in very many people's training. So there is a clear need to do something about those barriers.

Another very significant teacher for me was Charles Pinderhughes. He fostered and nurtured my interest in the connections between mind and body and helped me to expand and develop my thinking about psychosomatic medicine and particularly about the ways in which the burdens of life might be expressed in various organ systems. Charlie's impact was so strong that now, some 15 years later on three recent Saturdays, I have been conducting with colleagues a symposium on the ways in which anxiety manifests itself as seen in a systems review of the various organ systems of the body.

It all has to be integrated, whether it is Semrad's position about the sameness of people, or teachings about the problems in communication that we have across cultures, or the issues of how the mind and body connect. All of that is crucial to any health professional's training, and particularly to the training of the physician going into psychiatry.

Some idea of the manpower pool from which the medical schools draw is given by data on minority applicants to the Harvard Medical School (Table 13-1). There appears to be a reasonable pool to draw from, but actually, overall, it's going to turn out to be a very small pool of people nationally. In terms of understanding manpower needs and development, it would be helpful to know, for example, how the 25 Black applicants accepted in 1979 differed from the remaining 335 or so in that group. The Harvard applicant group contains a large number of people who probably applied to other medical schools as well, and it would be interesting to know a little more about them since they represent close to one-third of the total Black applicant pool to American medical schools. One can see that not every one who got accepted in turn accepted Harvard. Also there is probably a bit of a decrease or leveling off in the minority applicant pool size.

Table 13-1
Minority Applicants to Harvard Medical School*

Minority	1976	1977	1978	1979
Black				
Ap†	283	350	293	360
Ac†	21	28	24	25
Ma†	16	22	18	NA
Chicano				
Ap	93	94	57	93
Ac	9	8	8	5
Ma	6	5	8	NA
Puerto Rican (mainland)				
Ap	70	46	43	42
Ac	6	6	4	5
Ma	6	3	4	NA
American Indian/Alaskan				
Ap	19	12	9	21
Ac	1	1	1	0
Ma	0	0	1	NA

*Adapted from Admissions Committee Statistics (Oglesby Paul, MD, 9 May 1979).
†Ap = applied; Ac = accepted; Ma = matriculated; NA = Not Available.

Table 13-2 shows generally how minority applicants are reflected in the manpower pool. Approximately 6% of all the first-year students in this country are Black, and all minority applicants make up only 12.6%. Thus the roughly 350 individuals who applied to Harvard make up actually more than one-third of all the people who ultimately do get enrolled.

In Table 13-3 we can see who repeats the first year of medical school. Minorities are disproportionately represented, both in the first year and in subsequent years. This has a profound shaping effect on people. Basic science failures are almost always in the hard sciences (eg, microbiology, biochemistry, histology). In the later years, when there is repeating, it is usually not in the behavioral sciences of psychiatry, but rather in medicine, pediatrics, or surgery. When a student has a defeat and has to go back and work on it harder, the result of further exposure should yield a sense of mastery. Many students identify more strongly with those areas they find challenging but yet eventually master. This finding may have some influence on the eventual tracking of minority trainees. There may be something to the notion that easy courses are not ultimately valued (though they may be enjoyable). I am speculating on the theme, "easy come, easy go."

I look back on my own experience as a teacher (I taught college for 6 or 7 years early in my teaching career as well as teaching in medical school). I now work with trainees in psychiatry whom I saw as college

Table 13-2
Minority Enrollment in United States Medical Schools, 1977–1978 (%)*

Enrollment	Number	Percent
First year†		
Black (not of Hispanic origin)	956	6.0
Chicano (Mexican American)	216	1.3
Puerto Rican	229	1.4
Other Hispanic	164	1.0
American Indian/Alaskan	46	0.3
Asian or Pacific Islander	418	2.6
Total	2029	12.6
Graduate		
Black (not of Hispanic origin)	793	5.5
Chicano (Mexican American)	172	1.2
Puerto Rican	176	1.2
Other Hispanic	94	0.6
American Indian/Alaskan	47	0.3
Asian or Pacific Islander	319	2.2
Total	1601	11.0
Total		
Black (not of Hispanic origin)	3651	6.0
Chicano (Mexican American)	837	1.4
Puerto Rican	821	1.4
Other Hispanic	467	0.8
American Indian/Alaskan	205	0.3
Asian or Pacific Islander	1485	2.5
Total	7466	12.4

*Adapted from the Medical Education issue, *JAMA* 240:2824, 1978.
†First year enrollment data exclude repeaters from count.

Table 13-3
Students Repeating the Academic Year 1977–1978*

	First Year Class		All Other Classes	
Minority	Enrolled Total	Repeaters (%)	Enrolled Total	Repeaters (%)
Black (not of Hispanic origin)	1101	142(12.9)	2550	161(6.3)
Chicano (Mexican American)	238	22(9.2)	599	34(5.7)
Puerto Rican	231	2(0.1)	590	7(1.2)
Other Hispanic	174	10(5.7)	293	9(3.1)
American Indian/Alaskan	51	5(9.8)	154	8(5.2)
Asian or Pacific Islander	425	7(1.6)	1060	16(1.5)
All other students	13,914	225(1.6)	39,076	286(0.7)

*Adapted from the Medical Education issue, *JAMA* 240:2824, 1978.

students. They represent all races, with the exception of American Indians. Contact with these students early in their premedical education as college students had a considerable influence on their subsequent choice of training in psychiatry (and particularly our program). The recruitment process into psychiatric work is often influenced by the choices that one makes early on in life, but, even more often, it is influenced by the people to whom one gets exposed. If we want to make any significant impact on minority recruitment, it is going to have to be through psychiatrists having a greater teaching role in undergraduate or premedical education.

The data in Table 13-4 are very interesting to me. If we look at Massachusetts, for example, in 7 major teaching hospitals, there are 13 Black trainees — 13 spread across 7 hospitals. There are never enough in any given hospital to have a peer group, there are never enough for any kind of mutual support. I think that we dilute our minority trainees to such a great extent that some of their interests get lost, and the wish to be like everybody else gets supported. I have seen this regularly as a trainer. When we had classes of 25 residents, we might have one Black resident.

The service demands would be such that the Black community would demand the that Black resident work with the Black community. The resident almost invariably balked, and said, "I want the same experience and curriculum as everyone else." When we have a Hispanic resident in our program, who is then specifically asked by the Spanish Alliance to service the Spanish community, the result is very much the same. When there is only one trainee, that individual gets singled out, which I think is detrimental to training. The issue of critical mass must be addressed. I am not sure that by the competition we have among all of our programs to each get our one minority trainee from the limited pool, that we are doing anybody a service. I would think that that question must be addressed again. I am not suggesting that minority trainees should be segregated. There may have to be ways to coalesce trainees from various programs in a region to promote more formal efforts to support their minority identity within their graduate and postgraduate education. All trainees should work with the populations served by their program. Yet the last thing we want to do is single out and assign persons because of ethnicity or country of origin; they must get general training. Being singled out and identified from the start as different does not help trainees. If there are exceptions, I would like to hear about them, because the programs that I inquire about always have that as an uphill battle.

Only 4% (and it's actually less than 4%) of medical students are going into psychiatry today. We appear to be dealing with a shrinking manpower pool and at the same time wanting to improve and diversify our training programs. We are going to have to be very innovative and indeed go back in our recruitment if we are going to reverse this trend. Table 13-5 shows how Black trainees are distributed across specialties. Seven percent are in

Table 13-4
Black United States Citizens Serving in First Year Residencies,
September 1977*

State	Hospitals	First Year Residents
Alabama	2	5
Arizona	1	1
California	20	51
Colorado	2	2
Connecticut	4	8
District of Columbia	3	9
Florida	5	9
Georgia	5	18
Hawaii	1	1
Illinois	6	12
Indiana	2	6
Kansas	1	1
Louisiana	2	16
Maryland	11	27
Massachusetts	7	13
Michigan	3	5
Minnesota	1	1
Mississippi	2	2
Missouri	2	4
New Jersey	4	36
New York	20	66
North Carolina	1	3
Ohio	10	20
Pennsylvania	15	28
Rhode Island	1	1
South Carolina	2	2
Tennessee	3	6
Texas	5	16
Virginia	1	8
Washington	1	1
Wisconsin	4	5
Total	147	383

*Adapted from the Medical Education issue, *JAMA* 240:2841, 1978.

neurology and psychiatry. This represents 93 people, United States and Canadian graduates of whom about 75 are in psychiatry, a small number of people for the 300 or so programs across the country. Consider all of the programs which actually do spend dollars on affirmative action, all trying to recruit the same persons. It seems a rather inefficient exercise — one that I think is important, but one that probably needs to be structured in a different way.

If we were to correlate the weeks in clerkship (Table 13-6) with the subsequent choices of specialty, we can see that there is a reasonably high

Table 13-5
Black United States Citizens Serving Residencies
by Specialty as of September 1977*

Specialty	US and Canadian Graduates	Foreign Graduates	Total All Training Years
Allergy and immunology	1	...	1
Anesthesiology	20	20	40
Dermatology	6	...	6
Family practice	133	10	143
Internal medicine	345	34	379
Neurological surgery	20	5	25
Nuclear medicine	1	2	3
Obstetrics/gynecology	228	14	242
Ophthalmology	43	...	43
Orthopedic surgery	36	12	48
Otolaryngology	20	6	26
Pathology	23	16	39
Pediatrics	123	28	151
Physical medicine and rehabilitation	4	7	11
Plastic surgery	4	3	7
Preventive medicine	...	1	1
Psychiatry and neurology	93	61	154
Radiology	30	12	42
Surgery	161	23	184
Thoracic surgery	4	7	11
Urology	17	7	24
Other	18	30	48
Total	1330	298	1628

*Adapted from the Medical Education issue, *JAMA* 240:2841, 1978.

correlation. Namely, the areas in which one has exposure tend to be the areas that one chooses for specialization, not because of a hierarchy of importance in medicine, but rather that where skills, attitudes, and confidence are developed, identifications are made—all other things being equal.

That psychiatry is least represented in the required curriculum across the country may say a lot about why we find fewer and fewer people coming into our specialty. Compared with 10 years ago, there has been a substantial drop in the curriculum time for psychiatry, out of proportion

Table 13-6
Required Clerkships and Average Duration*

Clerkships	Average Duration (Weeks)	Schools
Internal medicine	12	119
Surgery	9	119
Pediatrics	8	118
Family medicine	7	43
Obstetrics/gynecology	7	118
Psychiatry	6	118

*Adapted from the Medical Education issue, *JAMA* 240:2826, 1978.

with other required clerkships. When I talk to students in college and minority students in particular about what they are going to do with their lives, one of the things that I hear regularly is, "Why in the world should I go into medicine—that's a low status profession." I hear it not only from white trainees but really from everybody. It is interesting. If one looks at what has happened to physician income over time compared to the consumer price index and the wholesale price index, the physician is not keeping ahead, even though physicians, I think, do well.

Many potential trainees have been more interested in law because they feel that they can be more effective in changing social policies through the law rather than through medicine. Some of the status of physicians has been lost, in general, and some of the attractiveness of psychiatry has been buried in the problems that we have had over the last several years.

BIOLOGICAL ASPECTS OF CULTURE

In contemporary psychiatry, when we focus on a culturally bound curriculum we cannot ignore the biologic component. Psychiatric service is not just therapeutic listening, and training is not just removing resistances so that those who have to do the therapeutic listening can listen better. Psychiatric services involve a comprehensive view of the individual with whom we work to understand not only environmental and intrapsychic but also his biologic antecedents. They may differ pharmacogenetically; they certainly may differ in their response to many of the medications we are likely to use in everyday practice. Significant work should be done to give us answers to many unanswered questions—questions that have not even been asked considering the vast numbers of people we serve.

Pharmacogenetics is an important dimension in research. For example, take acetylator phenotypes. When I was a medical student, among the first psychiatric patients I saw on a special medical-psychiatric ward at Bellevue were two Black women, each manifesting symmetrical facial rashes and psychosis. One of the important pharmacogenetic issues that has been learned in recent years is that cases of drug-induced systemic lupus erythematosus (SLE) appear to be more common in patients who show a slow rate of acetylation of marker drugs (Drayer and Reidenberg 1977). Acetylator status varies significantly among population groups according to racial background. For example, rapid acetylation occurs frequently among Japanese (approximately 45%, range 33% to 58%) and less frequently among caucasian Americans (9% to 27%), and least frequently among those in the South of India (approximately 6%) (Price et al 1960, Sunahara et al 1961, Ellard and Gammon 1977). Slow acetylation, for example, occurs in about 73% of Indians, 45% to 55% of caucasian Americans and 9% to 15% of Japanese. Black and caucasian Americans are said not to differ in proportions of rapid and slow acetylators. If a slow acetylator is given one of the many compounds that requires acetylation for its metabolism, there is a higher probability that the compound will affect him and his immune system and SLE will develop. How often anybody teaches that we ought to find out. As we work with different ethnic and cultural groups, we should find out what the patient's acetylator phenotype is before we give that patient a monoamine oxidase inhibitor. Again, cultural issues can be terribly important in the interventions that we make.

At least two drugs in psychiatry are commonly used, particularly across the world, that require acetylation as one of their major metabolic steps. One of these is phenelzine. It is now a very popular drug, prescriptions for phenelzine having gone up dramatically in the last 4 years, after about a 15-year period in which the drug was hardly used. The other drug is nitrazepam, which is one of the most common sedatives used outside of the United States.

Another area that is a known but rarely studied area is that people of Oriental background tend to have a great sensitivity to dopamine blocking agents. They require lower doses for efficacy and develop more extrapyramidal side effects at comparably lower doses. This has been known anecdotally for about 18 years. It has been observed in the Chinese, in Malaysians, and in the Japanese; yet, it has never gotten beyond the stage of anecdote—there has never been one published, prospective study that looks at dose responsiveness. And, again, why, I do not know. It may require somebody who has a cultural interest and motivation because it is close to his own heart to do that kind of work. So far no one has done it, and yet, we are treating people from different backgrounds all the time.

We rarely take into account, in treating a Black population where the incidence of hypertension is likely to be high, that it is essential to be careful about the selection of antihypertensives, because of how they may interact with various antidepressants. Again this interaction should be taught; it should be emphasized; it should be part of any reasonable curriculum.

Hereditary nonspherocytic and spherocytic hemolytic anemias occur in about 10% to 13% of Black Americans. Nonspherocytic anemias regularly are exaggerated or exacerbated by oxidants. Many drugs that we use in psychiatry are oxidants. Not one has ever been studied against red cell cultures taken from people with this problem to see whether they are going to increase hemolysis. It has never been done. Yet we have thousands of people out there who might suffer from drugs that we prescribe on a daily basis.

In sickle cell anemia, a major problem in many respects, we know that when somebody is in a sickle cell crisis, if we give a sedative-hypnotic, that any dose sufficient to decrease respirations at all (ie, that will produce any degree of hypoxia) increases the crisis. How often do we teach that to residents in emergency rooms? When a Black person comes in complaining of pain, and very often this happens in psychiatric settings, how often do we train physicians to check for sickle cell disease before they write that prescription? I think that as professionals with our emphasis on the cultural side, we have done a major disservice by neglecting part of our major mandate, which comes from our heritage as physicians.

Another problem is apparent in patients who are given lithium. The sickling process as sickle cells go through the kidney alters the currents in the medulla of the kidney, and, as such, the reabsorption and retention of reabsorbed water is modified in the presence of sickle cell disease, so that most people with any significant degree of sickle cell disease have a problem in taking back reabsorbed water. If you give lithium to somebody who is so compromised, lithium will affect the reabsorption of water in the distal tubule, then it is theoretically possible that these two diseases could be additive—another problem which has not been studied.

There is another important problem that has not been studied (I did not even know about it until I attended a conference in Washington, but no clinical implications were drawn from it at all—which again, shows that if one's awareness is not heightened and people from various cultural backgrounds are not looking for these kinds of things, these problem areas regularly get missed). Immature animals who are exposed to lead (and lead paint is certainly a problem in this country for people from poverty level backgrounds), when they are adults and given lithium, tend to develop more and irreversible central nervous system disease (Mailman et al 1978). I do not know whether anybody has ever taken a lead level of a patient before prescribing lithium, but I think if this animal-based observation could be substantiated as relevant for humans it would become a terribly important thing to do. This finding, presented in the context of a symposium on pharmacokinetic research from birth to death so that one could look at the influence of the aging process, this was presented as an anecdotal observation from which the researcher said that he could see no human application for the findings. We make a great mistake in emphasizing too much one dimension of what we are all about. If we are to make a contribution it would be in the area of taking a broader perspective in patient care.

BIBLIOGRAPHY

Drayer DE, Reidenberg MM: Clinical consequences of polymorphic acetylation of basic drugs. *Clin Pharmacol Ther* 22:251–258, 1977.

Ellard GA, Gammon PT: Acetylator phenotyping in tuberculosis patients using matrix isoniazid or sulphamidine and its prognostic significance for treatment with several intermittent isoniazid-containing regimens. *Br J Clin Pharmacol* 4:5–14, 1977.

Mailman RB, Krigman MR, Mueller RA, et al: Lead exposure during infancy permanently increases lithium-induced polydypsia. *Science* 201:637–639, 1978.

Price-Evans DA, Manley KA, MacKusick VA: Genetic control of isoniazid metabolism in man. *Br Med J* 2:485–491, 1960.

Sunahara S, Urano M, Ogawa M: Genetic and geographic studies on isoniazid inactivation. *Science* 134:1530–1531, 1961.

14 Relevant Generic Issues

Alexander H. Leighton, MD

The generic issues to be discussed in this chapter may be oriented according to two premises:

1. The mental illness field is heterogeneous, that is, not a scientifically defined subject matter area, but rather a somewhat borderless collection of many different kinds of human disorders that have become grouped together by medical and societal processes in the course of history. Consider for example that "mental illness" can be applied to conditions as different as psychoneurotic anxiety and organic brain syndrome; that the causes include many combinations of genetic, traumatic, infectious, degenerative, psychological, interpersonal, social, and idiopathic factors; that the recognized syndromes vary widely in the degree to which their causes are dependably known and clinically determinable, with paresis toward one end of the range and personality disorders toward the other; that degree of disability extends from slight to total; that duration varies from transient situational disorders to life-long psychoses; that frequency in populations ranges from the rare *fou savant* to common patterns of anxiety and depression which, like grippe, are found worldwide; and that

treatability extends from a potential for rapid and complete recovery to intractability in the face of every known remedy.

2. The clinical psychiatrist must be able to see his patient's disorder in terms of possible chemical, biological, psychological, and interpersonal factors operating both through his lifetime and at the cross-section of the current moment. These comprehensive requirements are in part derived from the heterogeneity that has just been described. If one specializes in a particular subarea, such as psychoneurosis, or in a particular kind of treatment, such as psychoanalysis, then the scope of the knowledge demanded may be reduced in favor of more detailed understanding of particular theory and methods. For the general psychiatrist and for the psychiatrist who is engaged in acquiring basic training, however, comprehensive, eclectic understanding is mandatory.

Topics and illustrative materials have been selected in what follows for psychiatric residents and directors of residency programs with two goals in mind: 1) to provide a clinically oriented introduction to concepts of culture; and 2) to make suggestions toward developing a curriculum.

The focus on psychiatric residency training naturally means an emphasis on psychiatry, but this should not be construed as an elite posture with regard to other mental health professions. Although there are many serious, unsettled questions as to the allocation of tasks among psychiatry, psychology, social work, and nursing, there is no doubt that each has contributions of major importance to make in the care and prevention of mental illnesses. It is my hope that members of the other medical health professions will find matters of interest to them in this chapter, but also that they will understand the primary intent to be instruction for psychiatrists in training.

Another intentional restriction is that of dealing only with what I conceive to be the primary business of the clinical psychiatrist: care for mental illnesses. Excluded are theories and methods for helping the "worried well," consciousness raising, personality enhancement, improving human relations, and so on.

An issue that might have been considered is the distinction between *disease* and *illness* that is recommended by some writers. According to Kleinman et al (1978):

> That distinction holds that disease in the Western medical paradigm is malfunctioning or maladapation of biologic and psychophysiologic processes in the individual; whereas illness represents personal, interpersonal, and cultural reactions to disease or discomfort. Illness is shaped by cultural factors governing perception, labeling, explanation, and valuation of the discomforting experience, processes embedded in a complex family, social and cultural nexus. Because illness experience is an intimate part of social systems of meaning and rules of behaviour, it is strongly influenced by culture: it is as we shall see, culturally constructed.

This viewpoint raises a number of complex questions. For example:

- Does the formulation contain new ideas or is it composed of old ideas with new labels?
- Is it mainly a pedagogic device or is it intended to be a representation of processes in nature? Does it imply that the scientific bases for the illness concept is on an equal footing with the scientific bases for the disease concept—in other words that biomedical science and social science have equivalent data so far as disease/illness are concerned?
- Is too much claimed for cultural anthropology at the expense of other disciplines such as sociology, psychology, social psychology, and liaison psychiatry? For instance, Kleinman et al (1978) say, "Medical anthropology is focussed on basic clinical questions to a greater degree than other social sciences."
- In this formulation, which of many possible models of culture is being employed, and is there danger of perpetuating myths about culture?
- Does the viewpoint run the risk of fostering habits of cultural stereotyping rather than attention to individual differences that are so important in psychiatry?
- Are important distinctions obscured among such concurrent processes as culture, culture change, sociocultural disintegration, social stratification, and minority group status?
- Is it a step forward or a step backward in understanding to dichotomize a field that is made up of such a vast number of complexly interrelated variables?

One final introductory note of explanation: The pronoun "he" and its variants is used in the indefinite sense to refer to human personages whether woman or man.

KNOWLEDGE OF CULTURE
APPLIED TO CLINICAL PSYCHIATRY

In arriving at a diagnosis, the heterogeneity of the mental illness field makes it necessary to distinguish carefully just which patterns of disorder are being displayed by a given patient. It also involves distinguishing normal behaviors and feelings.

In both these judgments the clinician has to take into account matters of context. A woman who feels depressed, weeps frequently, is full of self-reproach, and refuses food is not behaving abnormally if this is in the context of a recent bereavement. If an agnostic chemical engineer were to claim that a glass of wine served to him at dinner was not wine at all, but actually blood, there would be grounds for questioning his mental health. On the other hand, if he were a Roman Catholic and made the same statement about the wine served to him during the Eucharist, there would be no reason for such questioning. Some 700 million other people in the world would agree with him.

What this illustrates is that many of the behaviors of psychiatric interest that make up the recognized clinical syndromes have to be distinguished in relation to the context in which they occur. This sense of relativity is something that every psychiatrist learns as a fundamental part of his training. Age, sex, education, occupation, and religion are all background data that the diagnostician uses in defining particular behavior in particular patients as normal, questionable, or indicative of disorder.

Taking culture into account is an extension and development of this clinical sense of relativity. If a 35-year-old middle-class Episcopalian physician complains that someone is making him ill by witchcraft, a mental disorder is probably indicated. The same complaint from a 50-year-old Italian immigrant laborer, by contrast, might have no relationship whatever to any kind of mental disorder. The same would be true of persons of Spanish, Mexican, Pennsylvania Dutch, Nigerian, Eskimo, Navajo, Haitian, and many other cultures where belief in witchcraft is common.

Cultural anthropology, as the discipline concerned with culture, can add systematic knowledge and conceptual tools to the clinician's professional equipment, and so increase his capacity for discriminating and evaluating the context of verbal and other behaviors (Murphy 1965). The matter is of obvious importance in a multicultural population such as that found in North America where every psychiatrist is bound to encounter patients who come from cultural groups very different from his own. In some places, or for some psychiatrists, most patients will be of this kind. The study of culture therefore is valuable for two reasons: it can provide 1) understanding of general principles and 2) information about the specific content of those cultures most likely to be encountered. Such information can help the clinician put into better practice what he knows anyway, namely that for each patient he has to understand that individual's view of reality in the light of the belief system of the group to which the patient belongs, and not simply in terms of his (the physician's) own beliefs. He can, for example, come to appreciate more clearly that while it is correct to define delusion as false belief, the criteria of false must be culturally appropriate to the patient and his peers, not necessarily to the physician and his peers.

These points about diagnosis also apply to the identification of causative factors. Cultural practices that determine hygiene, diet, sexual activities, prenatal and perinatal care, and so forth can alert the clinician to possible organic causes. *Kuru,* a viral disease in New Guinea that destroys the brain, provides the most elegant demonstration so far of a direct link between a specific cultural pattern (in this case ceremonial cannibalism) and a specific mental disorder (Hornabrook 1968; Gajdusek 1977).

Culturally-connected psychological causes are less easy to demonstrate. Nevertheless, it is apparent on the basis of much clinical experience that an understanding of cultural processes in a patient's development and in the stresses of his current condition can reveal the nature of his disorder.

The same applies with regard to treatment. Comprehending culture as a process and knowledge of a given culture's content can aid in choice of therapy, in bringing about compliance, in mobilizing social support systems and other resources, and in general case management. The cultural orientation of a patient exerts a strong influence on his preceptions and beliefs regarding illness, disease, health, and healing, and hence on what he can accept or feels he must reject from the physician. Cultural understanding helps the psychiatrist appreciate the role of magical thinking in many patients and to distinguish between those beliefs and viewpoints that can be altered on a basis of reason and fact, and those that are affectively charged, ego-syntonic, and very difficult or impossible for a therapist to change.

A major benefit that can come to the clinician who studies at least one other culture is a greater comprehension of his own. This is clinically pertinent in at least two ways. First, the physician begins to understand better his feelings, perceptions, judgments, and actions as elements in a cultural system; and second, there comes an expanded understanding of what is going on among patients who share the physician's culture. Much of this is, of course, already known intuitively, but it can be rendered more cognitive and more at the command of the clinician by the experience of cultural comparisons.

A CLINICALLY USEFUL DEFINITION OF CULTURE

Up to this point I have avoided the problem of defining "culture," going on the dubious assumption that the reader would know what I was talking about. In actual fact the topic is complex, the writing about it prolix, and the popular ideas often misleading.

If one were to ask a random sample of 100 mental health professionals the meaning of "mental illness," the answers would not be notable for agreement. Some respondents might insist that there is no such thing.

The difficulty is parallel with regard to "culture." Kroeber and Kluckhohn (1952) report, after a search of the literature, 164 definitions. It is evident therefore, that the psychiatrist who thinks he can consult anthropological writing and quickly learn "the definition of culture" is in much the same position as an anthropologist who wished to find in psychiatry the definition of mental illness. Both would have a difficult time due to variations in the orientation and purposes of the many definers. A quotation from Leslie White illustrates the problem in anthropology.

> ...culture is "learned behaviour"; it is not behaviour at all but an "abstraction from behaviour"; it is "intangible," a "logical construct"; it is a "psychic defense system"; a "precipitate of social interaction," a "stream of ideas"; it "consists of n different social signals that are correlated with m social responses," etc. One anthropologist at least has gone so far as to question the "reality" of culture.

White proceeds to make a point that is important not only in understanding the word "culture," but also in understanding words like "mental illness" and the terms in the Diagnostic and Statistical Manual of the American Psychiatric Association (DSM) and International Classification of Disease (ICD) nomenclatures. He points out that there are two different types of questions that crop up in science: What is the chemical composition of the sun? and, To what class of phenomena should we apply the term bug? In the first question we are concerned with sensory exploration (with the aid of instruments) of the external, objective world (eg, does the sun's atmosphere contain hydrogen or doesn't it?). In the second we are concerned not with phenomena as such, but with the use of words, with arbitrary decisions regarding how they shall be applied to phenomena (eg, is a spider, which is distinct from insects, a bug?). The issue is not a fact of nature, but rather of conventional word usage in the interest of promoting more accuracy in thinking and communication as steps toward answering the first type of question.

Differences in answers to "What is culture?" are of this latter type and should be understood as due mainly to variations in purposes. Further, many of the purposes of anthropologists are unlike those of clinicians. In the main, the anthropologist is concerned with developing bodies of theory that will explain the known facts about culture and guide the search for more. The article "Functional Prerequisites" by Aberle et al in Appendix A illustrates such theory construction, but with the focus on society rather than culture. Our concern, in contrast, is to select a definition that best fits the clinical purpose of enhanced understanding of patients, their disorders, their resources, and their responses to life events and treatment efforts.

We may begin by taking note of just two meanings of the word "culture." These are in common use, and failure to distinguish between them has a potential for generating error. One refers to the ideas, beliefs, viewpoints, values, and feelings that are shared by any designated group of people. In such terms one can speak of the "culture" of the middle class, of a high school, of the medical profession, of a ship, or of a monastery, as well as of an Indian tribe or a nation such as Japan. In this usage there are as many cultures in the world as there are definable groups composed of individuals who to some degree share ideas and feelings.

The other meaning of culture is more restricted and encompasses a number of concepts among which **society, function, integration, adaptation,** and **duration** are central. An Indian tribe such as the Zunis or the Kwatkiutl can be used to exemplify the concept. In this view, the focus of a culture is in one or more self-sufficient social systems, each of which fulfills the definition of a **society** by Aberle et al (Appendix A). The notion is illustrated by Sharp's description of the Yir Yoront given in Appendix B. The main **function** of the culture is to preserve the existence of the society. The ideas, feelings, and perceptions of which it is composed serve to guide the behavior of individuals so that they can function together rather than dissolve into a "warre" of every man against every man, as Thomas Hobbes put it. The culture can be pictured as something like a computer program in that it tells people how to process information and how to respond to the input from events.

For people to do this, the various patterns and components of a culture must be linked together so as to constitute an **integrated** whole. They may not be (and usually are not) logically consistent in every way, but they must have an overall functional consistency if the culture is to perform adequately in the preservation of the society that carries it. All the cultures that have survived the processes of evolution and come down to us as going concerns have this attribute of wholeness. It does not follow that all are equally efficient in promoting the well-being of their respective societies, but it does mean that all are somewhat efficient and none consist in simply a miscellaneous collection of independent beliefs and behaviors.

Because of the changing conditions that surround and penetrate societies, cultures may vary considerably across time. That is to say, they have potentials for **adaptation** to change. This in turn implies that cultures, like the societies they guide, have **durations** that are longer than the human life span. Some anthropologists say that in order to be considered cultural a pattern must have functioned during at least three generations (Mead 1978).

If this holistic definition of culture is employed, it means that the patterns of a culture are conceived as functioning for the welfare of the society that carries them and are interlinked with each other so that a change in one has ramifications that extend widely through the culture. This is well demonstrated by Sharp in his "Steel Axes" for Stone-Age Australians"

(Appendix B). Realization of the functional significance of culture patterns has led many people to take the ethical position that members of a society have rights to the patterns of the culture they carry, and should not have changes (and the risks these entail) forced upon them by others. It has come to be thought that culture patterns should be respected.

When one employs "culture" in terms of the first, more diffuse and loose definition — shared ideas and feelings — the functional consequences of the second, holistic definition do not necessarily apply. There are many shared ideas and feelings held in groups that are not cultural in this sense. In such a case the patterns may or may not be socially functional, integrative, adaptive, and enduring. Indeed, under some circumstances the feelings shared by a group may be socially destructive as in states of panic, or in cult behavior as in the Manson family, Synanon, Jonesville, and, on a much larger scale, Nazi Germany.

If one looks at the shared ideas, feelings, and behaviors found among people in subgroups of societies such as a socioeconomic class, a high school, the medical profession, a ship, or a monastery, it is apparent that these are a mixture. Some are culture patterns in the holistic sense and pertain to the functioning and survival of the society of which the socioeconomic class, high school, or profession is a part. Others, though shared by some people, are much more limited in scope and lack any such significance. The risk of using the word "culture" in the diffuse sense is that it carries connotations derived from whole cultures and whole societies and applies them to subsets and fragments where they may not hold. For example, some of the shared ideas found in groups may be trivial and transient, or nihilistic, socially disruptive, and countercultural, signifying the splintering and demise of a society. It is important for the physician to be able to make these distinctions if he is going to take account of culture in his diagnostic and treatment procedures. He should be able to see fallacies in the following statement: if it is shared by a group, it is cultural; and if it is cultural, it contributes to social survival, well-being, and has ethical justification.

The dilution of the word "culture" so that it refers to virtually any kind of shared notion in any kind of group is remindful of what happened to "libido" in psychiatry. Beginning with a specific sexual reference, it spread until it came to mean in common usage virtually any kind of positive feeling toward an object. The more it became all-inclusive, the more it became vague and lost its conceptual utility.

The issue under discussion is not "the real nature of culture," but more or less useful ways to employ a word in order to deal with phenomena and concepts, and especially to prevent ideas from making nonlogical leaps from one category into another, by virtue of having the same name. The term "culture" is more useful and closer to anthropological traditions when restricted to the holistic and functional meaning I have outlined. For the more general, diffuse concept I would like to suggest the term "shared sentiments" (Murphy et al 1959).

Having distinguished the broad concept of shared sentiments from the more restricted notion of culture, it remains to point out that there are many phenomena that must be classified as lying between. As we shall discuss later, one of the features of modern life all over the world is the dissolution and breaking apart of cultures. Whole cultures guiding whole societies are becoming more and more difficult to find. The clinician, especially if he works in an urban area, will encounter few if any patients who are carriers of an intact culture. The question with regard to each patient, therefore, is whether he approximates a participant in a culture or more closely resembles a participant in some collection of diffuse shared sentiments, the functional significance of which is unclear.

The case vignette in Appendix B gives an unusually clear and terse account of what a culture can be like when it is an ongoing concern and independent of western influences.

The reader has now been presented with a general discussion of culture and with an ostensive definition through Sharp's account of the Yir Yoront. We shall turn next to the field of applied anthropology. Applied anthropology shares with clinical psychiatry the task of helping people adapt, and hence the conception of culture in this branch of anthropology has much to offer that is immediately pertinent.

George Foster begins his 1962 book with an Oriental parable that is highly relevant for all the helping professions, and which brings our attention once more to the importance of context.

Once upon a time a monkey and a fish were caught up in a great flood. The monkey, agile and experienced, had the good fortune to scramble up a tree to safety. As he looked down into the raging water, he saw a fish struggling against the swift current. Filled with humanitarian desire to help his less fortunate fellow, he reached down and scooped the fish from the water.

After this caveat, Foster (1969) goes on to make a number of definitional points from which I have selected four, and then added a fifth from Keesing (1958).

Culture is learned. The behavior patterns that constitute a specific culture are not genetically or biologically determined. Every normal infant has the potential to learn any culture.

Medicine's roots in biology lead us to expect a high degree of individual variation due to genetic factors and chance organic events that leave permanent traces. Foster points out other reasons for individual variation:

> Although everyone learns the culture into which he is born, the human environment and life experience of no two people are absolutely identical. The chance that determines [the society into which one is born] also determines one's statuses within the society, and these in turn affect the individual learning process. Consequently, although a culture/society produces similar products, these products are not absolutely uniform....Each person has an unique personality...and this personality in relation to the society and culture that goes with it, will determine the specific behavior of its owner.

Individuals in a given cultural group vary a great deal from one to another. The clinician, therefore, should expect considerable variation in the responsiveness he encounters to his questions and recommendations among people who support the same culture. His patient's belonging to a particular cultural group, which in general has certain characteristics, should not lead to cultural stereotyping and to overlooking the patient's individuality (Edgerton 1971; Goodman 1967).

> *A culture is a logically integrated, functional, sense-making whole.* It is not an accidental collection of customs and habits thrown together by chance. If the analogy is not carried too far, a culture may be compared to a biological organism, in that each of its parts is related in some way to all other parts. Each fulfills a definite function in relation to the others....To say that a culture is...a functional entity does not imply that its parts interact in perfect harmony, without stress or strain. In an absolutely static community this might be true. But cultures change, and the parts of a culture change at different speeds; consequently, perfect integration and perfect fit are impossible....Every culture, therefore, represents something of a compromise, an attempt to strike a balance between the stresses and strains that are inevitable consequences of unequal rates of change and the forces which work toward the unattainable goal of perfect harmony.

The notion of a whole that has problems because its parts are changing at different rates is, of course, familiar to the psychiatrist as a student of personality, especially adolescent personality.

> Significant change in any...phase of a culture cannot occur without accommodation in those phases that impinge upon it, and the degree of possible change is limited by the extent to which these accommodations occur. Conversely, any change in one (major phase) produces secondary and tertiary changes in others, of a nature and extent that cannot always be foreseen.

In other words, each individual who has grown up in a culture that is a going concern finds that he cannot easily, by his own individual act of will, undertake a practice or accept a set of ideas that is at variance with his culture, for to do so would invoke wide ramifications. Sharp illustrates this among the Yir Yoront in discussing the strength of ideas (Appendix B). The individual may not see all these clearly, but he feels them (often to some extent unconsciously) as dangerous to his sense of identity, to his place in his group, and to his coping abilities. In assimilating a culture as you grow, many of its orientations and values become ego-syntonic components of your personality. Hence, if in later life you are faced with a choice between a rational, fact-based decision that is contrary to your culture and one that is nonrational but in keeping with the culture, the latter is the likely choice.

All cultures are constantly changing: no culture is completely static. Although every culture produces inventors and discoverers, who are the ultimate sources of change, no group would progress rapidly if change could come about only through the ingenuity of its own members. If the opportunity for change were so limited, we should still all be in the Stone Age.

Thus it seems likely that the former remarkable stability of the Yir Yoront culture described by Sharp may be attributed largely to its isolation.

As far as a particular society is concerned, its proneness to advancement is the result of its members' exposure to the tools, techniques, and ideas of other groups, their readiness to recognize advantages in ways and forms not their own, and their opportunity to accept these ways and forms, should they wish to do so.

(This is known as diffusion. Mapping the diffusion of cultural patterns was at one time a major concern of anthropology and had to do with trying to reconstruct history.)

We may postulate an interactive process between the forces making for individual conformity and cultural stability on the one hand and adoption of advantageous new ideas and procedures on the other. Cultures therefore range in matters of change from the viscous to the fluid. None that have survived the forces of evolution are changeless. As we shall see later, most of those now extant in North America are fluid.

The changing character of cultures is sometimes lost from sight when people talk about "preserving" a culture. To the extent they have in mind the holistic conception, they are demanding the impossible, much as Kanut when he told the tide not to rise. There is no chance, for example, that the whole way of life of an Indian tribe in North America will be preserved. They have all been changing, at least since the earliest historical reports we have, and if archeology and linguistics mean anything, this was going on before the coming of Columbus (Driver

1969). The Navajos, to take one instance, came to the Southwest about the 10th century from the northern woodlands and picked up from the Pueblo Indians many of the traits we now think of as characteristically Navajo (Kluckhohn and Leighton 1946).

If, however, "preserving a culture" refers only to certain components such as language or religion, the case is different and perhaps more feasible, and it may be no more than just and fair to think that the people concerned should have the opportunity to control such matters.

> The complexity of our modern civilizations is due only in small part to the geniuses each has bred. It is due rather to the willingness of our ancestors, over countless generations, to see merit in the ways of other people and to adopt these ways as their own when they saw advantages in so doing.

Foster goes on then to quote Ralph Linton's well-known passage on America's debt to world cultures. This in part says:

> Our solid American citizen awakens in a bed built on a pattern which originated in the Near East, but which was modified in Northern Europe before it was transmitted to America....He puts on garments whose form originally derived from the skin clothing of nomads of the Asiatic steppes, puts on shoes made from skins tanned by a process invented in ancient Egypt and cut to a pattern derived from the classical civilizations of the Mediterranean, and ties around his neck a strip of bright colored cloth which is a vestigial survival of the shoulder shawls worn by seventeenth-century Croatians....He reads the news of the day, imprinted in characters invented by the ancient Semites upon a material invented in China by a process invented in Germany. As he absorbs the accounts of foreign troubles he will, if he is a good conservative citizen thank a Hebrew deity in an Indo-European language that he is 100 percent American.

> *Every culture has a value system.* All of us, to a greater or lesser extent, react emotionally to our culture....We classify the phenomena of our existence into good and bad, desirable and undesirable, right and wrong categories.

Cultures, molded by evolution, function as we have seen to ensure the survival of societies. One of the ways this is accomplished is through the inculcation and maintenance of shared values and shared perceptions of reality. This sharing, in turn, is dependent on the use of symbols, and for their elucidation, I shall now turn from Foster to Keesing (1958).

> *Cultures are transacted through the use of symbols.* A "symbol" is some form or fixed sensory sign to which...meaning has been arbitrarily assigned. As the signs are signalled between persons trained to know the form and meaning they have in the culture tradition concerned, these in-

dividuals share common understanding. A person outside that culture may see material objects or overt behaviors...or hear the signs of spoken language....He takes great risks in guessing from his own cultural meanings, though he may occasionally infer a general answer....A culture, looked at from this sign-meaning aspect, is sometimes referred to as a *symbol system.*

Shared values, shared perceptions of reality, and shared symbols by which thinking and interpersonal relationships are conducted constitute an interesting common ground between cultural anthropology and clinical psychiatry. Understanding a patient's feelings and values, perceptions of reality, and use of symbols is essential in diagnosis and treatment. When there is a cultural difference between patient and clinician it behooves the latter to grasp something about the culture in question and about culture as both a social and a psychological process.

The notion of function is central in the definition of culture I have emphasized. The value of this conceptualization has been questioned from several theoretical points of view (see for example Kaplan and Manners 1972); and there is no doubt that, like many other scientific ideas, it has suffered from uncritical enthusiasm and simplistic interpretations. But as an orientation it is of considerable utility to the clinician because it squares with observable phenomena and enables him to build on his grasp of biological and psychological functions and move toward an understanding of how social and cultural systems function (Leighton 1949). In particular it keeps him reminded of the interdependence of personality processes and sociocultural processes and enhances his ability to anticipate the consequences of his therapeutic endeavors. It also provides some protection against wandering beyond clinical issues into realms of philosophy, mysticism, nostalgia, romance and UPC.*

Appendix A is a classical statement on function in a society and I suggest that it be read in its entirety at this point.

ACQUISITION OF UNDERSTANDING OF CULTURE AND CULTURAL PROCESSES

When the physician belongs to one culture and the patient to another, problems of distinguishing what is significant and exercising clinical judgment are correspondingly increased, not only in diagnosis, but throughout the course of treatment and the mobilization of resources

---

*Coined by a John Robertson (1978) in an article in the *Lancet,* referring to medical pronouncements made by a British judge in a court of law. It stands for "unadulterated pseudoscientific codswallop."

for the patient's benefit. Understanding culture and distinguishing it from other kinds of group processes not only help to resolve some of these difficulties, but may also make the therapist aware of resources available in the patient's culture that do not exist in his own. Taking culture into account is an extension of what every clinician is expected to do: understand the patient's symptoms and underlying problems in the light of his particular current situation, life story, and panoply of perceptions, values, aspirations, and habitual modes of action.

The acquisition and practice of cultural understanding has two aspects: skill and knowledge. The skill takes shape as a style of interviewing and interacting with the patient that encourages him to explain what might otherwise be taken for granted. It is based on a reluctance to make assumptions (that might be all right in the clinician's own culture) without corroboration from the patient. Equally, there is reluctance to make assumptions too quickly based on the clinician's acquired knowledge of the patient's culture, since there is room here, too, for error. Starting then from a base that takes little for granted, but which is alert to many alternatives, the skill is to build an understanding of how things are for that particular patient, including the particular way in which cultural influences have been, and are, operating.

The above is an ideal which has to be adapted to realistic considerations such as the patient's age, sex, language fluency, and type of disorder. It is also important not to push questioning to the point of creating annoyance. One must recognize that for people in many cultures the act of questioning itself provokes reactions that limit its use. It can be considered insulting, irrelevant, or a mark of the physician's incompetence. The latter is likely to be true in cultures where the accepted mode of diagnosis is religious or magical. A Navajo friend in describing the great powers of a particular native diagnostician ended by looking quietly at me and saying, "He does it by knowing, not by asking questions and guessing." Nevertheless, the skill ideal stands, and ability in matters of balance and technique comes with experience.

The acquisition of knowledge can be seen as having a number of steps. First is reading scientific literature on the relevant culture. This is not a matter of light reading, but of study and committing to memory as one would with a psychiatric text. It is, however, a matter of selective reading since works by anthropologists and other social scientists cover many topics that have only remote relevance to the concerns of the clinician.

During the reading, several considerations should be kept in mind. One is that the very act of setting down a readable, generalized description of a culture reifies it; that is, makes it seem more of "a thing" than it actually is. One should be prepared to find that the people who support a given culture somehow do not take it quite so literally as the describer seemed to imply, and that, as was said before, there is much individual variation. Every clinician knows that it is rare to encounter in real life a case that fulfills the textbook description. The matter is similar with individuals in cultural groups: their behavior rarely matches the text. Also, it is likely that time has elapsed since the author's observations were made and written down, and that changes have occurred since then. It may be that the description now applies mainly to older members of the group, or even only to very old members.

For these reasons, and also to aid in selection, the readings should be done with the help of tutoring by a professional anthropologist who is currently expert in the culture and who understands the clinical task. Under such guidance, the reader would have the opportunity to ask questions and participate in discussions.

After a base has been established in the scientific literature, the clinician should expand his reading to novels, plays, and poetry, if these exist. This process must also be selective, if it is not to be a limitless task. It is important, however, because it gives affective quality and meaning to much of what has been acquired in only a cognitive form from scientific writings.

Learning to speak the language with fluency is another ideal, but may be a greater investment than most people would find possible. In such cases it is still worthwhile to learn about the language. With the help of a linguist, native speakers, or tapes, one can comprehend linguistic structure and acquire at least a small, basic vocabulary. This is not only good for rapport, but helps clarify aspects of the culture. For example, the distinctions made by the system of kinship terms may be illuminating with regard to family relationships. Or, grasping the syntax by which thoughts are put together can help with understanding the problems patients (or interpreters) have in expressing themselves in English, and can alert the clinician to areas in which loss of communication could occur (Marcos 1979).

Participation in events that are open to the public is another avenue to familiarity with the culture of a group. Opportunity can be taken to attend fiestas, carnivals, dances, concerts and so on, preferably in the company of someone who is a participant in the culture.

Friendships are a further step that may be pursued as the way opens. By and large, educational and religious organizations provide opportunities for securing introductions. Most important is to arrange to live with at least two different families over a period of several weeks each.

Finally, I would suggest the great desirability of obtaining from selected members of the cultural group the story of their lives. This should be done in the form of interviews with the physician writing down (or at least taping) for future review everything he is told. Where acceptable, questions seeking explanation and further elaboration may be interjected. The interviewees should, of course, be nonpatients, about eight or nine in number, and the selection should be of such a nature as to provide sampling of both sexes, the young, the middle-aged, and the elderly. This can yield a background of information that is of immense value when it comes to understanding the lives of patients and their "psychological reality" (Hallowell 1955). Indeed, of all the suggestions made here, this interviewing has perhaps the highest potential for enhancing the skill and knowledge of the clinician who has cross-cultural work to do.

It may seem that I have suggested an enormous task, much of it difficult. Certainly it is more than most residents would be able to accomplish in spare time, no matter how highly motivated. If, on the other hand, a program along these lines were developed within residency training, and suitable arrangements were made through the leaders of the relevant culture groups, a concentrated period of two months per culture would accomplish much. Such a curriculum would not turn out a cross-cultural psychiatrist, but it could provide insights not otherwise easily achieved and get the resident well started in a life-long career of continuous learning in these matters.

The study of a culture can in and of itself be a matter of great fascination with many intellectual, aesthetic, ethical, and warm human rewards. A genuine respect for another culture based on understanding it well yields not only knowledge that is clinically useful, but also perspectives on oneself, one's own culture, and the world.

APPLICATION OF CULTURAL KNOWLEDGE TO CLINICAL PSYCHIATRY

Overexpectation can lead to bad results and disillusionment. First of all, in terms of general experience, it is well known that the field of mental health is highly susceptible to fads and artifices of theory by which people get carried away. One of the recurrent tragedies in the care of mentally ill persons is the degree to which the theory-building component of science has time after time outrun the theory-verifying component. As a consequence, theoretical notions have frequently been treated as if they were factual discoveries and sold as nostrums. The history of mental illness care over the last 200 years contains a long series of boom and bust sequences in which ideas that doubtless contained some truth had their usefulness crushed by the collapse of overbuilt expectations. To a large extent this was the story of moral treatment, Dix's mental hospital movement, mental hygiene, child guidance, and psychoanalysis, and it may now be happening to social psychiatry and the community mental health center movement.

Similar examples of fads can be seen in the field of culture and personality. In the 1940s, the notion that Japanese national character was due to severe toilet training became popular. The basic idea was not ridiculous; on the contrary it involved an ingenious synthesis of psychoanalytic, learning and culture-functional theory (Gorer 1943). The defects lay in the insufficiency of the evidence, a matter which because of contemporary social-emotional factors, was disregarded. The Japanese were our enemies and we were engaged in hating them; hence it was very satisfying to believe that social science had proved them to have deformed personalities and had demonstrated the cause. Thus a theory spread itself widely in the guise of a finding.

Shortly after this, during the "cold war" it became popular to believe that the Russians had a national character based on the swaddling of infants (Gorer and Rickman 1962). One is reminded of Benjamin Rush's "observations" during the American Revolution, which asserted that the mental health of the Revolutionists was much superior to that of the Loyalists (Rosen 1969). Rush was, of course, a revolutionist and signer of the Declaration of Independence.

Over-reaching enthusiasm for theoretical notions has not been confined to the psychodynamic and cultural realms of psychiatry. In the 1920s, belief in foci of infection as the cause of mental illness went so far as to cause innumerable patients to undergo high colonic irrigations and to have tonsils, adenoids, other tissues, and all their teeth removed (Bunker 1944; Cotton 1922; Malamud 1944) — spectacular mass mutilation of the mentally ill masquerading as the contemporary version of "what we now know."

History suggests, therefore, that as a matter of general principle one should be suspicious of "new ideas" that purport to be major advances, especially if they appear both cognitively neat and well fitted to current social-emotional dispositions, particularly when the ideas are not supported by quantitative data, controlled observation, and experimental demonstration, or are cast in a theoretical form that is not susceptible to such challenge.

In addition to these general considerations, several more specific points can be made that relate to cultural theories. One is the belief that some cultures protect their participants from mental illnesses while others have a capacity for generating such disorders. It is often said that nonindustrial cultures, which emphasize being and spiritual values, belong in the former category, while the modern industrial culture of the West is in the latter. This theory of cultural determinism may contain some or even much truth, but it is advisable that it be treated with caution.

For one thing, the view that people in societies that carry a "primitive" culture are better off than we are may itself be a bias characteristic of western cultures. It has been a popular belief, at least among intellectuals, in Europe and North America for well over 200 years. Its prominence as a theme during the Enlightenment is attested by the writings of Kant and Rousseau. The former states explicitly "The primitive man is subject to very little insanity or stupidity" (Zilboorg 1941).

The origins of the idea are doubtless much older, very likely traceable to the belief of classic times that mankind had in a previous age experienced a Golden Era when the human way of life had been far better than the contemporary one. The story of the Garden of Eden is probably a still earlier expression of the same idea.

Benjamin Rush, who was an exponent of the Enlightenment, articulated the idea that "primitives" have it better (Rush 1821. Reprinted 1962), and it has been re-echoed by various successors in the 19th century such as Awl (Grob 1973), Jarvis (Rosen 1969) and Earl (Caplan 1969). Both Jarvis and Earl are quoted as saying that insanity is part of the price we pay for civilization. Freud, of course, carried forward and developed the theme in his *Civilization and Its Discontents* (1961). Very few, if any, of these writings were based on actual systematic study of "primitive" peoples.

A convergent stream did, however, come from the writings of some anthropologists and presented an idealized picture of non-Western ways of life (for example Benedict 1934, 1938; Mead 1928, Reprinted 1975; Diamond 1964; Opler 1967). These authors were impressed by the superb way some cultures take care of certain human needs, especially those which are affective. Such cultures appeared to constitute a less trouble-ridden and much happier way of life than the one we know, and from this it was argued that there must be little or no mental illness. Writers of many kinds in many media have picked up these ideas, circulating and utilizing them, until their sheer prevalence makes it seem that they must be true. The picture, however, is unbalanced; and it can, for example, lead us into visualizing the climate, easy life, and sexual freedom of the South Seas without awareness of the concomitant practices of slavery, cannibalism, and human sacrifice.

Another argument for cultural determinism consists in pointing to culture-bound syndromes such as *amok* in Malaysia, *piblokto* among the Eskimos, and *wihtigo* psychosis among certain Northern Indians. These, it is thought, help make a case for cultural determinism by demonstrating that some cultures not only produce mental illnesses, but produce their own particular kinds.

In the last 50 years a considerable body of theory has been developed by which to explain the role of culture in mental health and mental illness. Among the psychiatrists notable for such work are Harry Stack Sullivan (1953) and Abram Kardiner (1945). Some years ago Jane M. Murphy and I (Leighton and Murphy 1961) were able to extract from the literature 11 theories showing culture as causative of mental illnesses. Thus, the various motivations for believing in the power of culture have been matched by sets of systematic, plausible explanations.

Trouble comes when one begins to look for scientific evidence. Despite the generations that have believed that "primitives have it better," epidemiologic investigations have so far failed to demonstrate striking differences in mental illness rates that can be attributed to differences in culture (Murphy 1976). Differences are not ruled out, but if they exist they must be at a more subtle level than one would expect were this or that culture type prominent as a cause of mental illnesses. Above all, it is clear that no culture group has yet been found free of mental disorders.

Pertinent to this is an unpublished finding in our own work. When my colleagues and I compared the mental illness prevalence rates of three contrasting culture groups — Eskimos, rural Nova Scotians, and Nigerians — the differences among the group means were considerably less than the differences that occurred within each group in terms of population subsets marked by age, sex, and degree of economic, social, and psychological deprivation. This finding tends to support stress rather than culture-as-cause theory.

A cultural effect could, nevertheless, be implicated to the extent that culture patterns make certain subgroups in the population lead stressful lives. It may be theorized therefore that in the course of evolution, the cultures that have survived have achieved about the same level of controlling and preventing mental illnesses in their respective societies, and that no culture has yet emerged that avoids placing some subsets of people in psychologically noxious positions.

The finding can also be interpreted as compatible with theories of genetic causality. Thus, one can suppose that no culture has been able to prevent people handicapped by genetically-influenced mental disorders from aggregating in certain parts of the social structure.

The culture-bound syndromes do not stand up very well on close inspection as clear evidence in favor of cultural determinism. There is room for much doubt as to whether *amok* and *latah* are distinctive mental illnesses, or are states of excitement, rage, anxiety, or hysteria that have cultural coloring. In other words, if someone goes into a state of excitement and kills a number of people indiscriminately, is it called *amok* when it occurs in Malaysia, but something else when it occurs (as it does every year) in California, Texas, Chicago or New York? Perhaps the issue is again, basically, Leslie White's question as to whether or not a spider is a bug.

The epidemiologic work on these disorders, furthermore, is for the most part weak or nonexistent. The clinical descriptions are for the most part not by clinicians and the tabulations of frequency are vague. To the extent numbers are used, they are mostly numerators without denominators.

In instances where epidemiologic studies have been attempted, the results give little ground for crediting the common occurrence of culture-bound syndromes at the present time. As an example to illustrate this, let us consider *piblokto*.

According to one psychiatric text (Lehmann 1967) *piblokto* may be summarized as

> ...attacks lasting from 1 to 2 hours, during which the patient, who is usually a woman, begins to scream and to tear off and destroy her clothing. While imitating the cry of some animal or bird she may then throw herself on the snow or run wildly about on the ice, although the temperature may be well below zero. After the attack, the person appears quite normal and usually has amnesia for it. The Eskimos are reluctant to touch any afflicted person during the attack because they think it has something to do with evil spirits.

In 1954 and 1955, Murphy (1960) conducted a psychiatric epidemiologic study of the 178 individuals who made up the adult population of an Eskimo village in Alaska. Although 19% had one or another kind of mental illness (for the most part mild anxiety and depression), no case emerged that answered the description of *piblokto*. She extended the study retrospectively to include all those adults who had died during the previous 15 years. This was done by the aid of a key informant who systematically reviewed the health and behavior of each deceased person. Only one individual out of a total of 499 was described who might be considered to have *piblokto,* although this was uncertain.

Foulks (1972) has reviewed all cases of mental illness coming to medical attention out of a population of about 11,000 Eskimos from July 1969 through June 30, 1970. Among these he found "ten individuals who had manifested behavior similar in pattern to the Arctic Hysterias." While noting the importance of multiple factors, including culture, in shaping the behavior of these cases, Foulks also notes that "several subjects had epilepsy; several were diagnosed as having schizophrenia; most had low normal serum calcium levels, one had hypomagnesemia and possible alcoholism."

Numbers of authors comment that *piblokto* was very likely once more common than it is now. This could be so, but one must take into account that the farther back in time he goes, the less trustworthy do the accounts appear.

Finally, arctic hysteria-like behavior is not confined to the arctic. In my work among the Navajo I was told of individuals, particularly women, who at times ripped off their clothing, screamed, and ran off wildly regardless of weather. Synge (1909) has left us a description of similar behavior in a rural community in Ireland.

The facts regarding *wihtigo* psychosis are similar. The Lehmann text summarizes it as a psychiatric illness confined to the Cree, Ojibway, and Salteaux Indians of North America. They believe that they may be transformed into a wihtigo, a giant monster that eats human flesh. During times of starvation, a man may develop the delusion that he has been transformed into a wihtigo, and he may actually feel and express a craving for human flesh. Because of the belief in witchcraft and in the possibility of such a transformation, symptoms concerning the alimentary tract — like loss of appetite and nausea from trivial causes — may sometimes cause the patient to become greatly excited for fear of being transformed into a wihtigo. Yap considers this illness a good illustration of the effects of mythology and cultural environment on psychiatric manifestations and thinks that nosologically the disorder may be, like other demoniacal possession states, essentially hysterical in nature.

Teicher (1960) made an exhaustive review of sources regarding the *wihtigo* syndrome, citing some 70 possible cases. Honigman (1967) reviewed this material and concluded:

> Some of his cases described individuals whom famine had driven to cannibalism, but who felt no emotional compulsion to eat human flesh and came away from their desperate act without suffering any notable personality disorder....As for the other cases, I can't find one that satisfactorily attests to someone being seriously obsessed by the idea of committing cannibalism.

It would seem therefore that as with *piblokto,* the reason for the popularity of the *wihtigo* "syndrome" is its drama and theoretical appeal, not its factual basis.

Nevertheless, despite the inconclusiveness of the evidence about cultures as causes of mental disorder, at the level of clinical practice there can be no doubt that knowledge of the values, orientations, and customs encompassed by the word "culture" is of great importance. It is a necessary part of the framework for comprehending each person's particular mix of psychological, interpersonal, and social-environmental influences, what Murray called "press" (1938). Such knowledge can help the diagnostician choose the appropriate questions to ask, to interpret the responses, and to lay out a therapeutic and case-management plan that is adjusted to the relevant factors at work in the patient's life.

It is also important not to endow the cultural concept with properties it does not possess. As yet, no theory arising from studies of culture that might be a great leap forward in understanding mental illnesses has been established by scientific procedures. To take such theories literally as if they were real-life processes and apply them to real-life situations results in a kind of "culturizing" that can be just as intriguing and misleading as "psychiatrizing." The research challenge is great and important, but this importance should not obscure the fact that dependable results are not yet in.

Another cultural idea that needs to be treated with reserve is one which intimates that if a possibly psychopathologic item of behavior can be shown to be a cultural pattern, it is not a pathological disorder. For example, a complaint like suffering from witchcraft has cultural compatibility but does not ipso facto rule out the possibility of its having clinical significance too. When the Italian member of a witchcraft-believing culture says that he is bewitched, the cultural acceptability of the general notion does not negate the possibility that the complaint is nonetheless a manifestation of paranoid schizophrenia.

People suffering from mental illness express themselves in their culture's idiom. Thus, while the paranoid person in a culture that surrounds him with talk of microwaves and laser beams may very well report that it is by such means that "they" are harming him, similar disease in a member of a witchcraft-believing culture will lead him to complain in witchcraft terms. Consequently, even though the complaint of witchcraft in our immigrant from rural Italy is not as such clinically significant, the embedded complaint of being persecuted is. This calls for further inquiry and not immediate dismissal because the psychiatrist thinks he "understands the culture." The clinician must ask what other things go with the belief, what is the history of their development, and especially whether in the eyes of people in the same cultural group the belief seems normal, or has something odd about it. As the distinguished Sudanese psychiatrist T.A. Baashar (Savage et al, 1965) once said, you have to "look for the knight's move." By this he meant that it is possible for each component of a mentally ill person's delusion to be culturally compatible if considered separately, but that the way they fit together and into the individual's life situation could still have an eccentric turn that is not compatible with cultural expectation, and it is this that would suggest some kind of mental illness.

A popular tendency to idealize cultures, especially those that are non-Western, has already been mentioned. This now deserves a little further discussion since, from a clinical point of view, there is both good and bad care to be found among the cultures of the world.

My own studies of Navajo healing have led me to think that it is indeed powerful, and I have tried to summarize this in the description presented in Appendix C. It is important to realize, however, that this is not all of Navajo healing. There are other aspects having to do with witchcraft that do not seem right from a mental health point of view. They cultivate suspicion, hatred, and the persecution of innocent individuals.

Beyond witchcraft there are also other characteristics of healing, as prescribed in various cultures, that can be called into question. Let us approach this by looking first at an instance of the traditional healing in the West as it was practiced some 300 years ago. The patient is Charles II of England in his terminal illness, probably a cerebral accident.

According to Haggard (1929):

> As the first step in treatment the king was bled to the extent of a pint from a vein in his right arm. Next his shoulder was cut into and the incised area "cupped" to suck out an additional eight ounces of blood. After this homicidal onslaught the drugging began. An emetic and purgative were administered, and soon after a second purgative. This was followed by an enema containing antimony, sacred bitters, rock salt, mallow leaves, violets, beet root, camomile flowers, fennel seed, linseed, cinnamon, cardamom seed, saffron, cochineal, and aloes. The enema was repeated in two hours and a purgative given. The king's head was shaved and a blister raised on his scalp. A sneezing powder of hellebore root was administered, and also a powder of cowslip flowers "to strengthen his brain." The cathartics were repeated at frequent intervals and interspersed with a soothing drink composed of barley water, licorice and sweet almond. Likewise white wine, absinthe and anise were given, as also were extract of thistle leaves, mint, rue, and angelica. For external treatment a plaster of Burgundy pitch and pigeon dung was applied to the king's feet. The bleeding and purging continued, and to the medicaments were added melon seeds, manna, slippery elm, black cherry water, an extract of flowers of lime, lily-of-the-valley, peony, lavender, and dissolved pearls. Later came gentian root, nutmeg, quinine, and cloves. The king's condition did not improve, indeed it grew worse, and in the emergency forty drops of extract of human skull were administered to allay convulsions. A rallying dose of Raleigh's antidote was forced down the king's throat; this antidote contained an enormous number of herbs and animal extracts. Finally bezoar stone was given. Then says Scarburgh: "Alas! after an ill-fated night his serene majesty's strength seemed exhausted to such a degree that the whole assembly of physicians lost all hope and became despondent: still so as not to appear to fail in doing their duty in any detail, they brought into play the most active cordial." As a sort of grand summary to this pharmaceutical debauch a mixture of Raleigh's antidote, pearl julep, and ammonia was forced down the throat of the dying king.

It is difficult to see this performance as justified either from a biomedical (disease) or psychosocial (illness) point of view, and there is reason to be glad that western civilization has moved to the scientific medicine of our time despite all its faults. When the kind of treatment accorded Charles II occurs today, it is not made better if it happens to be folk medicine, or if its context is some nonwestern culture. These words, "folk" and "culture," include both beneficial and noxious practices.

Medicine has for long had to deal with an *antinomy* that hampers policy making, law enactment, and practice even when altogether within the confines of western culture. The antinomy arises in part from the medical belief that the expectations and emotional state of a patient can have a major influence in determining whether he will recover, become chronically ill, or die. The degree of this influence varies, of course, depending on many things, including type of illness, but it is generally thought to play at least a part in virtually all disorders, and in some it is considered major.

The other part of the antinomy comes from modern medicine's dedication to healing by means of scientific truth. What should one do when healing can be more effectively achieved by falsehoods that have a positive effect on the patient's expectations and emotional state? The issue is extraordinarily difficult, philosophically, ethically, legally, and practically and is responsible for much stumbling about in patient care among members of both the medical and legal professions. Efforts to avoid it often contribute to the rigidity of doctrinaire theories of biomedical cause, and encourage the suspicions and hostility with which some physicians view psychiatry because they think its methods, even if effective, are not based on scientific truth.

Often, of course, truth and helping the patient psychologically are not in conflict; while in other cases it may be more a matter of uncertainty than conflict, with the physician feeling justified in giving an optimistic rather than a pessimistic interpretation to the patient or going along with something the patient wants. Much of this is what has been called "the art of medicine" or more recently "Samaritanism" (McDermott 1974). The continuum extends, however, and ultimately one comes to the blatant lies of charlatans. That these through false promises betray, maim, and kill some patients, there can be no doubt; but, there can also be little doubt that some patients are helped either to more enjoyment of life while it lasts or in some cases to a recovery that might not otherwise have occurred.

The development of cultural understanding does not resolve the medical antinomy. Cultural knowledge adds resources for coping, but does not cause it to vanish. Overenthusiastic, mystical, indiscriminate belief in the virtue of a culture, however, can create such an illusion, but at high risk to the patient.

In terms of the clinical orientation that attaches importance to the well-being of every individual human being in a population, all known cultures are flawed. Although each culture that has survived to our time is generally functional for the societies that hold to it, and even though many cultures have admirable ways of providing some individuals with social supports, psychological refuge, and spiritual achievement, all impose stress and suffering on some categories of persons.

Slavery, for example, was an integral part of cultures right around the world, in Asia, Europe, Africa, the Americas and the Polynesian islands. Its disappearance as a legitimate practice is very recent, and it may be questioned whether as a shared sentiment it is altogether gone from all its old haunts.

Or, again, human sacrifice — the killing of selected men, women, and children with or without torture — for the greater good of the greater number was another worldwide practice that had notorious peaks among the Aztecs and the Phoenicians. Although it has lingered into the 20th century, it is probably now mostly gone as a mystical imperative. The values, however, which approve as natural or inevitable the labeling and execution of certain categories (religious or political) of persons for the supposed benefit of others have by no means vanished. The element of propitiating gods may have almost disappeared, but the sense of achieving salvation for some kinds of people by destroying other kinds has not. During my lifetime this pattern has reached secular magnitudes (in the Soviet Union, Germany, Indonesia, and Southeast Asia) that were probably never dreamed of by the Aztecs and Phoenicians.

Belief in witchcraft, which I have mentioned several times, is a stigmatizing and victim-creating pattern that is common from the northern, circumpolar coasts to the tips of Africa and South America. The core of the belief is that certain evil individuals—male and female—can and do through magical means secretly harm and kill other individuals. The details of how this supposedly works vary from culture to culture. In many it constitutes a main theory of illness and disease, and healing is largely devoted to countermeasures, including at times physical destruction of the suspected witch. One may theorize that witchcraft belief is able to confer some psychological relief on the alleged victim, such as absolving self from blame in the face of misfortune, and it can serve to exert social control, but this is at a cost of cultivating fear, suspicion, and hate among the people of a society toward each other on a false basis. Furthermore, it blocks realistic approaches and collective efforts toward recognizing and solving the actual, underlying problems. It fosters labeling, mistrust, prejudice, ostracism, and killing of persons who are guiltless of the crimes attributed to them.

In many, if not most of the world's cultures, the position of women and their value as human beings is clearly well below that of men. Sharp mentions this among the Yir Yoront and refers to it as "androcentrism." Even in matrilineal and matrilocal cultures, the headship roles and prestigious positions are occupied by males. Breeding and labor tend to dominate a woman's life in much of the world with a very narrow range of role choice and opportunity for self-realization and the development of special capabilities. A double standard in matters of sex is found to some degree almost everywhere and is very highly developed in some areas, with accompanying severe restrictions on personal freedom for women. The atrocities of clitoridectomy in Africa are well known.

Strong values and practices with regard to the care of family members exist in numerous cultures. This generally includes psychological support and guidance in life's difficulties and protection and provision of treatment in case of mental illness. Indeed, in some societies, the members of extended kinship networks will go to great lengths to provide money, personal care, and whatever else seems advisable to insure the best possible treatment of the individual.

There is, however, another side to these family-centered values, namely a lack of concern for people who are not members of the kinship network. In some cultural groups this line is sharply drawn so that people outside the network are treated largely in utilitarian terms, as if they were things rather than human beings. There may be no altruism for them and the notion of compassion for any human being who is suffering may be virtually without meaning, as it was not long ago among the Scottish clans.

So long as everybody in a population belongs to at least one functioning kin system, this pattern may not involve severe hardship. For the most part, however, such ideal conditions do not remain and there are people in mental and/or physical distress who have no one to help them. Such people, whether in the arctic or in tropical Africa may lead extremely miserable, wandering, and deteriorating existences until they disappear on the ice or are swallowed by the jungle. Even children can have such a fate.

This kin *vs* stranger orientation at a more extended level constitutes the "tribalism," which in Africa and among North and South American Indians, has made economic and political interaction so difficult and at times so bloody. "Ethnocentrism" is the same kind of pattern in still larger units, and it appears to be in some degree universal among the world's cultures. Individuals as geographically separated as Navajos and Eskimos each refer to themselves as "the people."

SOCIAL-ENVIRONMENTAL INFLUENCES AND CULTURE

There are four major social-environmental phenomena that are interwoven with culture or are affected by culture, but which are useful to keep in view as conceptually separate. These are culture change, sociocultural disintegration, social stratification, and deprived minority status. All are highly fraught with potentials for affecting human well-being.

In trying to understand the patient in this context, the clinician can be seriously misled if he construes as cultural a pattern of behavior that is actually an expression of too rapid change, or of loss of culture, or of class position, or of minority membership. Such patterns do not have the functional properties of culture and hence their clinical implications are not the same as those we have thus far discussed. They may, for example, be malfunctional, rather than functional for society, and they may be fragmented and detached, rather than part of a totality of interdependent symbols, meaning and shared values. Battered children and single parent households are common in some populations, but are not cultural in terms of this chapter. The same goes for general attitudes of apathy, hedonism, lack of interest in values, and unwillingness to plan for the future, which are also shared patterns in some groups.

Culture Change

As we have several times noted earlier, cultures have the function of enabling societies to survive. In doing this, they adapt to altering circumstances. Change, therefore, is in some measure part of the cultural process, even though it may have been exceedingly slow in some isolated societies such as the Yir Yoront and Eskimos.

The impetus to culture change is divisible into two types. One can be called endogenous because of arising within a society that supports a given culture. Population increase and technological invention are examples that have "domino" consequences that alter customs, values, and psychological reality (Hallowell 1955). Fire, the bow and arrow, the wheel, horse collar, the automobile, and the pill are all notable examples of technological inventions that have had such results.

The other type of impetus comes from contact with societies that have different cultures, and this can be called exogenous, or change by cultural diffusion. The items listed under endogenous also diffuse and so what is endogenous to one society may be exogenous to others. Exogenous cultural change can be further divided into the type that is imposed by conquest and dominance, exemplified by the way ancient Rome put its stamp on other cultures all around the Mediterranean, and the type that is elected because it seems desirable, as when Turkey did away with the veil.

In the multicultural population of North America, both these types of cultural change have been and are being transacted simultaneously, with two-, three-, and more-way exchanges occurring among cultural groups in contact with each other. This at best can be confusing to the participants and at the worst leads to intrapsychic and interpersonal strains, splitting families and creating isolated and alienated individuals who have severe problems of identity.

These points are important in clinical work. It is easy for a psychiatrist to mistake a problem due to culture change for one due to culture difference. He may think, for example, that a patient is anxious and depressed because his cultural values are at variance with those of western culture, whereas in actual fact the patient's problem is that his culture is changing under him and he no longer knows where he stands. Or, it may be that the patient wishes to give up his old culture but cannot understand the whirling inconsistencies of the new one he wishes to adopt. His cry may be for help in making a transition, rather than for encouragement and support in keeping to his former ideas and ways. In many cases successful therapy means aid toward achieving reconciliation and synthesis of the two. This is a special form of the common clinical problem of helping a patient work out a reconciliation and synthesis of his past life and its expectations with his present circumstances and their limitations.

Sociocultural Disintegration

As we have seen, any alteration in a sociocultural system calls for multiple readjustments, sometimes very widely distributed across the system. With sufficient time, however, these can take place without serious disruption to the functioning of the society, especially if the magnitude of any one innovation is not too great and there are not too many of them. When changes fall thick and fast, piling one upon another, the capacity for adjustment of a sociocultural system can be exceeded. The nine functional prerequisites postulated by Aberle et al (Appendix A) are not met and as a result discontinuities and conflicts become widely distributed and failures to meet both individual and societal needs take place. When these failures are severe and extensive, they create a physically hazardous and psychologically difficult environment for the people concerned.

We may conclude, therefore, that culture change per se is not necessarily harmful, whether endogenous or exogenous, but rather it is a question of its exceeding the adaptive capacities of human social systems. Many of these points are illustrated by Sharp in his description of the breakup of Yir Yoront culture (Appendix B). For a more quantitative investigation of the same processes among the Yoruba in Nigeria, see Murphy (1973).

A feature of western culture has been its rapid rate of change during the last 200 years. Not only has it been swift, but it has been accelerating at a pace without parallel in history. Furthermore, the other sociocultural systems of the world have been drawn more and more into this vortex. Ever since the 18th century, the speed as well as the content of the changes have been noted with misgiving by many writers, and the view advanced that the process was causing an increase in mental illnesses. For example, writing in 1857 John Hawkes (Rosen 1969) said:

> I doubt if ever the history of the world...could show a larger amount of insanity than that of the present day. It seems, indeed, as if the world was moving at an advanced rate of speed proportionate to its approaching end; as though, in this rapid race of time, increasing with each revolving century, a higher pressure is engendered in the minds of men.

Rapid change, therefore, is not something confined to third world countries, to American Indians or to recent immigrants, but has been a feature of western culture itself for generations. From a psychological point of view, cultural change for an individual would be manageable if it only meant moving from one well-defined and stable culture to another. In the world today, however, it means moving from one rapidly changing and consequently malfunctioning culture to another that is also rapidly changing and malfunctioning. A more extended discussion of these processes is presented in Appendix D. The diagram shown there and the text accompanying it are useful for understanding the dynamics of sociocultural disintegration. As can be seen, this process has the potential for remaining at a more or less chronic level of societal malfunction, but also for improving or getting worse. So far as the latter is concerned, the ultimate is the disappearance of the affected society when malfunction reaches a point that precludes survival.

The trouble experienced by a person caught between the conflicting values of two cultures is generally well recognized today. Less well recognized is the predicament of a person caught between two cultures that are both rapidly changing. These difficulties are increased again when the two cultures are not only changing but disintegrating in the process. At the present time, this latter phenomenon is, unfortunately, likely to be the one most common in cross-cultural clinical work.

Let us return now to the question of why sociocultural disintegration could foster an increase in the number of people seeking psychiatric help in populations so affected. Such empirical evidence as we have is all correlational (Kojak 1974). Numbers of studies have shown that sociocultural disintegration and high rates of mental disorders tend to go together. For explanation, two large bodies of theory are available: developmental and stress.

Developmental theory may be summarized as saying that as the child grows to adulthood, the sociocultural disintegration affects his family so that the mothering and fathering he receives is distorted. So too are later experiences, with the result that he does not pass in a normal way through such sequences as the Eight Ages of Man postulated by Erikson (Beiser 1965). The result is a distorted personality, which may be expressed as psychopathy or a predisposition to neurosis, psychosis, and so on.

Stress theory includes the notion of maldevelopment, but puts emphasis on the generation of disorder through the creation of severe and/or chronic affective states such as anxiety, fear, rage, apathy, and depression. It also postulates childhood as a high-risk period, but in addition holds that severe and/or chronic stresses in adult life can precipitate mental illnesses, which is to say patterns of feeling and behavior which are not then necessarily removed by removal of the stresses. Descriptions of battle and concentration camp reactions provide a model for this idea of cause and long term consequences (Arthur 1978; Murphy 1977). Sociocultural disintegration is conceived as working in a fashion comparable to war stresses, but more slowly and insidiously. The work of Selye (1956) and Wolff (1953) contributed to our frame of reference.

The word "stress" like "culture" and "mental illness" gives trouble because of its having a mixture of meanings. For example, according to *The Language of Mental Health* (Fann 1977) it stands for "An over-load that the organism cannot handle; may be caused by inadequacies in the organism, extreme environmental in-put, or both."

First of all this definition is confusing because it is tautological: "over-" and "cannot handle" mean the same thing. More important, however, is that it allows the word to mean both an environmental event ("-load") and the organism's reaction ("cannot handle"). In some contexts therefore, it may refer to both a cause and its effect. This can be a prime source of confusion, and in order to avoid it I shall employ in what follows "environmental stress" to represent environmental factors, and "strain" (Langner 1963) to represent their mental, emotional, and physiological consequences in the individual.

Sociocultural disintegration is a condition in which cultural symbols, signs, and signals have become unreliable and difficult to interpret. This is illustrated in Figure 14-1 and may be summarized as environmental stress composed of misleading, contradictory cues (Sharp, personal communication 1950).

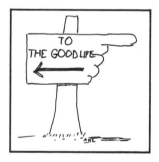

Figure 14-1

Much clinical observation and experimental work with humans and other animals suggest that higher organisms experience strain when subjected to prolonged exposure to a field of contradictory cues in which they must nevertheless act. The feeling of strain may be represented in terms of three components.

Torn in two or more directions   This is the perception of being dragged against one's will by ineluctable yet incompatible forces (Figure 14-2).

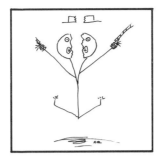

Figure 14-2

Frustration   Achievement is blocked (Figure 14-3). No matter how hard the individual tries, he repeatedly fails to reach completion, closure, and a feeling of success.

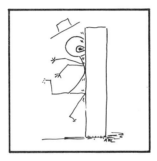

Figure 14-3

Disorientation   This is a state of not knowing where one is, or indeed, who one is (Figure 14-4). As David Landy (1958) has expressed it, "blind groping in an unknown labyrinth."

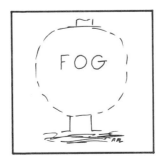

Figure 14-4

The affective state that results from these experiences, sensations and perceptions is some commingling of anxiety, fear, rage, apathy, and depression which may ultimately become molded into one of the clinical syndromes in which the effects of stress are probably combined with genetically determined predispositions.

The theoretical underpinning of the ideas summarized in the cartoons can be found in Leighton (1959).*

Social Stratification

Different levels of socioeconomic class are well recognized in North American society, particularly in cities, and the noxious mental health consequences of life in the lower strata have given much concern. This class structure is a particular instance of the general phenomenon of stratification found in all societies. Aberle et al (Appendix A) observe:

> Stratification is that particular type of role-differentiation which discriminates between higher and lower standings in terms of one or more criteria. Given the universality of scarcity, some system of differential allocation of the scarce values of a society is essential. These values may consist of such desiderata as wealth, power, magic, women, and ceremonial precedence...[Rank] order must be legitimized and accepted by most of the members...of a society if stability is to be attained. Allocation of ranks may be on the basis of ascribed (as in a caste system—AHL) or achieved (as in a democracy—AHL) qualities or both.

> Some individuals will thus receive more than others. These privileges are usually made acceptable to the rank and file by joining to the greater rights of the elite a larger share of responsibilities. The Brahmins stand closer to other-worldly non-existence than do the members of any other Hindu Caste, but they also have to observe the most elaborate ritual obligations. The Trobiand Chief enjoys a multiple share of wealth and wives; he must also finance community enterprises and exhibit at all times more generosity than anyone else.

In North America, living in the lowest levels of stratification tends to be exceedingly stressful due to the limitations imposed by poverty, lack of education, and various forms of discrimination. The experience is similar to that in a disintegrated society. Contradictory cues, chronic frustration, powerlessness, being torn in different directions, and a general sense of disorientation are common, and so too are reactions in terms of anxiety, apathy, and resentment.

---

*See pages 135–159, and 306–315 together with the chapter notes. I am particularly indebted to Gantt (1944) for his interpretations of Pavlov's work and for his own studies.

There are, for each socioeconomic class, attitudes, opinions, and customs that are more or less characteristic. In the lower strata these tend to be dominated by reactions and adaptations to living amid stressful conditions. They are sometimes referred to as the "culture" of the lower class, but this is "culture" in its more diffuse sense and runs the risk of imputing functional significance and capabilities which the patterns often do not have. Such patterns, even though reactive and widely shared, can very well be maladaptive and self-defeating so far as relief from stresses is concerned. Some examples are hedonism, disinterest in values, authoritarianism, passivity, and unwillingness to plan for the future, together with single-parent households and battered children.

It is safer to refer to these as shared sentiments and common practices rather than culture. Moreover, "culture" as defined in the more restrictive sense cannot logically be applied across the board to all the behavior patterns and sentiments characteristic of a socioeconomic class. This is because class is not a society, but a part of a society. Far from being more or less self-sufficient, it is dependent on the rest of the society. Class V, for instance, (the lowest in the Hollingshead system [Hollingshead and Redlich 1958]), is highly dependent on the other four classes for jobs, welfare, and medical care. Within itself a class has no unitary political structure, but is rather a categorization that cuts through such structures.

A reason for emphasizing these distinctions is that a particular culture in the more restricted sense may on occasion be a feature of people in a lower socioeconomic stratum. This is because both foreign immigrants and Native Americans have a tendency to collect at these levels in cities. Such comes about when the individual arrives in a city without the capital, occupational skills, or family connections that would enable him to begin at levels higher than unskilled labor. As a consequence, a physician may find that the behavior of a patient is the product of both a distinctive culture and of living in a low socioeconomic environment, and that the psychological significance of each is considerably different.

For instance, as we have seen earlier, little solid evidence exists that high or low prevalence rates of mental illnesses are associated with one culture as compared to another. The case is quite different with regard to socioeconomic class. One of the most consistent findings in psychiatric epidemiology across many different societies is that the lower levels of socioeconomic status have high rates of mental illnesses (Schwab and Schwab 1978).

Deprived Minority Status

There are, of course, privileged minorities such as the Brahmins, as well as deprived minorities, but it is the latter that concern us as most relevant to cross-cultural psychiatry in North America. The members of deprived minorities experience prejudice and discrimination from the majority population and are more or less barred from access to the goods and privileges (what Aberle et al call the "scarce values") that are otherwise available. Particular features are low prestige, and being the object of hostility, tragically exemplified at present by the Chinese in Southeast Asia.

The economic, social, and psychological factors that contribute to the creation and maintenance of deprived minorities in all probability overlap to a considerable degree with those responsible for slavery, serfdom, and the treatment of outsiders as things rather than as persons — as excluded from the ethical framework that pertains to one's own kind. At any rate, the phenomenon is found widely distributed across the world, particularly in large, complex societies, and is visible outside North America in such groups as the Untouchables of India and the Eta of Japan.

The general topic of deprived minority status and the stressful consequences for individuals is vast. The only point I should like to make, therefore, is the desirability of drawing a distinction between noxious influences that stem from cultural differences and those that stem from deprived minority group status.

The two are easily confused because many minority groups are identified by the name of a culture. This can be the case even when the culture has largely disintegrated so that it is no longer a functioning whole but is rather represented by certain surviving traits such as language (which may not be well spoken) and religion (to which adherence may be indifferent). Such surviving cultural patterns, even though no longer part of an integrated whole way of life, may nevertheless be highly regarded by the members of the minority and serve as symbols to enhance group identity and "we-feeling."

The members of the larger society may also take cognizance of the culture label and interpret it to mean that the group does in fact have a whole culture. This can lead to "over-culturalizing" — that is, mistaking reactions to poverty, discrimination, and injustice for cultural patterns, and considering them just some of "the cultural peculiarities of those people." I have many times heard government policy makers and news media writers say of Indian tribes and Japanese American communities, "They do so and so because of their culture," when culture was little more than coloring for the reactive apathies, anxieties, hostilities, and despair that were being expressed.

The stresses, and reactions to them, that have been sketched in discussing sociocultural disintegration and low socioeconomic status apply to people in deprived minority groups even when there is no major cultural difference from the larger society. My colleagues and I have observed this in studies that we have made in rural Canada and I suspect that the same could be said of the Eta in Japan. Many of the deprived minority groups in North America, however, do have to cope not only with minority status, but also with cultural differences, rapid culture change, varying degrees of sociocultural disintegration, and low socioeconomic class position. For the psychiatrist with a patient who is Black, Spanish speaking, Asian, or Native American it is important to think in terms of these multiple, interactive factors and not interpret from a cultural frame of reference only.

ACKNOWLEDGEMENTS

I am greatly indebted to Jane M. Murphy for guidance and criticism in the preparation of this chapter. Appreciation is expressed to the Department of National Health and Welfare, Canada, for support under National Health Research and Development Projects 602-7-148(29) and 603-1042-22(48). Appreciation is also expressed to Linda Pereira for help with the references and to Vivian Crowell for preparing the typescript.

BIBLIOGRAPHY

Arthur RJ: Reflections of military psychiatry. *Am J Psychiatry* 135(suppl):2–7, 1978.

Beiser M: Poverty, social disintegration and personality. *J Soc Issues* 21(1):56–78, 1965.

Benedict R: *Patterns of Culture.* Boston, Houghton Mifflin, 1934.

Benedict R: Continuities and discontinuities in cultural conditioning. *Psychiatry* 1:161–167, 1938.

Bunker HA: American psychiatric literature during the past one hundred years, in *One Hundred Years of American Psychiatry.* New York, American Psychiatric Association (Columbia University Press), 1944, p 247.

Caplan RB: *Psychiatry and the Community in Nineteenth-Century America.* New York, Basic Books, 1969, p 22.

Cotton HA: The etiology and treatment of the so-called functional psychoses. *Am J Psychiatry* 79:157–194, 1922.

Diamond S: *Primitive Views of the World.* New York, Columbia University Press, 1964, pp vi–vii.

Driver HE: *Indians of North America.* Chicago, University of Chicago Press, 1969, pp 3–24.

Edgerton RB: Anthropology, psychiatry, and man's nature, in Galdston I (ed): *The Interface Between Psychiatry and Anthropology.* New York, Brunner/Mazel, 1971, p 41.

Fann WE, Goshen CE: *The Language of Mental Health.* St Louis, Mosby, 1977.

Foster GM: *Traditional Cultures and the Impact of Technological Change.* New York, Harper & Row, 1962.

Foster GM: *Applied Anthropology.* Boston, Little, Brown, 1969.

Freud S: Civilization and its discontents, in Strachey J (ed): *The Standard Edition of the Complete Works of Sigmund Freud,* vol 21. London: Hogarth, 1961.

Foulks E: *The Arctic Hysterias of the North Alaskan Eskimos.* Washington, DC, American Anthropological Association, 1972, p 117.

Gajdusek DC: Unconventional viruses and the origin and disappearance of Kuru. *Science* 197(4307):943-960, 1977.

Gantt WH: *Experimental Basis for Neurotic Behavior.* New York, Hoeber, 1944.

Goodman ME: *The Individual and Culture.* Homewood, Ill, Dorsey, 1967.

Gorer G: Themes in Japanese culture. *Trans NY Acad Sci* 5, 1943.

Gorer G, Rickman J: *The People of Great Russia, A Psychological Study.* New York, Norton, 1962.

Grob GN: *Mental Institutions in America.* New York, Free Press, 1973, p 73.

Haggard HW: *Devils, Drugs and Doctors.* New York, Harper, 1929, pp 334-335.

Hallowell AI: *Culture and Experience.* Philadelphia, University of Pennsylvania Press, 1955, p 434.

Hollingshead AB, Redlich FC: *Social Class and Mental Illness: A Community Study.* New York, Wiley, 1958, pp 37, 387-397.

Honigman J: *Personality in Culture.* New York, Harper & Row, 1967.

Hornabrook RW: Kuru—a subacute cerebellar degeneration, the natural history and clinical features. *Brain* 91:53-74, 1968.

Kaplan D, Manners RA: *Culture Theory.* Foundations of Modern Anthropology Series. Englewood, NJ, Prentice-Hall, 1972.

Kardiner A: *The Psychological Frontiers of Society.* New York, Columbia University Press, 1945.

Keesing FM: *Cultural Anthropology: The Science of Custom.* New York, Holt, Rinehart & Winston, 1958.

Kleinman A, Eisenberg L, Good B: Culture, illness, and care, clinical lessons from anthropologic and cross-cultural research . *Ann Intern Med* 88(2):251-258, 1978.

Kluckhohn C, Leighton D: *The Navaho.* Cambridge: Harvard University Press, 1946, pp 3-4.

Kojak G: The American community in Bangkok, Thailand: A model of social disintegration. *Am J Psychiatry* 131(11):1228-1233, 1974.

Kroeber AL, Kluckhohn C: A review of culture: A critical review of concepts and definitions. *Papers of the Peabody Museum of American Archeology and Ethnology,* vol 47, no 1. Cambridge, Harvard University Press, 1952.

Landy D: Cultural antecedents of mental illness in the U.S. *Soc Sci Rev* 32:350-361, 1958.

Langner TS, Michael ST: *Life Stress and Mental Health.* New York, Free Press, 1963, pp 6-8.

Lehmann HE: Psychiatric disorders not in standard nomenclature, in Freedman AM, Kaplan HI (eds): *Comprehensive Textbook of Psychiatry.* Baltimore, Williams & Wilkins, 1967, pp 1156, 1158.

Leighton AH: *Human Relations in a Changing World*. New York, Dutton, 1949.

Leighton AH, Murphy JM: Cultures as causative of mental disorder, in *Causes of Mental Disorders: A Review of Epidemiological Knowledge*. New York, Milbank Mem Fund Q, 1961.

Malamud W: The history of psychiatric therapies, in *One Hundred Years of American Psychiatry*. New York, American Psychiatric Association (Columbia University Press), 1944, pp 308, 311.

Marcos LR: Effects of interpreters on the evaluation of psychopathology in non-English-speaking patients. *Am J Psychiatry* 136(2): pp 171–174, 1979.

McDermott W: General medical care, identification and analysis of alternative approaches. *Johns Hopkins Med J* 135, 1974.

Mead M: *Coming of Age in Samoa.* New York, Morrow, 1975, pp 206–207, 216–217. (Originally published 1928.)

Mead M: Knowing, reaching and serving the wounded, disadvantaged and vulnerable of our world, in Beiser M, et al (eds): *Today's Priorities in Mental Health. Knowing and Doing*. Miami, Symposia Specialists, 1978.

Murphy JM, Hughes, CC, Leighton, AH: Notes on the concept of sentiments, in Leighton A.H. (ed): *My Name is Legion*. New York, Basic Books, 1959. (The concept of sentiments is mainly derived from the writings of William McDougall and Adolf Meyer.)

Murphy JM: *An Epidemiological Study of Psychopathology in an Eskimo Village,* thesis. Cornell University, 1960.

Murphy JM: Social science concepts and cross-cultural methods for psychiatric research, in Murphy JM, Leighton AH (eds): *Approaches to Cross-Cultural Psychiatry*. Ithaca, Cornell University Press, 1965, pp 251–284.

Murphy JM: Sociocultural change and psychiatric disorder among rural Yorubas in Nigeria. *Ethos* 11(2):551–561, 1973.

Murphy JM: Psychiatric labeling in cross-cultural perspective. *Science* 191(4231):1019–1028, 1976.

Murphy JM: War stress and civilian Vietnamese, a study of psychological effects. *Acta Psychiatr Scand* 56:92–108, 1977.

Murray HA: *Explorations in Personality, A Clinical and Experimental Study of Fifty Men of College Age*. New York, Oxford University Press, 1938, pp 40–41.

Opler MK: *Culture and Social Psychiatry*. New York, Atherton, 1967, p 271.

Robertson AJ: Malingering, occupational medicine and the law. *The Lancet,* October 14, 1978.

Rosen G: *Madness in Society, Chapters in the Historical Sociology of Mental Illness*. New York, Harper & Row, Torchbook, 1969, pp 176, 186–187.

Rush B: *Medical Inquiries and Observations upon the Diseases of the Mind*. Hafner Publishing Co., 1962, pp 65–66. (Facsimile of the Philadelphia 1812 edition, under the auspices of the Library of New York Academy of Medicine).

Savage C, Leighton AH, Leighton DC: The problem of cross-cultural identification of psychiatric disorders, in Murphy JM and Leighton AH (eds): *Approaches to Cross-Cultural Psychiatry*. Ithaca, Cornell University Press, 1965, pp 48-49.

Schwab JJ, Schwab ME: *Sociocultural Roots of Mental Illness. An Epidemiologic Survey*. New York, Plenum, 1978, p 1-2.

Selye HS: *The Stress of Life*. New York, McGraw-Hill, 1956.

Sullivan HS: *The Interpersonal Theory of Psychiatry*. New York, Norton, 1953.

Synge JM: The oppression of the hills, in Wicklow S (ed): *The Complete Works of John M. Synge*. New York, Random House, 1909.

Teicher MI: Windigo psychosis, in *Proceedings of the 1960 Annual Spring Meeting of the American Ethnological Society.*

White LA: On concepts of culture, in Manner RA, Kaplan D (eds): *Theory in Anthropology, a Source Book.* Chicago, Adline, 1968.

Wolff HG: *Stress and Disease.* Springfield, Ill, Thomas, 1953.

Zilboorg G: *A History of Medical Psychology.* New York, Norton, 1941, p 308.

15 Discussion: Relevant Generic Issues

Edward F. Foulks, MD, PhD

Dr. Leighton points to the danger of "susceptibility to fads" in psychiatric training. With the rest of the medical profession, psychiatry has shared high prestige and status in American society until this decade. Unlike other medical specialties, psychiatry has increasingly expanded its domains and has, at times, assumed a rather uncritical, all-knowing attitude toward not only mental illness, but also problems of living and even conflicts of national and international scope. Psychiatry began as a medical specialty that focused on "mental illnesses" found predominantly in seriously afflicted hospitalized patients. The concern of the field in the late 1800s and early 1900s was focused on organic dementias, the psychoses, and mental retardation. Treatment methods were largely custodial, often involving fresh air, recreation and exercise, and application of methods such as cold packs, and social isolation from the stresses of everyday life. A short time later, the discoveries offered through psychoanalysis brought powerful new treatment methods to psychiatry. Psychoanalytic theory embraced almost all aspects of the human condition. Psychoanalysis was not confined just to helping the psychiatrist understand the apparent ramblings, delusions, and word salads of the psychotic patient, but also offered great insight into the symptoms of many others. As psychoanalysis was embraced by American psychiatry, the scope of the field broadened.

However, there has been growing disenchantment for the past decade among the public, within the profession of psychiatry and, more generally, from medicine itself, with many aspects of psychiatry. The psychiatric profession has suddenly pulled in its wings. Psychotherapy, to be sure, is still valued. However, as practiced by psychiatrists, it is of a "conservative" brand, which would include traditional psychoanalysis, psychoanalytic psychotherapy, group therapy, family therapy, sexual and marital counseling, and behavior modification. "Other" psychotherapies extant today, such as EST, Reikian therapy, Jungian therapy, T-groups, sensitivity groups, social network therapies, and the meditative and transcendental therapies are for the most part considered exotic and not part of the practice of psychiatry.

Psychiatry is attempting to return to the house of medicine. Increasing attention and allegiance have been shown for the recent psychopharmacologic and psychobiologic discoveries in psychiatry. Psychiatrists are now donning white coats and spending greater periods of time in consultation and liaison work within general hospitals. In many departments across the nation, there has been a strong backlash and disavowal of psychodynamic and social understanding of mental illness. I fear that the psychiatric profession, in its attempt to become as rigorous and scientific as general medicine, may also become as mechanistic, chauvinistic, and dehumanized, as have many aspects of American medicine.

Herein lies the importance of Alexander Leighton's directions for the training of not only future psychiatrists but those in all branches of medicine. To be sure, biologic and physiopathologic processes occur in people whatever their culture or society. On the other hand, how an individual experiences, identifies, interprets, and communicates such biologic dysfunction is determined to a large extent by culture.

Leighton begins his chapter by stating two premises of clinical psychiatry. He emphasizes psychiatry's commitment to eclecticism; that is, the premise that human behavior is determined by biologic, psychologic, social, and cultural factors. In order to be accredited, psychiatric residency training programs must be eclectic in their offerings. Psychiatric residency education is now 4 years in duration. Four months of the first year must be spent in medicine or pediatrics. The remaining 44 months are usually spent in clinics and in hospital wards treating patients with mental illnesses. In this educational process, the biologic, psychologic, and social aspects of human behavior are supposed to be covered by didactic seminars and individual supervision.

In most training centers, cultural issues in psychiatry are either not dealt with at all or, at best, given token acknowledgement. The importance of understanding culture needs to be given practical clinical relevance before the psychiatric teacher or trainee will have it included as a regular part of his curriculum. Physicians and psychiatrists generally are becoming more aware and involved with treating American ethnic minority groups. In addition, there are many ethnic groups in America that are not considered minority (such as Irish, Italian, Polish, Jewish, Appalachian), for whom cultural factors between patient and treating physician would be important in the healing process. The advent of community mental health and the increased awareness of minority group issues have brought a special focus on the practical relevance of culture in serving the physical and mental health needs of these populations. Leighton offers us the guidelines by which we might proceed in developing a curriculum of clinical relevance to the subject of culture.

He begins by asking, "How may knowledge of culture be applied in clinical psychiatry?"

1. Behavior is necessarily normal or abnormal depending on its context—social and cultural.
2. Delusions must be understood and identified in context.
3. Life history is determined by cultural context, and life history has obvious relevance for the shaping of mental disorder.
4. Support systems, choice of therapy, compliance, and general case management all depend on understanding cultural context.
5. Finally, understanding another culture often results in a psychiatrist's understanding his own culture and makes him more sensitive and insightful generally.

After discussing the complexities in the definition and scope of the concept "culture," Leighton then outlines how an understanding of culture and cultural processes might be acquired.

He proceeds to provide an overview of how much can be expected from the application of cultural knowledge in clinical psychiatry. Most of us have found Leighton's theories regarding the lack of social integration and mental disorder to be highly useful clinically. They form a theoretical basis for milieu therapy practiced in most hospital inpatient units today. They have application for family and social network therapies as well as vocational and social rehabilitation approaches with psychiatric patients. Other applications of Leighton's theories may be found in primary prevention approaches used by public health or casework efforts in community education and enhancement of community organization.

His argument for the value of culture in the education of the psychiatrist and his suggestions for acquiring some educational background in cultural psychiatry are most timely. Such a curriculum could and should be built into the first years of training. In addition, during the third and fourth postgraduate years, the psychiatry resident should have some patients from cultural backgrounds other than his own in ongoing, supervised treatment.

Increasing efforts have been made recently in psychiatric residency education to develop an explicit curriculum. In this regard, the work of the American Association of Directors of Psychiatry Residency Training, the Liaison Committee on Graduate Medical Education (1978), and other agencies has resulted in increasing uniformity in the curriculum and clinical experience now offered by residency education programs.

The American Psychiatric Association has recently created a Task Force on Multiethnicity and Cultural Psychiatry. This group has been charged with heightening the awareness of the importance of understanding the specific cultural, national, or ethnic backgrounds represented in our culturally diverse, pluralistic society, emphasizing specific culturally differentiated diagnostic and treatment techniques for the various ethnic groups. They will attempt to generalize and correlate a multiethnic and culturally appropriate mental health approach with other medical specialties. This group is also charged with conducting an inventory of the curricula of the residency training programs with respect to the inclusion of this subject matter or to develop model courses and bibliographies for use in psychiatric residency programs in the future (Spiegel, personal communication 1978).

Many training centers have had difficulty developing a formal approach to the teaching of cultural psychiatry, which may reflect the difficulties inherent in the medical model of mental illness. This model is sometimes interpreted with assumptions that schizophrenia is schizophrenia, depression is depression—no matter what the cultural background. There is, at times, an ethnocentric assuredness that an accurate diagnosis determines prescription of an inevitable treatment process. Clinical experience often demonstrates, however, that how an individual experiences, identifies, interprets, and communicates psychic function is determined, to a very large extent, by his culture. When, how, and to whom he seeks relief, what treatments he understands and accepts, how long and to what extent he will comply are further obvious functions of his background and culture. The value of an accurate scientific diagnosis is diluted when a patient does not appear for a follow-up appointment or cannot take blue pills for a "cold illness," or feels that the malady is due to being out of grace with God.

Culture plays a major role in shaping how people think, behave, and feel. Culture determines how and by whom children are raised; how they are cuddled and fed; how they acquire rules of behavior; how they are punished; how they learn about sex, gender roles, and marriage. Culture may affect personal psychology and shape character. Culture provides standards and values from which one evaluates the self, one's group, and outsiders. Culture provides guidelines and rules for recognizing or diagnosing emotional illness, and for its management and sometimes treatment. When psychiatrists raised in one culture encounter people raised in another, some conflict and misunderstanding may result regarding many issues such as how children should be raised, rules of behavior, gender roles, marriage patterns, standards and values from which one evaluates self and others, and how mental illness is perceived and dealt with (Foulks 1977).

PROPOSED CURRICULUM

Cultural Sensitivity Groups

Sensitivity and insight into one's own attitudes, reactions, and biases toward others has always been an important aspect of residency training. Many residents seek or are directed to their own therapy or personal psychoanalysis to gain a better understanding of themselves and to increase their degree of objective empathy with their patients. Pinderhughes and Pinderhughes (see Chapter 16) have proposed the usefulness of cultural sensitization and introspection in psychiatric residency training through the use of special short-term sensitivity groups in which each member is given the opportunity of talking about and exploring his own ethnic background, and the assumptions and stereotypes attributed to other ethnic groups. Actively exploring one's own cultural heritage with its own unique values often brings to the fore many attitudes toward members of other ethnic groups that had been implicit in their thought and action but outside the awareness of the resident. The group experience is designed to render the resident more sensitive and appreciative of differences between his own culture and that of his patients and others.

Course Content

Favazza (1978) has recently outlined major works in cultural psychiatry that relate the concept of culture to the practice of psychiatry and psychiatric theory. The scope of these studies includes cross-cultural comparisons; emics and etics*; subjective culture; culture and personali-

---

*Following the distinction in linguistic studies between phonemics (a system of describing sound in a culture) and phonetics (a system of describing sounds in all cultures), from Pike K: *Language in Relation to a Unified Theory of the Structure of Human Behavior*. The Haque, Moulton, 1966.

ty; culture, mental health, and mental illness; the culture of mental hospitals; and folk beliefs and rituals, which include folk classifications and causes of mental illness, folk diagnosis, folk treatments, the nature of folk healers; and psychiatric epidemiology. Residency programs in Canada have been developed according to a set of educational goals and objectives, which include the contributions of the sociocultural services to psychiatry (Thompson 1979). The final objectives determined most relevant to residency education include the following:

1. To attain an understanding of some of the various concepts of culture and the idea that cultures have arrived at a variety of greatly diverse solutions to the problems of survival and the achievement of satisfaction.
2. To learn the range and diversity of marital and family patterns across cultures and the ecologic forces that may determine them.
3. To have an awareness of some of the research concepts related to the mental health aspects of culture change and migration.
4. To become familiar with some of the main concepts and terms used by sociologists when considering psychiatric phenomena.
5. To attain an understanding of what is meant by social class and how social class position may be related to psychiatric disorders, psychiatric treatment, and attitudes of psychiatrists.
6. To become familiar with research findings concerning relationships between various ecologic factors and differential rates and patterns of psychiatric disorders.
7. To attain an awareness of some of the studies and findings concerning the social systems of psychiatric wards and their indications for reform.
8. To have an awareness that all cultures generate psychiatric disorders, but that their forms may vary from culture to culture in a way that is linked to cultural symbols, belief systems, or modal personalities.
9. To learn that the prevalence, age of onset, duration, and outcome of psychiatric disorders may vary across cultures and that variations are often best explained in cultural terms.

This outline, with accompanying enabling objectives, provides the initial framework for basic courses in cultural psychiatry for residents. Such a course would obviously be more theoretical than clinical, but would have application and relevance to the field of psychiatry. Further topics, which might be developed in a basic didactic course, include medical anthropology, basic theoretical approaches to understanding disease and illness; social integration-disintegration in relation to psychiatric symptomatology; sociocultural change, modernization and psychiatric disorder; poverty and psychiatric disorder; stress-coping–adaptation in relation to class and ethnicity; alternative healing systems; and cross-cultural issues in psychiatric assessment and treatment (Croog 1979). The Society for Medical Anthropology has also recently published a curriculum guide of undergraduate, graduate, and medical school courses in medical anthropology (Todd and Ruffini 1979). Many of these topics are relevant to training in psychiatry programs as well.

Field Experience

Residents, however, learn material best when it is closely related to clinical experience. Therefore, a didactic course would be ideally accompanied or followed by an opportunity to apply the knowledge to the clinical setting. Leighton has proposed guidelines for developing clinical applications in cultural psychiatry. Such experiences are intended to provide the resident with an understanding of culture and cultural processes. His recommendations are to develop a curriculum in cultural psychiatry which would foster, among other things, the interviewer's learning to refrain from making assumptions based only on his own values, without collaboration from the patient, and learning to be sensitive to cultural values that might inhibit, embarrass, or intimidate the patient. He recommends that curriculum development should proceed first from identifying an ethnic group commonly encountered in the clinic and reading scientific literature relevant to that group. He suggests that residents spend time acquiring their language or idiom with some fluency, or at least learn about the language. Residents should enter relationships and friendships with people representing the culture. Residents should be assigned to obtain the story of their lives from selected members of the cultural group, ideally from eight to nine nonpatients representing both sexes and various ages. A course of this nature would lend itself naturally to the basic science curriculum of the early years of psychiatric education.

Study Groups

In Philadelphia, we have extended seminars throughout the entire 4 years of residency training by offering an elective weekly evening study group in cultural psychiatry. The group is composed of Anglo and

Hispanic residents, staff psychiatrists, psychologists, social workers, and other therapists who work in clinical settings serving a predominantly Puerto Rican population. Special topics related to clinical care such as family structures, the role of women, and eating behavior are subjects for study.

Clinical Experiences

For cultural psychiatry to attain a high level of educational importance to the resident, it should be directly linked to problems encountered in the actual diagnosis, treatment, and management of psychiatric patients. Psychiatric residents should have some patients from cultural backgrounds other than their own. Special problems in the treatment of these patients are frequently encountered. Initially, the psychiatric resident might profit from supervised experiences in interviewing mentally ill patients from cultures other than his own. Supervision of interviewing should focus on developing style which is as free as possible from implications or subtle slips reflecting cultural biases or ethnic or racial stereotyping. Cultural differences between clinician and client often generate many misunderstandings on the part of both parties. True understanding of one another is made difficult, not only by possible language barriers, but also by the use of different body postures and expressions, the holding of different value systems, and the different modes used to communicate distress and affect. The Anglo clinician sometimes mistakes the Puerto Rican act of pointing with puckered lips as having sexual overtones. The Anglo clinician sometimes considers obesity in a married Puerto Rican woman as a sign of emotional problems, while the woman feels a strength and certain pride in herself as a complete woman. The Anglo clinician, at times, misinterprets and misdiagnoses an *ataque de nervios* as an acute schizophrenic episode when, in fact, it is an expression of social, usually marital, turmoil. The Anglo clinician working with certain Native American patients might receive no reply from a patient regarding questions of how his mother or father might think or feel, and might begin to wonder about the patient's ability to empathize with the feelings of family members. This patient may be manifesting a high regard and respect for his elders by not presuming to speak for them. The western clinician treating the Asian American patient might be presented with a series of complaints regarding belching and, after finding no organic disorders, wonder about the hypochondriacal nature of such complaints. The patient, on the other hand, may be expressing the loss of *chí* which is equivalent to life energy. The American clinician treating a patient from a Middle Eastern background may likewise be impressed with the high degree of hypochondriasis, particularly complaints regarding the area of the heart, and not fully appreciate that the patient is directly communicating distress in which he/she recognize to be the seat of emotions. The locus of affect in many people from Iran, for example, is in the heart and not in the mind as in the Western world.

The congruence of the patient's explanatory model(s) of illness vis-a-vis the clinician's explanatory model(s) of illness often creates additional misunderstandings. Patients who believe that the cause of their problems and illness lies outside of themselves and their control are often considered lacking in insight and not easily reached in psychotherapy. Implicit in this setting is a real difference between the patient's model of illness and the physician's model of illness. One maintains that the locus of causation is social or environmental, the other that the locus of causation is within the psyche of the patient. The converse also occurs in psychiatric practice. Patients feel that the causes of their problems are in their childhood experiences or in their current manner of relating to others and do not want to be "drugged," but the physician recognizes symptoms of manic-depressive illness and prescribes lithium.

Noncongruence of explanatory models frequently leads to impasses in therapy, noncompliance, and reinforcement of clients' stereotypes of clinicians and clinicians' stereotypes of clients.

CONCLUSION

Many difficulties encountered in psychiatric treatment relate precisely to the differences between the scientific medical model of diagnosis and treatment of disease according to the realities of our modern empirical world versus other models of the world and human emotion and functioning that are frequently found in our patient populations. Many of these models are not fully translatable into the medical model. In fact, many are difficult for the physician to understand. At best, by explicating them to their fullest, we should be able to appreciate the power of culture in determining what the patient feels is an illness, what treatment the patient respects, and provide reasons for why the patient will or will not comply with prescribed psychiatric treatments. When folk models are at gross conceptual variance with standard psychiatric models, true understanding in the doctor–patient relationship is precluded and treatment will be made more difficult accordingly. Cultural psychiatry provides possibilities for more efficient implementation of medical treatments in such populations. If the cognitive realities of the folk system are well understood, aspects of the folk system might actually be fruitfully used and incorporated into the delivery of adequate medical treatment. Also, when discrepancies exist between the folk model and the medical model, programs might be instituted to acquaint patients with the medical model—to attempt to adapt their systems to those that we are more familiar with.

The work of Kleinman (1978), Fabrega (1974), Snow (1974), Kleinman et al (1978), and others in medical anthropology provides the theoretical framework for designing effective therapeutic approaches in cultural psychiatry. These approaches focus on the effect of diagnostic and therapeutic processes of patients' conceptions of their illness, the psychosocial problems associated with their illness experience, patients' requests and expectations from specific clinical interactions, and negotiations aimed at establishing therapeutic goals. A comprehensive discussion of cross-cultural patient–clinician interaction is too extensive to be dealt with here, but these issues deserve special attention in the supervision of psychiatric residents' interviewing and conduct in treating psychiatric patients.

BIBLIOGRAPHY

American Medical Association, Liaison Committee on Graduate Medical Education: *Directory of Accredited Residencies 1977–1978*. Chicago, AMA, 1978, pp 361–362.

Croog S, Ness R, Wintrob R: Seminar in Social and Cultural Psychiatry, postgraduate program syllabus. Farmington, University of Connecticut School of Medicine and the Institute of Living, 1979.

Fabrega H: *Disease and Social Behavior*. Cambridge, Mass, MIT Press, 1974.

Favazza A: Overview: Foundations of cultural psychiatry. *Am J Psychiatry* 135(3):292–303, 1978.

Foulks E, Wintrob R, Westermeyer J, et al: *Current Perspectives in Cultural Psychiatry*. New York, Spectrum, 1977.

Kleinman A: Clinical relevance of anthropological and cross-cultural research: Concepts and strategies. *Am J Psychiatry* 135(4):427–431, 1978.

Kleinman A, Eisenberg L, Good B: Culture, illness and cure. *Ann Intern Med* 88:251–258, 1978.

Pike K: *Language in Relation to a Unified Theory of the Structure of Human Behavior*. The Hague, Moulton, 1966.

Snow L: Folk medical beliefs and their implications for care of patients. *Ann Intern Med* 81:82–96, 1974.

Thompson M: *A Resident's Guide to Psychiatric Education*. New York, Plenum, 1979.

Todd HF, Ruffini JL (eds): *Teaching Medical Anthropology*. Washington, DC, American Anthropological Association, 1979.

16 Perspective of the Training Directors

Charles A. Pinderhughes, MD
Elaine B. Pinderhughes, MSW

TRAINING PROGRAM REQUIREMENTS

A psychiatric residency training director has the overall objective of producing an attractive training program that meets the standards set forth by the Liaison Committee on Graduate Medical Education, the American Board of Psychiatry and Neurology, and the Joint Commission on Accreditation of Hospitals (AHA 1978; AMA 1978). These agencies define the requirements and minimum standards to be met in training programs. Staff, resources, equipment, organization, records, affiliations, resident selection, policies, and administration of didactic instruction, supervision, and clinical assignments are among the training director's responsibilities.

The Liaison Committee on Graduate Medical Education stipulates that the trainee should be provided an educational experience of quality and excellence that assures that graduates will possess mature clinical judgment and a high order of knowledge about the diagnosis, etiology, treatment, and prevention of psychiatric disorders and the common neurological disorders.

> The curriculum must provide a thorough, balanced presentation of the generally accepted theories, schools of thought, and diagnostic and therapeutic procedures in the field of psychiatry...recognized as significant both in this country and abroad. In addition to basic sciences relevant to psychiatry and neurology, sufficient material must be included from the social and behavioral sciences (such as psychology, anthropology, sociology) to help the resident understand the importance of economic, ethnic, social, and cultural factors in mental health and mental illness.

Residents must have experience in the care of patients of both sexes, patients of various ages from childhood to senility, and patients from a wide variety of ethnic, social, and economic backgrounds.

> All residents must have communication skills needed to treat effectively the patients for whom they have clinical responsibility.

> The program should provide instruction about American culture and subcultures and about the attitudes, values, and social norms prevalent among the various segments of contemporary American life.

The Liaison Committee on Graduate Medical Education further stipulates that the faculty should include representatives of all the other major mental health-related disciplines and should be sufficiently varied to provide instruction and supervision in all the major types of therapy including individual psychotherapies, family therapies, crisis intervention, group therapy, pharmacologic therapies, physiologic therapies, and selected special techniques such as behavior therapy, hypnosis, and biofeedback.

It is notable that in the content areas most closely related to cross-cultural psychiatry, there is little discussion and virtually no consensus about what material should be presented to residents and in what kinds of courses. An unusual amount of variation exists from one program to another. There are no reliable texts and no generally known model courses available as in the basic sciences and various areas of clinical psychiatry.

Information in this area has remained scattered and poorly synthesized. Often materials available are borrowed from other behavioral science fields such as sociology and anthropology. Because of unfamiliar language and concepts or problems in clinical application, or biases of one kind or another, these materials are sometimes avoided. Training directors sometimes avoid them because they too may have difficulty in applying them to areas of clinical practice with which they are most familiar.

Transmission of Bias From Trainers to Trainees

Training directors and faculty members are less likely to be involved significantly in intercultural, interethnic, and interracial therapy than the residents they train. When faculty members speak positively of their private patients and only supervise but do not treat the public ward or clinic patients, residents are being trained in prejudices and patterns of discrimination that have been institutionalized in medical care for a long time. Usually residents identify with and follow the footsteps of one or more of their more valued teachers. These issues should not only be addressed, but corrected, or cross-cultural psychiatric instruction will be a sham with one thing preached and the opposite practiced. If a training director cannot alter entrenched, institutionalized patterns involving large numbers of people, he or she may ensure that residents have the opportunity to analyze the situation, learn how it came about, learn what perpetuates it, and define options and sequences of steps for producing constructive changes.

Cross-Cultural Psychiatry and Systems Concepts

A training director is administrator of a sizeable system with many subsystems, each of which is part of and interacting with a variety of other systems. Each system or subsystem in a medical center's training complex forges its own distinctive patterns in the course of time and may be thought of as having its own culture or subculture that interfaces and interacts with other cultures and subcultures of the medical center. In the different subcultures at the medical center, people speak different languages, have different values, different backgrounds, and different behaviors and sometimes experience difficulty in understanding and getting along with one another.

Each resident psychiatrist whose assignments are rotated employs personal coping mechanisms in the interactions experienced in the various subcultures, but rarely receives any formal training in the principles and practices that make these "cultural exchanges" work most favorably.

Time and again old responsibilities and relationships may be carried over from one assignment to another. Invariably, this interferes with development of relationships and assumption of roles and activities in the new assignment. The dynamics are as predictable as those encountered by the person who carries his previous culture to his new environment.

While there has been little formal education developed in these areas, the gap is filled partly by the informal education that residents develop. They discuss various assignments, various faculty members, and personnel, and define what they are like and how to interact with them. They can be more honest and forthright in this search jointly with their peers than they can be with faculty members who might be offended or protective of valued relationships. Generally, it is quite difficult for faculty members to discuss themselves or fellow faculty members with the kind of objectivity used when discussing patients. The whole area of dynamics of interaction of different personnel and faculty and of one medical center subsystem with another is closely related to dynamics of intercultural, interethnic, and interracial interactions. Who identifies with whom and who projects upon whom is the name of a game in which most people participate, while rarely discussing the issues professionally in a formally structured manner.

In most large training programs, diverse personalities with varied backgrounds interact, sometimes harmoniously, sometimes competitively, and sometimes with misunderstandings and conflicts. Rarely are the excellent first hand data examined and discussed as part of the resident's training. The training culture that the resident is part of and the personalities within it (which influence the training culture), by implication, are off limits so far as formal training discussions are concerned. Faculty members and training directors retain their privacy and protect cherished relationships, behavior patterns, beliefs, and narcissism. Residents are taught to look at certain things and certain people and to avoid looking at others, when faculty members silently participate in institutional systems that provide much to some and little to others with the same problems. Frequently, interpersonal dynamics contribute to the silent acceptance of discrimination within an institution. People are reluctant to "make waves" unless they have support of a group and positive rewards for doing so.

It is possible that one or more competitive or exploitive persons can subvert and abuse people who communicate in an open manner about themselves and others. Open, forthright communications are adaptive only where alliances, trust, and goodwill are strong and where group processes and leadership are adequately strong, considerate, wise, and protective. Otherwise, what one says may be used against one.

In every medical center, as well as in other social orders, some are favored while others are deprived. This results in different standards of care, different classes of patients, and the use of different values and different behavior with people in different categories. What can training directors do about such pervasive problems? They can use and can advocate a clinical approach that includes observing, collecting, and organizing data, understanding the history, the dynamics, and the forces perpetuating the problems, approaches to the problems, and resistances and obstacles to their solution. The training director may lack the constituents, the support, the resources, the personal attributes, and necessary conditions and other factors required for constructive change or reform. However, he should not lack the interest, the motivation, and the sense of responsibility to teach and encourage use of a clinical psychiatric approach with social structures, family structures, and personality structures.

Training directors should exercise some responsibility in making sure that trainees develop understanding of social and organizational dynamics beyond traditional psychologic, interpersonal, family, and social dynamics. Residents' input into advisory, planning, and policy making groups can offer additional learning opportunity to a few residents. Effort should be made to evaluate, analyze, diagnose, and formulate corrective approaches to problems in the various social contexts with which residents have contact. This is seldom done, and residents often complete their traditional training feeling powerless to understand and deal with problems in the social systems in which they function.

Problems in the Definition of Cross-Cultural Psychiatry

Cross-cultural psychiatry deals with the identification, treatment, and prevention of psychiatric problems in social fields that involve representatives of two or more different cultural systems. The prefix *cross* implies a meeting and interaction of lines or forces going in opposing directions, and included among its dictionary meanings are an opposition, a frustration, a thwarting, a misfortune, trouble, mixing, betraying, interbreeding different species, ill-humored, and angry. With so many negative meanings attached to the word *cross,* there should be little wonder that *cross*-cultural psychiatry is not popular. The term *cross-cultural* may even activate unconscious resistances in some minds.

In sociology the term *culture* is applied to the total of ways of living built up by a group of human beings and transmitted from one generation to another. At present there are few purists who think of cross-cultural psychiatry exclusively in relation to culture defined in this manner. More often than not, the term *cross-cultural* is applied to a conglomerate including intercultural, interethnic, interracial, and other intergroup phenomena in which the dynamics within and between the groups are analogous.

Since *culture* in the United States includes both interaction and a blend of components from many cultures, psychiatrists should be able to relate effectively to intrapsychic and interpersonal dynamics in people with a common culture and to intrapsychic and interpersonal dynamics in people from different cultural backgrounds.

Conclusions

1. The field of cross-cultural psychiatry is poorly defined and underdeveloped.

2. The term *cross-cultural psychiatry* has been used as an umbrella term under which intercultural, interethnic, interracial, interclass, and other intergroup behaviors are classified. Only in recent years have psychiatrists in large numbers focused attention on various social systems with which individuals interact. There is need for practical principles for classifying and organizing information about social systems so that psychiatrists can apply it effectively.

3. Since cross-cultural psychiatry currently is dealt with in a somewhat sloppy manner and probably will not be systematized and well-organized in the immediate future, training directors should plan their efforts as transitional steps toward the clearer, more systematic, and better organized intersystems psychiatry we can expect will evolve in the future.

Recommendations

1. Cross-cultural psychiatry should be broadened in definition to include behavioral phenomena in any social system, together with a set of norms developed by people living and working together over time, when successive generations being affected by that social system have their behavior programmed or strongly influenced by the system and its norms. Cultural, ethnic, caste, class, family, institutional, organizational, occupational, political, educational, religious, ideologic, and other social systems that "process and program" a succession of "generations" could be examined in light of common principles and analogs in dynamics. Information and concepts developed in one area could be more easily translated and applied in other areas. Advances in preventive psychiatry would be fostered by better delineation of pathogenic processes and principles of behavior in the various social systems.

2. Since so much information, and so many approaches, schools of thought, and courses involving many disciplines must be included in a 3-year psychiatric residency program, often to the exclusion of important underdeveloped areas like cross-cultural psychiatry, it is recommended that there be a clear and official specification of the minimum requirements for cross-cultural psychiatric training necessary for accreditation.

3. We would recommend that, for accreditation, each 3-year program include the following five minimum requirements for training in cross-cultural psychiatry:

First year An insight-inducing, behavior-modifying group seminar on cross-cultural, cross-ethnic, cross-racial, cross-class, and cross-occupational interactions (see A Small Group Experiential Training Method for Therapists Engaged in Cross-Cultural Psychiatry).

Required readings and lectures on psychiatric epidemiology around the world (primary emphasis on work of Alexander Leighton).

Required readings and lectures (at least two) on factors in biologic psychiatry, which may vary according to race or culture, including unique factors in physiology or pathology that should be taken into account when treating certain conditions in particular patients. (Shader has spoken of the great importance of this area. As an example he has cited the importance of knowing whether a Black patient had sickle-cell anemia before contemplating the use of medication or other treatment that may lower oxygen tension in the blood, see Chapter 13).

First and second years Instruction and supervision in an interviewing technique which systematically corrects the biased thoughts occurring in the interviewer about any patient (see Requirements for Reliable Interviewing in Cross-Cultural Evaluation and Treatment Interactions).

Second year A seminar (readings, at least three didactic sessions, and at least three evaluative sessions) on institutional racism and class discrimination in the affiliated institutions in the training program.

Third year Seminar (readings and at least two meetings) on common principles in the dynamics of intercultural, interethnic, interracial, and interinstitutional interactions. Hypotheses concerning relationships between biologic, psychologic, and social behaviors that have relevance in cross-cultural interactions should receive some attention. Charles Pinderhughes' (1979) hypotheses about differential bonding attempt to integrate concepts in these areas and may be used to stimulate discussion.

Each year Required readings and lectures providing blocks of information about various cultural groups around the world with participation by representatives from those groups (at least one lecture for each continent).

Seminar on uses of individual and family interviewing techniques with representatives of various cultures (at least three meetings).

These requirements could be offered in group meetings for 1 hour a week for 20 months or its equivalent divided between 2 years or between 3 years.

Having these requirements would improve the personal attributes, knowledge, and skills applicable in general as well as in special areas of psychiatry. The requirements could foster more rapid development and organization of the field of cross-cultural psychiatry and serve as a transition toward more scientifically based, preventive psychiatry. Experience over a few years with these minimum requirements and with other innovative program components in cross-cultural psychiatry could offer a basis for appropriate modifications of training in this field.

Residents trained along these lines should not only know, but be able to apply, Bradshaw's general principles (1978) for therapists in cross-cultural interactions as paraphrased below:

1. Use continuous introspection and self-analysis.
2. Learn about the culture of the patient to comprehend what represents normality and ego-syntonic behavior within that culture.
3. More actively ask what the patient means by a particular word, phrase, statement, or anecdote.
4. Offer some acknowledgement of the therapist's awareness of external environmental pressures.
5. Experience empathy appropriately.
6. While remaining aware of the risk of infantilizing the patient, consider helping the patient to deal with external problematic realities before, or simultaneous with, the internal conflicts.
7. Recognize and become comfortable with aggression in oneself and in the patient.
8. Perceive the adaptive value of autonomous, constructive, assertive action, thought, and feeling and do not be frightened by it although it is at variance with inclinations of the therapist.
9. Be prepared to deal appropriately with maladaptive expression of aggression including resistance to treatment.

A SMALL GROUP EXPERIENTIAL TRAINING METHOD FOR THERAPISTS ENGAGED IN CROSS-CULTURAL PSYCHIATRY

Background

Members of one group in the presence of members of another group are likely to hide and deny any attitudes, thoughts, and feelings they deem offensive to the other group. The unspoken, denied attitudes and thoughts may interfere with development of trust and may promote both conscious and unconscious behavior that interferes with development of alliances. This can cause major problems in intercultural, interracial, and interethnic treatment interactions.

Often this reluctance poses a dilemma for training directors, for they, too, are social beings and have similar feelings about discussing attitudes and thoughts that prove offensive to some groups. They may assist trainees to be alert to resistances shown by patients with backgrounds different from the therapist's. There is great variation in the activity recommended beyond being alert. Some encourage exploration of the resistances to treatment without assuming that some cultural, racial, or ethnic issue is the cause. Some encourage that patient attitudes about the cultural, racial, or ethnic differences be reviewed where resistance appears. Some encourage that patient attitudes about the existing cultural, racial, or ethnic differences be discussed in the initial contact or early in treatment, whether there is resistance to treatment or not. We do not know of any reliable study of these options and have heard of successes and failures with each.

What is most notable is that problems in the attitudes of the patient are likely to be explored at one time or another while problems in the attitudes of the trainees and faculty members are likely to remain unexplored. This occurs for many reasons. In any heterogeneous faculty, there is likely to be great variation in the cultural, racial, and ethnic backgrounds and in the attitudes, ideas, and prejudices associated with each. Some faculty members may even reinforce destructive prejudices in the trainees. Trainees regularly adopt some of the prejudices of teachers with whom they identify.

How can we explore attitudes of the trainees (and faculty) for beliefs and biases that can foster problems with patients? Are special training or special attributes required in the instructor? Is there any reliable method for doing this in a systematic way? What outcome can be expected when the method is used?

In the course of dealing with these training questions at Boston's Solomon Carter Fuller Mental Health Center, a useful training technique was developed for individuals working with persons from a variety of ethnic backgrounds. This training technique has been used with first-year residents in psychiatry for 4 years, with social work students for 3 years, with ward personnel in a mental health center and a state hospital, with personnel in a child guidance center, and with administrators and teachers in a public school system.

The ethnic groups represented in these training-teaching seminars include Americans of the following ethnic backgrounds: African, American Indian, English, French, Italian, Scottish, Jewish, Welsh, Polish, Czechoslovakian, Lithuanian, Russian, Greek, Norwegian, Danish, Swedish, Swiss, German, East Indian, Chinese, Portuguese, Cape Verdean, Puerto Rican, Cuban, Jamaican, and Barbadian. Also included have been natives of the following countries: Ethiopia, Canada, Czechoslovakia, Yugoslavia, Columbia, India, and Pakistan.

The training process was developed because of an observation that clinical programs failed in focusing on the culture of clients, defining it, understanding its norms, beliefs, and values, and in assessing the implications for treatment. The underlying assumption often appeared to be that all cultural groups should be basically the same, the yardstick for conformity being based on a white, American, middle-class value system. In addition, the focus on transference and countertransference omitted a consideration of stress resulting from environmental pressures, cultural value conflict, and so on. An examination of mental illness on a cross-cultural basis makes clear some factors that should be better understood:

1. Symptoms and behavior viewed as pathologic (by American, middle-class, cultural values) but considered normal in a subculture.
2. Excessive stress due to conflict between American values and those of the subculture.
3. Environmental stress related to ethnic identity, (ie, poverty, racism, oppression).
4. Values in the subculture that program childrearing in a "pathological" direction (these values serve or may have served an adaptive function).
5. Values of the subculture that define illness.

Recently there has been recognition of a need for greater focus on cultural issues in training. Programs now may include some focus on different cultural norms and values, acknowledging the significance of differences and the need for consultants who understand specific ethnic groups. However, such information is less useful if the training fails to include a *focus* on *the therapist's awareness of his own culture, norms, and values, and their effect on the client's.* The paradox is seen especially in the cross-racial encounter where Blacks and people of color are defined by race and whites are defined by country of national origin and religion. A Black views his therapist as a white person, not as English, Italian, or Jewish. This confusion can be clarified in an experiential process that throws the conflict and contradictions into bold relief and lays bare the resistance of the therapist to perceiving himself as his patient sees him.

The Experiential Process

The process (E. Pinderhughes 1979) focuses on the student's understanding of 1) the values of his own ethnic group and 2) the relative power or lack of power he associates with his ethnic group status.

After all participants are introduced to one another, they are asked to discuss their goals for participating in the process and to agree on a code of behavior that will 1) guarantee respect for the point of view of each group member, 2) encourage the building of trust within the group, and 3) enable each individual, when possible, to attain his objectives. Interest in understanding biases toward various groups is usually prominent in the goals described by participants.

The following questions are used as a beginning focus for discussion which includes, as far as possible, participation from every member.

1. What is your ethnic background?
2. What is the locality in which you grew up and what other ethnic groups resided in that community?
3. What are the values of your ethnic group?
4. How did your family see itself as like or different from other ethnic groups?
5. What are your earliest images of color as an ethnic factor?
6. What are your feelings about your ethnic identity? How might they be influenced by the power relationships between your ethnic group and others?

Identifying Ethnic Background

Students share comparatively easily their self-awareness and early experiences as ethnic persons (items 1 through 4). The process in which they become involved generates enthusiasm for most and anxiety for some as the approval of discussion of ethnic identity and ethnic experiences encourages them to reveal parts of their lives and themselves not usually revealed in a classroom or educational setting. Being listened to with respect while explaining significant aspects of self and recalling incidents of importance and meaning in one's life is usually experienced positively by the participants. Some examples of their statements follow:

> The majority of people in our community were French-Canadian, so I rarely experienced the prejudice that is often directed to us. But we looked down on the Italians and the Poles.

> I don't have any ethnicity except American. My people have been here so many generations, I guess you'd call me a WASP; but I don't know what that is.

> I came from a Polish-Russian background in a farming community and my family taught us not to mix with the others (non-Polish), as they felt they were better than us. I still remember how they burned down our barn one night.

> As a Hispanic, this color thing has me all confused. In Puerto Rico, color is not so all-important, but here we have to be Black or white, and we don't consider ourselves either one.

The opportunity for review of early ethnic experiences can put participants in touch with feelings and incidents long-forgotten though still influential on their perceptions and behaviors. The process appears similar to the uncovering that occurs in psychotherapy. There also

emerges a growing awareness of the complexities involved in the understanding of color and ethnic identity, for it becomes clear that while Black
is considered an ethnic identity, white is not usually so considered, since
identity for whites is viewed in terms of national origin, while identity for
peoples of color is viewed in terms of race. Glazer and Moynihan (1963)
say that since color has become a marker for groups, "Perhaps most
significantly, the majority group to which assimilations should occur,
white, has taken on the significance of an ethnic group also." This incon-
sistency may be seen as a major contributor to misperception and misunderstanding between whites and minorities. Minority immigrants
experience particular sensitivity to this issue.

The articulation of one's ethnic group values in the context of this
process offers the students the opportunity to 1) appreciate their own
clarity, or lack of clarity, concerning ethnic identity, and 2) appreciate the
similarities that exist across ethnic groups and the differences that exist
within them. Some examples of statements from this stage of the process:

> As an Irish Catholic girl, I was taught to strive for purity and goodness.
> The nuns at school taught us well.

> Italians are expressive, express feelings openly, and are very giving. We
> also respect the elderly, especially the grandmother. When a WASP
> client told how her 10-year-old daughter treated her grandmother, I
> knew Italians would see that as deviant behavior.

> My parents taught me that Jews must achieve and conquer their prob-
> lems. When my Puerto Rican client tells me she believes, "What must be
> must be," I have to try hard to understand that.

In addition to values, one's perceptions are influenced by behavior
and feelings in oneself and others. Therefore, the process that has up to
now been largely descriptive and intellectual is shifted to a focus on the
emotional aspects of ethnicity.

Understanding Ethnic Behavior in the
Context of the Power Differential

Feeling responses are more difficult for most to describe than mere
description of incidents. However, describing provides participants an
opportunity to become more comfortable with 1) their own feelings about
self and others, and 2) the process of exploring and understanding feelings
and attitudes in others. Examples of statements from this stage follow:

> If I'm honest, I'll admit that in our town the WASPs felt superior. We
> were taught that we had to assume a lot of responsibility for those not so
> fortunate.

My father was a Northern Irish Protestant and we were a minority in our town. We were taught that we were better than the Irish Catholics who lived around us. Now I wonder if my father didn't use that superiority thing to bolster himself since he was not faring as well as some of his brothers.

My mother was Black and my father Portuguese. I still remember the anger I felt at being called a "nigger" by a Portuguese kid who was even darker than me.

I grew up feeling bad about being poor. The only people poorer than us were Blacks, and I was glad I was not Black too. I guess it made me feel a little better that they were in worse shape, but the people the community excluded the most were Jews.

Being white is very comfortable and secure. It means being like others, being accepted and not having to spend a lot of energy dealing with how society beats you down.

As a white, I was ashamed of my kinky hair as a child; it was too close to the kind of hair Blacks have. I idolized my blond friend and used to dream I would return in the next life with long, blond straight hair.

As students discuss their feelings and behaviors, it is suggested that they be viewed in the context of the power accorded them as ethnic persons and persons of color. This enables them to see the connection between the relative power of their groups and their feelings, perceptions, and behavior with self and others. It is established that one usually does perceive his own ethnic group and that of others as existing in a complementary hierarchical relationship in which one group has more power and the other less, and that when members of these groups relate to one another, their feelings and behavior tend to be complementary and are influenced by their power position. For example, the more powerful ones tend to take initiative and feel competent, whereas the less powerful tend to comply and feel less competent.

Often the discussion of power focuses on the individual as a person of power or nonpower within his family. Intrafamily role behavior is intimately linked to cultural factors and may differ greatly from one culture to another. Power and powerlessness are common experiences for everyone regardless of background and are thus readily understood in the context of family and other relationships. Whether entitled or scapegoated as a family member or an ethnic group member, the participant comes to understand his own "power gestalt" and to comprehend it as a major determinant of his perceptions, feelings, and behavior.

With encouragement from each other and supported by an atmosphere of trust, participants share and compare their perceptions, becoming able to understand how their own perceptions may be deemed as bias by others. They become more comfortable with the concept of bias and understand how it originates and is maintained. Their ability to perceive self and others more accurately is enhanced at the same time that they develop more tolerance for differing perceptions in others. Mirelowitz and Grossman (1975) state that

> the opportunity for face-to-face encounters and a chance for sharing experiences and thinking as freely as possible within a neutral milieu can help students with their identity struggles as well as with their more generalized irrationalities and stereotypes.

Understandings about power behavior are often applied to sex status issues. When it has been difficult to initiate a discussion of feelings regarding ethnicity, a beginning can be made with a focus on how it feels to be male or female. Placed in the context of the power differential, the feelings and behaviors identified with a male social role are usually similar to those of the underpowered group (Lowenstein 1976).

Implications for the Helping
Relationships: Building Empathy

Therapists find that an experience structured in this manner is of practical value in clinical work.

The group experience of discussing thoughts and feelings about ethnic status in a matter-of-fact way offers a background experience that helps residents to discuss similar questions with patients in a matter-of-fact way when appropriate.

The helping relationship is in itself a power relationship wherein the dynamics of power and lack of power are operating. Kadushin (1972) and Siporin (1975) discuss this issue. For the therapist and patient alike, the expertise of the therapist and the neediness of the patient place them in positions of power and lack of power, respectively. The cross-cultural and cross-ethnic encounter compounds the consequences of this power differential. For the patient, intervention by a member of a group he regards as his oppressor may offer a reinforcement of the powerlessness he is experiencing in his moment of need. Intervention by a therapist whom the patient sees as inferior may also reinforce the client's sense of helplessness. On the other hand, power issues related to differences in ethnicity, class, sex, or age may exaggerate the power inherent in the helping role in such a way that the worker misperceives and misunderstands the patient and his reality. With awareness of the meaning and influence of power in complementary relationships, the student is better prepared to guard against occurrences that may result in a destructive use of the therapist's power or the patient's lack of power.

Empathy, the essential ingredient of the helping relationship, which neutralizes the patient's powerlessness, requires accurate perception of the patient. Essential in building trust and developing a relationship that will enable growth and change, empathy becomes, for the patient, an anesthetic for the pain of his loneliness, feelings of abandonment, and powerlessness. Keefe (1976) analyzes empathic behavior as requiring the therapist to 1) be receptive, and 2) transmit accurately to the patient his awareness of the patient's state of being (ie, he must perceive accurately the patient's gestalt and be able to feel with the patient at the same time that he understands wherein his own feelings are different and holds in abeyance any cognitive distortion such as stereotyping or value judging).

This process of receptivity requires the therapist to "take in" the patient's behavior (verbal, postural, affective) without distortion. It also demands that the therapist be aware of the feelings within himself set in motion by the patient's behavior, recognizing which feelings represent judgments and stereotyping according to the worker's values and which feelings are like those of the patient.

The student's awareness of his power gestalt in relation to ethnicity, race, class, or sex enhances this necessary ability to perceive the patient of another ethnic group accurately and at the same time be able to understand which of his own feelings are similar to or different from those of the patient. This more accurate perception of self and patient protects against stereotyping, which is itself a mechanism for reinforcing power. Persons unclear about themselves as individuals and as ethnic persons have difficulty developing this skill. This process helps identify such a deficiency, and at the same time, enhances the skill.

REQUIREMENTS FOR RELIABLE INTERVIEWING IN CROSS-CULTURAL EVALUATION AND TREATMENT INTERACTIONS

The Need for Objectivity in Interviewing

The ability to recognize and label the cultural background of a person promotes the illusion or delusion that one knows some meanings associated with that person in the minds of other persons. In fact, one does not know what is in other minds without some method for objective study and validation. An interviewer may know what content and meaning are associated in his own mind with particular cultural attributes but can only speculate and project his own ideas on the other person until informed by the other person.

With great frequency, therapists hold delusions about their patients, and patients hold delusions about their therapists of which both are unaware. This is often accentuated in cross-cultural interactions. Significant amounts of interview time may be devoted to ideas being expressed or suggested by one party and then corrected or modified by the other party.

Objectivity-Focused Interviewing

In 1972, interest in this issue led (C.A. Pinderhughes) to describe the minimum requirements for a reliable medical model for interviewing involving a modification and adaption of Felix Deutsch's Associative Anamnesis interview technique (1939). Combining the principles of scientific method with associative interviewing can offer more reliable interviewing in cross-cultural clinical activity.

Central nervous system (CNS) tissues have characteristics which enable experience to influence the patterning of psychological processes. Imprinting, conditioning, and learning are all based upon physiological changes in CNS tissue. The revival of a particular CNS pattern associated with earlier experience may activate additional tissue responses referred to as "psychological defense mechanisms." Psychoanalysis or psychoanalytically-oriented associative interviewing offers one method of studying how experience has affected the CNS tissues of a patient.

Associative interviewing—which neither directs nor limits—encourages more spontaneous unfolding of the CNS tissue patterns (memories, feelings, fantasies, and thoughts) associated with the patient's complaints. Evaluative interviewing should begin with associative interviewing and later shift to directed questions to develop more comprehensive data.

The interviewer registers, in his or her own CNS tissues, impressions produced by postural, gestural, motor, verbal, affective and vegetative communications from the patient. The interviewer has the task of defining what messages and meanings are being received and how these differ from those being spoken by the patient.

Formulations about patients may be conceptualized in terms of relationships concerning body parts and body processes. These are universal, shared features of all humans, and they comprise the early basic components of the CNS representations to which all subsequent mental representations become linked in what is commonly called the body image.

Example In 1972, while interviewing a 20-year-old single Norwegian female during a symposium on psychotherapy in Norway, according to C.A. Pinderhughes, the interviewer was unable to understand some Norwegian words the patient included as she talked. In response to inquiry about why she sought treatment, she said what sounded like, "I was a student under a lot of pressure and thought I had developed—I don't know how to say it in English but the Norwegian word is *mave saar.*" Simultaneously she rubbed her abdomen in a circular motion with the palm of her right hand.

She was asked to leave the room so the interviewer might share his thoughts with doctors in the audience. When she was two rooms away and unable to hear, the interviewer stated to the audience his speculation that she was concerned about pregnancy. He indicated that even though the word *mave saar* was pronounced in a way that reminded him of the English word "motherhood," he would have suppressed this thought had not she used a gesture suggesting a well-rounded stomach. Norwegian doctors in the audience indicated that the patient had used the Norwegian word for ulcer and that her problem had nothing to do with pregnancy. The interviewer suggested that he would wait for further data, but would not discard his thought until there was at least some data opposing the thought. He clarified that his thought was a speculation or at best a hypothesis that was not even partially validated, and that he would not accept it as applicable to the patient until there was substantial supportive and confirmatory data and no data to the contrary.

The patient was invited to return and she eagerly picked up where she had left off, saying, "I was so upset I thought I had what we call *mave saar*. My boyfriend and I had been having sexual relations without contraceptives and I was getting more and more upset about becoming pregnant." With this particularly open and expressive patient, confirmatory data had emerged quickly. The meaning received by the interviewer was validated as the meaning being conveyed by the patient. By conceptualizing the patient's communications in terms of body parts and body processes, the interviewer was quickly alerted to an underlying concern.

Systematic Approach

An interviewer functioning in the framework of a medical model should proceed through the same systematic sequence of steps with each patient. At a minimum the sequence should include:

A. Evaluation
  1. Establish a relationship that facilitates communication.
  2. Associative interviewing, which encourages expanding discussion of thoughts, feelings, persons, and situations that, in the mind of the patient, are connected with his or her concerns. There should be no interruptions and no introduction of any content from the mind of the interviewer. (The associative interviewing process will be described in greater detail.)
  3. Directed questions about the patient's concerns.
  4. Directed questions to develop a comprehensive history.
  5. Directed questions to assess the mental status.
  6. Examination (physical, psychological, laboratory, special examinations and consultations).
B. Formulation of issues in intrapsychic, interpersonal,

biological, and behavioral terms; development of problem lists; diagnosis.

C. Recommendations, prescriptions, proposals, referrals as indicated.

D. Development of contract and goals for treatment.

E. Development of a relationship designed to achieve progress toward treatment goals.

F. Development of actions and interactions designed to achieve progress toward treatment goals. Actions may include use of psychotherapy, family therapy, behavior therapy, pharmacotherapy, electroconvulsive therapy, physical medicine, occupational therapy, and other therapies.

G. Periodic review, assessment of progress, adjustment of plans if indicated.

H. Termination process.

I. Follow-up as indicated.

Associative interviewing provides maximum opportunity for the patient to communicate as fully as possible the concerns and the mental, emotional, somatic, and interpersonal content associated with the concerns.

Associative interviewing can be useful during the evaluation process or during the treatment process. By initiating each treatment interview with the question, "How are things?" the interviewer may induce an initial associative interview process that reveals the concerns, mental status, experiences, and organization that prevail on that day. Upon locating the treatment issues in the material of a particular day, the interviewer may use this emotionally meaningful material to assist the patient toward treatment goals.

Transcultural psychiatrist–patient relationships often increase opportunities for imperception and for false perception. For this reason psychiatrists in transcultural contacts should employ methods and behavior that support clear and complete transmission, open attentive reception without alteration, discover erroneous perception, correct erroneous perception, and prevent erroneous perception.

Although some of the communication problems in transcultural exchange may exist in the patient, it is most useful for the psychiatrist to assume full responsibility for the generation of satisfactory communication. As long as communication is inadequate, it is of great practical value for the psychiatrist to assume responsibility for the inadequacy. Instead of imputing inadequacy to the patient and withdrawing, the psychiatrist should continue communication efforts with empathy and with increased resourcefulness.

Above all, the psychiatrist should be aware that behavior, information, assumption, beliefs, interpretations, and perceptions that seem absolutely valid and appropriate to the psychiatrist may seem absolutely false or inappropriate to the patient. By employing principles of scientific method with associative interviewing, the psychiatrist can increase opportunities for a meeting of minds and correct the misunderstandings that develop in his own mind.

Recommended Principles for Scientific Associative Interviewing

1. The psychiatrist meticulously should behave as if he is totally ignorant. In fact, he is totally ignorant of the meaning in a patient's mind until the patient conveys the meaning to him. Any and all responses constitute data including words, gestures, body movements, and secretory activity. If a body part opens or closes or stiffens or becomes limp after a question is asked, that reaction should be considered as part of the answer fashioned by the person and expressed in the body part. Expression in verbal, motor, and autonomic modes varies from person to person and within the same person under differing circumstances.

2. When the patient is talking, the psychiatrist meticulously should observe, listen, take in the information conveyed by the patient and carefully note sequences, patterns, and relationships.

3. The psychiatrist should assume that unfolding behavior in associative interviewing is an externalized expression of internal relationships in the body image and that the mechanism of projection is central in all verbalization and thinking. As a listener, the psychiatrist projects on the perceived auditory stimuli a set of highly individualized meanings. Each psychiatrist trusts and believes in the meaning he imputes to the patient's expression — unfortunate because the meaning the psychiatrist trusts may be erroneous. These projective and other subjective processes in psychotherapists present the biggest obstacles to objective scientific medical psychotherapy. They are responsible for the introduction of such false information and unreliable meanings in transcultural psychiatry that a scientific attitude and method should be combined with associative interviewing to discover and correct errors.

4. In his own mind and quite silently, the psychiatrist should speculate broadly and wildly about unconscious and body image meanings that might be associated with the patient's words. The broader the range of speculations, the more likely it is for the psychiatrist to think beyond his own hangups and socially reinforced meanings. Speculations should be acknowledged as the interviewer's own private thoughts, having nothing to do with the thoughts of the patient.

5. Should some thoughts of the patient seem analogous or similar to the psychiatrist's speculations, and if there are no data from the patient

that oppose the speculations, then the speculations may be elevated to hypothesis status and examined in the light of data from subsequent associative interviewing.

6. If any data from associative interviewing opposes the hypothesis, the hypothesis should be discarded. An hypothesis supported by substantial data from associative interviewing and not inconsistent with any data should be considered to be partially validated. An hypothesis that is consistent with all data, that is supported by substantial data, and has been used repeatedly to predict successfully data in advance in associative interviewing may be accepted as a validated hypothesis. The validated hypothesis may be useful as an index of aspects of organization and tissue patterning within the patient. The validated hypothesis can contribute to reliable formulation and diagnosis and to appropriate treatment.

What the Scientific Associative Interview Method Accomplishes

Charles A. Pinderhughes teaches this method in videotape seminars involving first- and third-year residents. Residents rotate in providing videotapes of their interviews once a week for 6 months. Each resident must learn to 1) listen, 2) elicit and take in and register the patient's meanings, 3) scientifically validate perceptions and understandings of the patient's meaning, and 4) recognize and control his or her own projections.

Each resident is taught this method for developing in the interviewer's mind a replica of content and relationships that exists in the patient's mind. The resident thus learns about the culture, the familial, the personality, and individual experiences of the patient as they are registered in the mind of the patient. Since few patients have had textbooks written about them, each patient becomes the textbook, which the interviewer studies to learn about the cultural, familial, and individual experiences that play a part in the patient's concerns. With this method we are able to demonstrate that the tissue patterning expressed in verbal, motor, and vegetative behavior is as constant and recognizable for each individual as fingerprints, and is thus capable of objective study.

Residents must be warned repeatedly not to halt prematurely their exploration and not to jump to conclusions. They are encouraged to recognize and distinguish their knowledge from their partly validated hypotheses, from their assumptions, from their speculations, and from their fantasies.

Without rigorous training of this kind, many residents unknowingly mix knowledge, partly validated hypotheses, speculations, and fantasies into their psychotherapy in a manner that makes them indistinguishable from each other. Unfortunately, many trained psychiatrists do this also.

Most patients are only partly understood. In fact, it would be quite uneconomical and impractical to have "complete understanding" as the therapist's objective. There should be sufficient understanding to delineate any psychiatric and other medical problems that are present and to generate appropriate responses to the problems. Knowledge of individual, familial, and cultural experiences of patients is as important for satisfactory evaluation and treatment in psychiatry as are physical, laboratory, and special examinations.

ILLUSTRATIVE EXAMPLES OF TYPICAL TRAINING ISSUES IN CROSS-CULTURAL PSYCHIATRY

[Note: The following examples represent selected experiences of C.A. Pinderhughes in medical centers in the United States unless otherwise indicated.]

Example 1 A vigorous, muscular, athletic man 58 years of age came to the psychiatric clinic complaining that he was having difficulty controlling his temper. He lived with his wife and children. Although the family had eaten together for many years, he had begun to eat separately to avoid getting into intense arguments with his children. His department store business was falling off and in the red at a time when financial needs for college and graduate school tuitions were at their height. He was aware of mild depression but had no morbid thoughts and no loss of weight. In recent weeks he had jeopardized his relationship with his best friend because of frequent arguments. He was especially concerned by these eruptions because he had always been a very disciplined person. He sought psychotherapy after receiving repeated recommendations from family and friends. He was strongly opposed to use of any drugs.

When told that there was no need to consider hospitalization and that one of our psychiatrists would evaluate him for treatment in short-term psychotherapy, he replied: "You cannot refer me to a woman psychiatrist and the psychiatrist must have gray hair." When asked why, he replied, "Although I am American, I am American Lebanese. Before my distinguished military career, I was reared in Lebanon where respect and trust were reserved for men and for older persons." He indicated that it was sad but true that he had such prejudices, but that he was quite set in his ways and could respect and trust only an older man. He was assured that the same basic knowledge and skills were employed by any to whom he might be referred and that the ability to listen, understand, and empathize were not dependent upon age. He indicated that he would like to believe this but that he could not really feel reassured.

He then said, "You have gray hair. I could be treated by you. Where are you from?" (Being a 60-year-old Black male American, I wondered if the patient was stating that my age was all right, but that he had some question about my background. Having experienced this question many times, I have learned, for reasons to be discussed shortly, that it can be quite helpful to ask the patient, "Where would you say I am from?" I did so.) The patient then said, "You are from India. I am sure you can help me."

I explained to the patient that I would not be available but might be able to confer with and supervise other doctors he saw. He indicated that such an arrangement would be quite satisfactory.

Discussion   Culturally bound attitudes similar to this can be found in many societies and in many cultures. A director of training for psychiatric residents must deal with such attitudes in two ways. First, he must insure that opportunity be provided in the training program to develop knowledge and sensitivity to such attitudes in patients. Second, he must develop methods for dealing with these attitudes in the trainees themselves, since many programs include trainees with different cultural backgrounds.

The patient in Example 1 had lived one-quarter of his life in Lebanon and three-quarters in the United States but was firmly attached to some important Lebanese cultural patterns. Societies differ in the nature and amount of cultural pressure they impose and in the rigidity or flexibility of roles permitted or required. In addition, variations in cultural pressure exist among individuals and families of a given culture and in the ease or difficulty with which they relinquish or modify old cultural programs in a new situation.

As a Black American psychiatrist, I have frequently had patients question my background. I am convinced that important transference attitudes that are useful to explore are regularly contained in such questions. Always I wonder, "What do I mean to this patient?" "Can the patient be using thoughts and questions about me to avoid painful issues for which he seeks assistance?" "Does the patient have some thoughts or feelings about me or what I represent to him which may cause problems in the development of a therapeutic alliance?"

Invariably I explore the questions first and give answers to the patient's questions only after I have data that enable me to understand better the meaning of the questions. I would emphasize that I do not explore such questions in a defensive or adversary fashion; but, with an understanding smile, I am apt to explore by asking, "What have you taken me to be," or "Where would you guess I am from." Should the patient again request an answer before responding further, I am apt to say, "I will be happy to answer your question directly and will do so when we gain some understanding of your questions and doubts. I consider it to be an important responsibility of mine to examine with you the doubts and questions and conflicts in your mind rather than attempt to answer questions before clarifying the issues associated with them."

During such discussions much can be learned about presenting problems, personality patterns and traits, transference issues, and resistances that may be encountered.

Example 2   A young woman seeking assistance for unexplicable inability to speak at times in a job that required fluent verbal communication repeatedly asked if I believed in Freud. She indicated that Freud had associated psychiatric problems with sexual matters and that if I were Freudian, her priest would not permit her to come to see me. The question so dominated early interviews that I suggested that discussions with her priest could be clarifying since she was relying completely upon her fantasy of what her priest would say and do. She consulted her priest, who happened to know me and to think favorably of me. He advised her that I was trustworthy and encouraged that she discuss everything, including sexual matters, with me. In the next few meetings she cried profusely, first at a sense of being abandoned by the priest and left vulnerable to the Freudian psychiatrist. Very shortly, her tears were related to a sense of guilt and inability to control the intense affectionate and aggressive feelings and sexual thoughts she sometimes experienced. We learned that conflicts about these feelings and her periodic inability to speak were linked to close but conflictful relationships with her father and her God whom she viewed as very punitive. Improvement occurred in speech, in management of emotions, and in relationships (especially with father and with God) during therapy. Although she continued a very religious life without physical sexual activity, she became more comfortable with her sexual thoughts and feelings and aware that attacks she had feared came primarily from her overly strict conscience.

Discussion   Religious feelings and beliefs within individuals and the religious pressures and practices within a society vary from culture to culture and may strongly influence behavior. The early and repeated association between religion and experiences with strong feelings and important relationships leaves religion in a central position in the lives of most of the earth's people. It is important that psychiatrists be able to take up a patient's relationship with religion in a sensitive, skillfull, constructive, and respectful way.

Example 3   A young adult male patient referred to me for treatment of an obsessive compulsive neurosis quickly noted, "I am convinced that there is no way a Negro psychiatrist could understand me." When asked what he meant he replied, "My family is and has been one of the wealthiest in this country and your background experiences would not permit you to understand what I have experienced. Certainly I shall have to have another psychiatrist." When asked what I might not be able to understand he replied, "You could not imagine all of the protection, the bullet-proof cars, and every conceivable isolation to protect me from the harm which could come to children of wealthy people." My capacity to explore, understand, and empathize with his sense of isolation, separation, and loneliness paved the way toward the development of an ambivalent but viable therapeutic relationship. Disappointment and anger at me emerged in numerous criticisms, which gradually spread to include his disappointments and anger at many other persons in his life. No more was heard about the patient's concerns that class differences, racial differences, or cultural differences might make treatment impossible. Cultural, racial, and class issues stimulated by the patient's perception of differences in race and background between him and the therapist resulted in early mobilization of outspoken resistance which might have continued unrecognized in more subtle resistances in treatment with a therapist with whom the patient identified.

Discussion   At one and the same time, criticism of or resistance to a therapist of differing background may express the patient's 1) conscious responses to the perception of differences, 2) expression of unconscious issues connected with his problems (in Example 2, the excessive protection and isolation that the patient felt was a description of his obsessional defenses against affects and close relationships, which he felt no freely emotional, or Negro, person could understand), and 3) ambivalence about and resistance to treatment or to anyone getting close.

Meticulous use of a clinical approach is recommended at such times. Generally, one should assess the meanings of the criticisms and resistances before answering questions or making decisions or offering recommendations or taking actions. Answers should be given only when there is a sound rationale for doing so (ie, to facilitate communication when it may not develop otherwise, to help an excited person to manage his fears and behavior). It is a therapist's responsibility to evaluate, formulate, diagnose, recommend and prescribe, jointly establish a contract and goals, take appropriate actions to produce progress toward the goals, periodically review, and finally to terminate the process. Questions or complaints about the therapist should not be answered only because the patient wants a response. Usually they reflect anxieties, doubts, and concerns within the patient or associated with other persons. If the therapist immediately offers an answer or reassurance about a complaint, the underlying anxiety and conflict remain unknown and are temporarily put aside to return again and again in various forms.

Naturally, a patient has the right to discontinue work with one therapist and to choose another. A patient also has a right to a consultation or second opinion while in treatment. The consultant should also explore and evaluate carefully before responding. In one instance, a Black youth was showing resistance in his treatment with a white psychiatrist. The white psychiatrist suggested to the youth and his parents that possibly the youth would show more progress with a Black psychiatrist. A Black psychiatrist was consulted. In two evaluative consultations he found that the Black youth was very fond of the white therapist and would look upon referral to another psychiatrist as abandonment by someone he trusted. He had reached a point where further change in his thinking and behavior threatened his status in his neighborhood peer group and resistances in treatment resulted. Among some therapists there is a tendency to assume that having a therapist of the same background generally is preferable to having a therapist of a different background. Differences in personality, training, and experience are usually more important than background, and there are so many variables that each case should be studied carefully and judged on its merits.

Example 4 Difficulty was experienced in eliciting information from a young adult female psychiatric resident from a remote area of the Far East. A series of unusual experiences had led to her training in Boston, and she found herself unable to ride subways or take taxis to her assignment. If not picked up by a friend, she would call in sick, and she was jeopardizing her appointment. Attempts to understand what bothered her were met with absolute passivity and silence. In discussions with her after the seminars, I persisted in asking questions and in trying to discover what would facilitate communication with her. Gradually I learned that she was quite comfortable in the office with me and was neither anxious nor fearful; in fact she said she found me much like her husband on whom she depended for direction and guidance. It was her impression that such a role relationship existed between the women and men in her family and among people in her home community. She described feeling lost rather than depressed, and it became clear that her mood became elevated and she functioned better if I assumed a more advisory and directing role. She began to take public transportation to her assignment. After a short time I saw no psychiatric syndrome in evidence. It appeared that independent autonomous functioning was extremely difficult for her as a result of her background, but that she functioned very well if a family were available to her. Once this assessment was made, psychotherapy was not recommended, and her excellent functioning was maintained in her newly developed role as a friend of my family who visited with us a couple of times a month.

Discussion In some cultures independence and autonomy are encouraged only in certain specified roles. Persons whose prescribed roles require that they remain dependent and accommodative may have problems functioning in cultures where they are expected to function independently. At one university a dormitory for students was organized so that all students rotated the various housekeeping chores. Students from countries where men were not permitted to do housekeeping and where women insisted on doing all housekeeping usually had problems, as male students refused their designated assignments and female students assumed that duty for any male. These patterns may be so ingrained that refusal to comply with other schemes takes place. It is as if the patterns are non-negotiable and inaccessible to reason, to counseling, and to psychotherapy. Placement in circumstances that better fit the individual's patterns is a common solution.

Example 5　A young adult, married, Indian psychiatric resident born and reared in Kenya was being evaluated in a conference that included the resident, her two clinical supervisors, and me. After strong endorsement of her knowledge and technical skills, the clinical supervisors and I informed her that her progress was good and that our only concern had to do with what her supervisors described as a feeling of distance that had not interfered with the excellent quality of her work. The resident revealed that, although her husband and children were with her, she had felt a sense of difference and loneliness in her work as a resident. She had wished for a more hospitable relationship but felt that she should wait for some sign of this to be initiated by others. The supervisors acknowledged that they had behaved in a rather cool way toward her, having assumed that she was more comfortable with a somewhat distant relationship. We all laughed at the way we had misperceived her and from that moment on, much more open and warm interactions prevailed, including some interactions with the resident's family.

Discussion　When two persons relate to one another with perception of differences in their appearance and background, they may relate in a hesitant, tentative, and cool manner as they wait for warm, positive feedback and encouragement instead of relating more openly and spontaneously as they would with persons seen as similar to themselves. Under these circumstances, both parties are inclined to be aware of their own respective wishes for relationship and generally unaware of the coolness of their own behavior. At the same time, they are inclined to be aware of the coolness of the other person and unaware of the other person's wish for relationship. While some measure of this behavior is common to all newly developing relationships, there is a much stronger tendency to project the negative behavioral attributes on the other party in intercultural and interethnic interactions.

Example 6　A psychiatric resident from Iran was hardworking, very competent, and able to show considerable empathy in appropriate ways. She had unusual capacity to form businesslike, warm, and empathic relationships with her patients and colleagues and had demonstrated excellent therapeutic skills. Her supervisors considered that the one area needing improvement involved functioning with greater objectivity, with more assertiveness, and more systematic functioning in some instances in which this was more appropriate than her passive, relaxed style. The resident did not change. The supervisors modified their appraisal as they associated her patterns of functioning with a longstanding, deeply ingrained role behavior that did not significantly interfere with her progress or with a satisfactory outcome for patients. With supervisors she never asserted herself in a direct or outspoken way, but usually in a passive aggressive way. Exploration of her passive aggression regularly revealed that she had excellent grounds for her resistance and was opposed to something that needed to be changed. Her passive aggressive resistance made her supervisors aware of the problem, and offered a stimulus for changes.

Discussion We tend to accept our own behavioral styles and role relationships as good, proper, and adaptive and seldom question them. Intercultural interactions offer greater opportunity to observe and compare other ways of doing things. However, the prevailing power relationships generally influence judgments more than reason. Training directors and supervisors generally must work harder to get deviant resident behavior to fit their expectations, whether it deviates from expectations because of characterological or cultural factors. Often, resistance to our efforts can force us to look critically at our own behavioral styles and role relations with which we are comfortable, and can lead to discovery that ours are not always good and proper and adaptive. Unfortunately, such discovery seldom leads to more than minor transient change, since we and the many influential persons around us are tightly bonded to cherished patterns and are unwilling to change significantly unless a sufficiently powerful movement for change can be generated.

Example 7 A psychiatric resident from Brazil functioned excellently with one exception. She related to patients primarily in a passive-receptive way and used nondirective interviews. It was difficult to get her to develop an interview technique that included direct questions to elicit a comprehensive history and satisfactory mental status. Exploration revealed no relationship to cultural background but a clear relationship to having been in psychoanalysis for several years. The activity of her analyst had been incorporated and was being used inappropriately in the evaluative interviews, which required more activity and direct questions than she was comfortable using. She improved greatly after active supervision of her videotaped interviews.

Discussion Because a resident from another culture shows a training problem, the problem need not bear a relationship to cultural factors. Psychiatric residents reared completely in the United States with lengthy experience in psychoanalysis or in the family of a psychoanalyst with prominent passive behavior traits sometimes have shown this same training problem.

Examples 8 and 9 A male resident from Peru and a female resident from Chili functioned with excellent knowledge and skills and with excellent clinical effectiveness. However, they were so devoted to very structured activity roles with considerable directive questioning that nondirected interviewing and associative interviewing concepts and skills were difficult for them to develop. In both instances they had not had exposure to these methods, as many North American students do. It may well be that interviewing methods employed in a particular culture tend to be those compatible with prescribed roles for doctors, for men, for women, for upper- or middle- or lower-class people. In Examples 8 and 9, residents were from social groups in which taking initiative and active mastery were strongly reinforced.

Example 10   A young male resident repeatedly asked questions in an aggressive but dependent way and in a manner that evoked provocative adversary relationships with supervisors. This pattern appeared to be part of a search for an intense interaction with some parental figure. Since it happened more with male supervisors than with female ones, it was assumed that this tactic might be related to wished-for interactions with male parental figures. The frequency and persistence of these interactions interfered with his opportunity to learn and in some instances disrupted seminars or conferences. Moreover, his use of projection and criticisms increased in the context of these adversary relationships and they often produced discomfort for him and for others. He attempted to rationalize his behavior as culturally determined since he was born and reared with a strict upbringing in a middle European country. Although his supervisors felt that cultural factors might be reinforcing the character traits he displayed, they were sufficiently maladaptive to warrant direct activity on the part of supervisors. This included counseling, a series of discussions of the psychodynamics in relation to training, and emphasis on the importance of changing the pattern whether he wanted to or not. A combination of insight and behavior modification was the objective. Considerable progress was made during a 2-year period.

Discussion   Again, the point is made that training problems related to maladaptive character traits in a resident from another culture should not be looked on or dealt with as some unchangeable expression of culture. In the context of a considerate and caring relationship with the resident, a mixed program of instruction, counseling, referral for psychotherapy, and behavior-modifying administrative activity can often result in successful outcomes where there had been serious, deeply ingrained problems. In the few instances when I have encountered such problems, the residents have always been highly intelligent and they greatly valued being right and using power and control in relationships. Changing them in a 2- or 3-year period requires strong mutual affection, mutual respect, wise special training strategies and tactics, effective use of power and behavior modifying administrative practices, close coordination of the resident's instructors and supervisors, and frequent review meetings of the resident with all supervisors. An integrated program for the individual resident should include all of the items listed.

Attempts to modify behavior in the context of mutually affectionate and mutually respectful teacher–pupil relations result in cooperative effort, though not without resistance. Attempts to modify behavior without mutual affection and respect foster a sense of persecution and rejection and increase resistance to change. In addition, the resident should understand that the changes are related to an objective desired by the resident and not just requirements arbitrarily imposed. It may be useful to assess the use to which a resident intends to put his training and where. Is the resident interested in clinical, administrative, research, or public policy roles? Some character attributes that may be maladaptive in one area may be highly adaptive in another.

Finally, training directors have a responsibility to produce sound, effective, useful, safe products. A sound selection process is the first step. Sound training of faculty, and sound program, resources, and training methods follow. Each resident should participate in frequent two-way evaluations that clearly delineate the training objectives, the progress toward those objectives, what needs to be done to achieve the objectives, and the chances of reaching them. If successful completion of training depends on certain changes or accomplishments, both the resident and the faculty should know it in sufficient time to produce the necessary changes and accomplishments. If not possible, the resident and faculty should change their objectives and plans in a considerate process that assists the resident to consider various occupational alternatives.

Example 10 has led to a general discussion of kinds of training problems experienced by residents regardless of cultural, ethnic, or class background. The same general principles are applicable to any of the serious training problems that may be encountered. It should also be underscored that what is considered to constitute a training problem differs greatly from culture to culture just as that which is considered appropriate in various role relationships differs greatly from culture to culture.

Example 11 A young Black female resident from a Caribbean island was so convinced by and devoted to her own ideas and values that she sometimes had difficulty relating to ones that differed, whether presented by patients, supervisors, or others. She was often defensive or assertive toward ideas or values that differed and was quite reactive against interference and suggestions from others. This left her using assertive, relatively nondynamic approaches with patients. With supervision, remarkable improvement occurred in the course of the year. She came to function with warmth, sensitivity, more openness, and ability to build therapeutic alliances with patients and with persons in the patients' lives. She began to manage her assertive and oppositional traits well. From the beginning she had shown good administrative skills and good common sense and judgment. She became able to employ these in a perceptive, responsive, psychodynamic framework at a time when she developed a rewarding relationship after a disappointing period without one.

Discussion   In this case there was a shift from frustrating life circumstances to very gratifying life circumstances associated with the shift from a rather rigid, passive-aggressive pattern to a more flexible, warm, open pattern. With the lifting of her disappointment and her mild depression associated with it, together with the development of some gratifying relationships, the inclination toward aggressive responses greatly diminished. Her remarkable progress was related to such factors as well as to training factors.

Example 12   An 88-year-old man entered the hospital seeking repair of his umbilical hernia. Medical workup revealed a large mass on the right side of the colon, diagnosed as probable cancer. He insisted on an operation for his hernia but refused an operation for the cancer. Psychiatric consultation was requested. In the interview the man emphasized that a sister and his wife had died following operations for cancer.

Interviews with the patient and family members revealed him to be a prideful Italian patriarch of a large family who was determined to have his own way. When it became clear that the psychologic and possibly physiologic integrity were linked to his initiative-taking, masculine, patriarchal role, we could not feel sure that his belief he would die in a cancer operation was false. He continued to insist, with his right hand on his umbilicus: "Repair this hole and leave my lump alone!" We hypothesized that a feminine fantasy or fantasies of defects associated with the hole in his abdominal wall felt threatening to him, but not as much so as taking away his lump would be. (We assumed the lump symbolized for him his penis, his masculinity.)

Example 13   Residents from South American countries, European countries, Mexico, Canada, and India have been trained in programs with which I have been associated without encountering training problems of any kind. Cultural factors have played little role so long as the ability to communicate in English, the ability to identify with interests of patients and colleagues, ability to empathize, and well-organized, fairly healthy personalities were present. Usually residents from "foreign" countries experienced difficulties when a combination of maladaptive personality traits reinforced by and seemingly validated by cultural experience resulted in relatively inflexible use of these personality traits where they did not fit well with the patterns of patients, colleagues, and supervisors. It is important to separate the problem patterns of personality and bring to bear on them such insight-evoking and behavior-modifying activity as is appropriate for a teacher-pupil relationship. In addition, recommending evaluation for psychotherapy may also be appropriate.

Example 14   Four young psychiatrists applied for psychoanalytic training and were rejected because of their "inclinations toward spontaneous action and emotional expressiveness rather than thoughtful reflection and more deliberate action." All were from the same South American country where their behavioral attributes had been reinforced by sociocultural factors. Since all were well-trained and respected psychiatrists, since no psychiatrists with backgrounds in those countries had been accepted by this institute for psychoanalytic training, and since the same selection committee members voted for acceptance and the same ones voted for rejection in each instance, it seemed likely that a cross-cultural psychiatric issue existed here. Sociopolitical and administrative processes usually are employed to resolve questions of this kind, and open-minded inquiry following the voting is rare. Selection committee members may have had the illusion that they were relating objectively to the individual merits of each applicant because the four applicants were scattered over a 6-year period. The majority who supported rejection of the applications described the applicants as inclined toward action instead of reflection, as if these qualitites were mutually exclusive. The minority who advocated acceptance described the applicants as thoughtful and reflective as well as active persons, as if these qualities were not mutually exclusive. Wherever the gateway to an institution is controlled primarily by members of one background, they tend to admit easily persons like themselves and to resist admission of persons who appear quite different.

However, this generalization should be qualified, for it depends much on the general thinking and behavioral styles of the people involved. Persons with a generally affiliative and affectionate style are more inclined to be accepting and less inclined to be rejecting than persons who are generally differentiative and aggressive in behavioral style. In a paper entitled "Ego Development and Cultural Differences," C.A. Pinderhughes explored this issue in some depth.

Often minority group members in western societies have affiliative and accommodative roles reinforced in complementary relationship to the differentiative and initiative-taking roles reinforced in members of more powerful groups. To improve their adjustment and self-esteem in a competitive society, persons in minority groups develop initiative and often employ accommodative and initiative-taking roles alternatively and comfortably. Members of more powerful majority groups find their initiatives encroached upon and have no motivation and no positive reward for accommodating, so they resist the role changes and the advances of less powerful minority groups. The basic dynamics, ethics, and behaviors associated with social class interactions are analogous to those found at ethnic and cultural group interactions.

Example 14 occurred before 1968. During the social changes of the late 1960s and early 1970s, there was a heightened awareness of the unconscious bias and discrimination against some groups being exercised at gateways to institutions. Changes in attitudes, criteria, and admissions processes resulted in more appropriate openness in selecting candidates for training in psychoanalysis. In some instances affirmative action was employed to recruit more actively members of groups with little representation in this field.

Concluding examples and discussions   While providing psychiatric treatment in the city of Boston, I have been identified by patients as Black, American, Jamaican, Mexican, American Indian, a native of India, and Arabian. The identity imputed to me has depended on several factors, including the meaning that 1) "Black American" has for the patient and the degree of comfort or discomfort the patient experiences by associating these meanings with me, and 2) other labels the patient tends to associate with me. The nature of the feelings and thoughts a patient associates with me sometimes has governed a patient's perception of me. This has been most noticeable in circumstances where a white patient has developed a strongly positive transference and observes with surprise that I seem to be white. One such patient in psychoanalysis would see me as white on some days and Black on others and on some occasions would turn around on the couch to test the validity of his perception.

The previous experience of the observer is a powerful determinant of perception. A mixture of impressions from past experience, from related fantasies and wishes, and from present stimuli tend to be projected upon any individual being perceived.

Example 15   I once talked with a Chinese resident physician who insisted I was Jamaican and refused to believe me when I said I was not. When I asked her how she could be so certain that I was Jamaican, she informed me that she was born and reared in a large Chinese community in Jamaica and could recognize Jamaicans easily.

Example 16   While I was at the University of Ife in Nigeria, two well-dressed men approached me, begged my pardon for their intrusion, and asked if I might settle an argument they were having about me. One had insisted that I was Nigerian while the other insisted that I was Egyptian. Of interest is that the man insisting I was Nigerian was a light-brown-skinned Egyptian whose complexion was similar to mine. He had lived in Nigeria for several years. The man insisting that I was Egyptian was a dark-brown-skinned Nigerian. Each was renouncing me as a member of his own group and insisting that I was a member of the other group as if to say: "He's not mine, he's yours."

This example illustrates the following principles: the context in which an observation occurs is an important determinant of the associated perception. A perception is usually a composite interpretation of stimuli from persons and objects, from interactions, and from the contexts in which the persons, objects, and interactions appear.

Example 17   Sometimes supervisors and residents of common background have problems establishing a satisfactory training alliance.

For one reason or another they may frustrate or disappoint each other, or perhaps provoke or antagonize each other. Once hostile or adversary relations develop, they may escalate, and training may be jeopardized. Under these circumstances it is useful to enlist assistance from an experienced consultant from within the program. When problems of this kind have unfamiliar cross-cultural features, or when several of the key faculty members are embroiled in conflict with a resident, it can be useful to invite an experienced consultant from outside the program to evaluate, recommend, and assist with the training problem.

One unusually bright immigrant frequently challenged rules and regulations and showed little respect toward supervisors. Discussion of characterological and cultural aspects revealed that he greatly valued "the intelligent, brave, and highly organized people like the Germans, Dutch, Norwegians, Swiss, Danes, Austrians, Rumanians, Hungarians, and high-caste Indians who deal more with respect, show more authority, more hostility, less appreciation, and less empathy." They were viewed as similar to his ideal view of masculine behavior. He devalued the "emotional" French, Italians, Spanish, and various low-caste people "who use authority less, deal less in respect, tend to be more pleasing and to show more appreciation, more empathy, and more affiliation." He viewed these people as similar to his view of feminine behavior.

The dilemma of the instructor with such a student is one that is not encountered with students who share the instructor's background and value system. First, the instructor must identify and acknowledge the differences in background and value system and assess the impact of these differences on various aspects of training. Second, the instructor should differentiate and give special attention to those values and personality traits that impair ability to learn or to practice psychiatry effectively and ethically in a humanitarian way. It is possible that some values and personality attributes may have an unfavorable effect on the interaction of the student with instructors or supervisors but not with patients. Handling this question may be unsettling, since it is extremely difficult to predict that a trait responsible for problems with supervisors will not cause a problem with some patients. Third, I have favored the full and open discussion of these kinds of problems with the residents so that I can be up-to-date in my appraisal of work and progress and better able to make a valid evaluation of the resident. Thus far in instances in which I have detected such problems, I have used behavior-modifying approaches that have included 1) nonnegotiable directives and ultimatums, 2) confrontation in group settings with their peers and with their supervisors, 3) use of the resident review board to reinforce the pressures applied, and 4) vigorous alliance-forming activity with frequent meetings in which I attempt to use and role model the behaviors I am encouraging the resident to learn. At points where the resident and I identify a problem or persistent personality trait that interferes with training or clinical work, I recommend evaluation for psychotherapy.

Example 18   When a minority resident is identified with particular patients in the clinical units of the training program, these patients may be referred to the resident with unusual frequency. More Black patients may be referred to a Black resident than to his or her non-Black colleagues. More Spanish-speaking patients may be referred to a Spanish-speaking resident than to non-Hispanic colleagues. More Chinese patients may be referred to a Chinese resident than to non-Chinese residents. This practice may compromise the training of the minority resident with nonminority patients and may compromise the training of nonminority residents with minority patients. For this reason the caseload of minority residents should be monitored whenever referrals of this kind are likely to occur. It is often useful to encourage the minority resident to offer consultant services to fellow residents treating minority patients with whom the minority resident identifies. Supervision and training should be offered for consultative services of this kind, which the minority resident is apt to encounter for the rest of his professional career.

Example 19   As a Black psychiatry resident training in a Massachusetts hospital, I was surprised when three white male patients from Alabama, Georgia, and Kentucky respectively, separately and independently requested that they be assigned to me for psychotherapy. Each had been in Massachusetts for a very short time; each felt uncomfortable living in the North; and each felt he would be less anxious and more comfortable with a Black psychiatrist who sounded as if he were from the South than with a strange northern psychiatrist with unknown attitudes.

HOW WILL THE TEACHERS BE TAUGHT?

One reason for training program inadequacies are the inadequacies in the training programs that produced present faculty members. Since Doctor Gaw conceived and began to develop this project, his colleagues and fellow faculty members at the Edith Nourse Rogers Memorial Veterans Administration Hospital in Bedford, Massachusetts, have had their consciousness about cross-cultural psychiatry elevated in discussions related to the project. In a meeting of 16 instructors and supervisors of residents on March 12, 1979, after receiving an outline of this chapter, numerous suggestions were offered for a model curriculum. The following paragraphs, which conclude this chapter, represent a summary of their suggestions.

Residents should learn that emotional acceptance and a sense of affiliation and affection may be present even when minds and meanings are far apart. In cross-cultural interactions this happens frequently. There may be an early sense of understanding and closeness based on eye contacts, smiles, and other nonverbal interaction. Later, there may be a painful recognizition of differences and even an unwillingness to go through painstaking efforts to learn each other's language, meaning, and background experience, enough for a meeting of minds to occur.

In view of the vast number of interactions among different cultures since the industrial revolution, and since migration of large numbers of people from one continent to another, and from one country to another, serious attention to cross-cultural psychiatry is quite warranted. Cross-cultural marriages and cross-cultural dating produces bicultural families, bicultural personalities, and often multicultural families or personalities. Cross-cultural interfaces thus have been produced in many families and within many personalities.

Even in the most homogeneous traditional society, there can be sufficient variation in individual background and experience to produce persons who differ from culture mates in thinking, feeling, and behavior patterns. Within a culture, diverse subcultures may be produced. This is more likely to occur in westernized and nontraditional societies. Interactions among subcultures, castes, and social classes frequently are the site of problems analogous to problems at cross-cultural interfaces. Greater differences often exist between the classes or castes within a given culture than between analogous classes or castes of different cultures.

Within a given culture, different castes and different classes may be programmed into complementary roles with initiative required of one and accommodation required of the other. Such role relationships may appear unequal but harmonious.

Wherever people live together over generations and long enough to develop a dependably-structured culture, tasks and roles and responsibilities are divided and assigned in ways that control and fit together component persons, families, organizations, and institutions into an integrated whole.

Affects, role relationships, thinking patterns, and physical activity are dealt with differently in different cultures. Residents should be instructed about these differences and their meaning in relation to various methods of treatment. It was noted that in some strongly religious cultures alcoholism is not tolerated, and persons from these cultures may have great difficulty in understanding alcoholism in the United States. One resident from such a country had difficulty accepting and relating to alcoholic patients as a result of this.

It was recommended that residents be instructed in demographic patterns in the United States. It was stressed that residents have opportunity to discuss in a seminar the relationship of various clinical services in the medical center to the people in the immediate environment. This discussion should include the history of institutional biases concerning different groups. Discussions of this kind and courses in cross-cultural psychiatry should begin in the first year and should deal first with groups served in the community of the medical center. Since medical students as well as residents learn and develop skills with a population that is usually different from the one they will later serve, curricula on cross-cultural interactions should be included in medical school training as well as in residency training.

Physicians should be instructed about some of the differences in doctor–patient relationships that exist in surgery, medicine, pediatrics, psychiatry, and other fields. In some instances, patients rely primarily on physicians for their knowledge, judgment, and technical skills. Empathy for the patient and identification with the patient are not critical factors for medical practice in some fields, as they are in psychiatry. In this connection it may be useful to conceptualize different disciplines in medicine as having "cultural differences." The ability to develop a realistic and balanced appraisal of each patient regardless of his background was stressed as the soundest professional goal to strive for. Inability to identify with a patient can foster negative projections on the patient, and an overly strong tendency to identify with patients can foster the projection of positive attitudes on the patient. In either case an objective and balanced view is likely to be compromised.

Detailed advance knowledge about cultural aspects of the patients one serves merely provides the psychiatrist with a block of information to be projected on these patients. These are still projections of content from the therapist's mind upon the patient, although they may be more accurate and more charitable than the content the resident would have projected before receiving advance information about the patient's culture. Thus, in the final analysis, the development of relationships and interview techniques that insures the faithful replication in the resident's mind of concerns, related content, and background information existing in the patient's mind, and use of thinking methods that detect and correct misinformation and bias are the single most important elements relating to cross-cultural psychiatry in a residency training program.

The problem of defining a curriculum in cross-cultural psychiatry may prove to be far easier than implementing it. The first generation of teachers will be largely self-taught. Attention should be given to a set of recommendations and procedures for tooling up the faculty so that they can meet their responsibilities and put out attractive, sound, and effective products. Materials and methods for teaching them should be defined, used, evaluated, and redefined until reliable effective courses are developed. As early as possible, participating faculty, and eventually all faculty, should be involved in small-group experiential training as an important part of their preparation for teaching cross-cultural psychiatry.

BIBLIOGRAPHY

American Hospital Association Joint Commission on Accreditation of Hospitals: *Accreditation Manual for Hospitals 1978*. Chicago, AHA, 1978.

American Medical Association Liaison Committee on Graduate Medical Education: *Directory of Accredited Residencies 1977-1978,* Chicago, AMA, 1978.

Bradshaw WH: Training psychiatrists for working with Blacks in basic residency programs. *Am J Psychiatry* 135(12):1520-1524, 1978.

Deutsch F: The associative anamnesis. *Psychoanal Q* 8:354-381, 1939.

Glazer N, Moynihan D: *Beyond the Melting Pot.* Cambridge, MIT Press, 1963.

Kadushin A: *The Social Work Interview.* New York, Columbia University Press, 1972, p 228.

Keefe T: Empathy: The critical skill. *Soc Work* 21:10-15, 1976.

Lowenstein S: Integrative content on feminism and racism into the social work curriculum. *J Ed Soc Work* 12:91-96, 1976.

Mirelowitz S, Grossman L: Ethnicity: An intervening variable in social work education. *J Ed Soc Work* 11:76-83, Fall 1975.

Pinderhughes CA: The minimum requirements for a medical model for psychotherapy. *J Nat Med Assoc* 64(2):129-144, 1972.

Pinderhughes C: Ego development and cultural differences. *Am J Psychiatry* 131(2):171-175, 1974.

Pinderhughes CA: Differential bonding: Toward a psychophysiological theory of stereotyping. *Am J Psychiatry* 136(1):33-37, 1979.

Pinderhughes EB: Teaching empathy in cross-cultural social work. *Soc Work* 24:312-316, 1979.

Siporin M: *Introduction to Social Work Practice.* New York, Macmillan, 1975, p 205.

SUGGESTED READINGS

Allport G: *The Nature of Prejudice.* New York, Doubleday, 1958.

Bromley D, Longino C: *White Racism and Black Americans.* Cambridge, Schenkman, 1972.

Clark K: *Dark Ghetto.* New York, Harper & Row, 1965.

Coles R: Children of affluence. *Boston Globe,* Sunday, Sept 25, 1977, p B-1.

Crompton D: Minority content in social work education — Promise or pitfall? *J Ed Soc Work* 10:9-18, 1974.

Erikson E: *Identity, Youth and Crisis.* New York, Norton, 1968.

Greer C: *The Divided Society: The Ethnic Experience in America.* New York, Basic, 1974.

Grier W, Cobbs P: *Black Rage.* New York, Basic, 1968.

Guterman S: *The Black Psyche.* Berkeley, Glendessary Press, 1972.

Kagwa W. Utilization of racial content in developing self-awareness. *J Ed Soc Work,* 12:21-27, 1976.

Knowles L, Previtt K: *Institutional Racism in America.* Englewood-Cliffs, NJ, Printice-Hall, 1970.

Leichtenberg P: *Research in the Service of Mental Health.* US Dept HEW Pub. No. (ADM), 1975.

Miller J: *Toward a New Psychology of Women.* Boston, Beacon, 1976.

Orcutt B: *Poverty and Social Casework Services.* Metuchen, NJ, Scarecrow, 1974.

Ordway J: Some emotional consequences of racism for whites, in Willie CV, Kramer BM, Brown BS (eds): *Racism and Mental Health.* Pittsburgh, University of Pittsburgh Press, 1973.

Papajohn J, Spiegel J: *Transactions in Families.* San Francisco, Jossey-Bass, 1975.

Pinderhughes C: Racism and psychotherapy, in Willie CV, Kramer BM, Brown BS (eds): *Racism and Mental Health.* Pittsburgh, University of Pittsburgh Press, 1973, pp 61–121.

Turner JB: Education for practice with minorities. *Soc Work* 17:112–118, 1972.

Watzlawick P, Beavin J, Jackson D: *Pragmatics of Human Communication.* New York, Norton, 1967.

17 A Resident's Perspective

Adela G. Wilkeson, MD

In 1971, five Black psychiatrists who had recently completed their residency training described the numerous problems they encountered concerning minority mental health issues during their training (Jones et al 1970). Their description is similar in many ways to the problems I encountered in my training program. Questions regarding the specific effects of different cultural backgrounds and race on psychic dysfunction, diagnosis, and treatment were not systematically addressed and were rarely asked. At the same time, a review of inpatient and outpatient treatment selection practices within their programs demonstrated marked discriminatory practices. The resident's own different cultural background was usually ignored by peers and supervisors while residents felt an implicit, strong expectation to reaffirm "the white institution's concept of itself as liberal, unbiased, and nondiscriminatory. Should their attitudes, actions or views be perceived as challenging, threatening or contrary, they may be considered unsuitable for the system or if they are accepted, they may be in for a difficult time." Personal struggles of the residents who had internalized attitudes of inferiority associated with race added further to the difficulties of approaching such problems in a constructive manner.

It is not clear to me how much of the inattention to cultural issues by current psychiatric educators stems from lack of knowledge or lack of exposure to training experience with minority individuals. The years of residency training are certainly most formative in terms of the theoretical framework each psychiatrist assimilates and the supervisory staff that provide crucial role models.

All of us who have been raised in our contemporary American culture have been exposed to and have inherited attitudes of racial discrimination that have very deep historical and psychosocial roots. It thus does not seem to me that a discussion of cultural issues in psychiatric training would be complete without simultaneous exploration and education regarding the forces that have perpetuated selective inattention to race and culture within our profession and society. I have tried to present the topics I have found relevant in an integrative fashion so they can be more easily incorporated into the multiple levels of resident education. My hope is that future generations of psychiatrists will be more informed and attuned to these issues and will not consciously or unconsciously perpetuate existing patterns of ethnocentric bias.

THE FACTS

One out of 5 Americans is a member of an ethnic or racial minority group: 24.1 million are Black; 11.1 million are Hispanics; 1.2 million are Native Americans (both Indian and Alaskan); and 2.5 million are Asian. A task force on mental health for children (Shapiro 1974) stated:

> Racism is the number one public health problem facing America today. The conscious and unconscious attitudes of superiority which permit and demand that a majority oppress a minority, are a clear and present danger to the mental health of *all* children and their parents.

At the same time, it is clear that the mental health services provided for minority individuals today are inadequate (Fiman et al 1975; The President's Commission on Mental Health 1978; Senate Bill S.2373 1977; Sabshin 1970). Recording of statistics of mental disorders by race still hampers efforts to understand these complex issues (King 1978, Sabshin 1970, Willie et al 1973). Numerous reports indicate (King 1978) that Black minority individuals:

> emerge from the diagnostic process "appearing" (quotes added) more disturbed and more pathologic than whites who have shown this same behavior; that the same behavior in black women is called schizophrenic

while in whites it is called neurotic; that there is a greater frequency of depression labeling in whites and a greater frequency of personality and character disorder labeling in blacks, and that black hospital admission rates are much higher than those of whites and of these groups, blacks are heavily concentrated in the category of psychosis to the relative exclusion of other categories.

Race has also been found to influence the diagnosis and type of referrals from psychiatric emergency rooms (Gross et al 1969). Blacks are more often seen for diagnosis only (Jackson 1974). Blacks are more likely to be seen by paraprofessionals (Stanley 1977). And minority groups receive "qualitatively inferior" or "less preferred" forms of treatment (Yamamoto 1968).

Though a complete review of the literature regarding American psychiatric approaches to mental health in minority populations is beyond the scope of this paper, the above references are representative of the evidence gathered by Sabshin et al (1970) and Thomas and Sillen (1972) to document the existence of institutional racism in psychiatry. The Thomas and Sillen book provides a comprehensive and at times quite poignant review of how American psychiatric thinking has paralleled the process of racism and de facto racism within American culture since the slave trade through to modern times (Kerner et al 1968). Identification of and attention to the reality that ethnocentric attitudes influence all aspects of psychiatric care, research, and thinking does seem to be a necessary precondition to the hopes for substantial change.

Active recruitment of minority individuals into psychiatric training programs seems to be at least one possible partial solution to the existing inequities. As of 1972, however, only 12 of 162 approved training programs reported active recruitment efforts (Rosenfeld 1976). While the early 1970s showed a modest increase in the number of women and minorities entering psychiatric residencies, minorities are still significantly under-represented (Pardes 1978; Rosenfeld 1976). A 1972 NIMH survey showed 1.4% of American psychiatrists were Black, 1.5% Hispanic, and 1.3% from other minority groups. Combining these figures with overall population statistics shows that there is 1 Black psychiatrist per 73,000 Black Americans, while there is 1 white psychiatrist per 10,000 white Americans. Due to the slow rate of increase of minorities in institutions of higher education, it is clear that in the next several decades the mental health care of American minority groups will be met only if white psychiatrists actively participate in service delivery as well as research.

Will this occur? A recent report prepared by the APA Task Force on Racism in Psychiatric Research has documented awareness and interest of minority residents to questions relating to minority mental health but no concomitant concern on the part of the majority residents surveyed

(Thomas, unpublished data). Will education make a difference? In principle, the psychiatric educators who prepared a recent APA publication on psychiatric education (Rosenfeld 1976) support and repeatedly emphasize that psychiatrists have a broad base of knowledge not only in the biologic and psychologic aspects of mental illness but also of the socio-cultural context in which the patient and physician interact. They also note that there is considerable diversity in currently existing training programs and that major difficulties exist in establishing priorities for resident education, considering the broad range of knowledge that ideally would be mastered by all psychiatrists during their formal training.

Since there is no systematic study of current residency curricula to ascertain whether cultural issues are being addressed, I sent a brief questionnaire to the residency training directors of 14 residency programs in the Boston area. Ten questionnaires were returned. The program directors reported overall approximately 27% of the patient population served were minorities. Two programs had a seminar or course that specifically addressed minority issues. One of these programs, from a catchment area where 90% of the population was from an identified minority group, dedicated 20% of its didactic teaching time to minority cultural aspects of mental health. The remaining programs reported only 1.6% of the total didactic time was used for this purpose. Four of the 10 programs attempted to assign supervisors with expertise in this area to as many residents as possible. Except for one of the programs that reported already having a seminar on cultural issues, all expressed an interest in reviewing and potentially utilizing the curriculum developed by this panel.

THE RESIDENT'S LEARNING EXPERIENCE

Setting priorities for learning is a problem that faces each psychiatric resident as well as resident training directors and faculty members. The first-year residency work in psychiatry has been described as the single most difficult period of training for any physician. Residents generally begin their psychiatric experience on inpatient units where they are expected to manage the most disturbed and psychotic patients while simultaneously receiving didactic and supervisory instruction about the medical and psychologic aspects of major mental illness for the first time. The personal stress of being intensely exposed and subjected to the most primitive of psychotic behavior and affects is not to be minimized nor is the necessary shift in professional identity from being a direct provider of patient care to learning to facilitate patients' growth through psychotherapy (Semrad and Van Buskirk 1969).

Thereafter, different types of learning dilemmas face the resident in general outpatient clinics, where both short-and long-term individual and group psychotherapeutic experiences are to be mastered, on medical consultation services, in emergency rooms, walk-in clinics and psychopharmacology clinics, during rotations through community mental health clinics, and in inpatient or outpatient child psychiatric experiences.

In addition to the intensity and diversity of these training experiences, it is clear that the recent cutbacks in federal fundings for residency training have made it necessary for programs to require greater and greater service commitments from residents. This situation is understandably resented by many residents and can, at least transiently, reinforce resistances to learning. When community mental health clinic rotations are not fully supported as integral parts of residency training and when appropriate concomitant didactic seminars and supervision are not provided for this work, it can indeed be experienced as one more unrewarding service requirement. This was in fact a predominant attitude toward the community rotations in the psychiatry program I recently completed. Poor Irish Catholic, Italian, and Hispanic populations were served by the clinics where residents rotated. The sense that these rotations were primarily a service commitment was further fostered by the clinic staffs who in fact very much valued the residents' time because of chronic problems of insufficient staff (particularly psychiatric staff) to meet the needs of the patient populations. Also, despite some members of the relatively large faculty's having expertise in minority issues, no effort was made to assign supervision by these faculty members to residents during their community rotation. In fact, the actual patient contact during the community rotations went largely unsupervised.

Despite my fluency in Spanish I was unable to communicate with a relatively well-educated Puerto Rican store owner undergoing psychotherapy for what appeared to be a problem of sexual dysfunction. He reported having difficulty not believing his problems in some way had to do with spirits, even though intellectually he disavowed their existence. Without knowing the deep-seated cultural beliefs of many Latins in such phenomena, I certainly would have been more likely to attribute this complaint to an incipient psychosis. Other aspects of the patient's cognition and function were intact, however, and the problem of the evaluation seemed more to do with the patient's difficulty in candidly discussing his concerns about sexual dysfunction with a female physician. Though I have great uncles and aunts in Puerto Rico, I was raised in the United States and did not feel sufficiently in touch with this man's immediate cultural background to discuss my awareness of this impasse in a way that was useful to him. This one case provided a potential for learning about how to deal with a heritage of beliefs in supernatural forces as well as what to anticipate with regard to sex role stereotypes in Puerto Rican men. Unfortunately, without supervision or any specific instruction in these areas, I continued to wonder about what I might have learned. Similarly, many patients had a combination of real day-to-day living problems secondary to their low economic status plus chronic anxiety and depression. It seemed group psychotherapy would be of significant value to these individuals. When presented to them initially by myself and my Honduran paraprofessional co-worker, the recommendation was accepted by each. However, only half showed for the first session and none thereafter. Why?

I left my community rotation with many unanswered questions. How could I translate and transfer the skills I was acquiring on the Boston side of the bridge to this impoverished and largely illiterate group of Hispanics in Chelsea? Are different, initially more open, and personal styles of interacting during evaluation interviews indicated because of cultural expectations of greater mutuality among Latins? On the other hand, was the pull I experienced to be more open a reflection of a potentially detrimental overidentification? How much did the difficulty I encountered in trying to engage these Latin clients in treatment reflect their socioeconomic status rather than cultural differences? What aspects of their distress related to the difficulties caused by their recent immigration (migration from Puerto Rico) to a very different American culture? What type of adaptations and conflicts occur for second-generation American Hispanics whose familial culture differs from the educational and peer culture they experience? In what ways did the cultural expectations of Cuban patients differ from those of Puerto Ricans, Mexicans, and other Latin American ethnic groups? Is there any easily accessible summary of psychiatric literature that could provide answers to these and other questions that continue to arise as I encounter minority individuals in the general hospital outpatient clinic, emergency room, and consultation service?

Providing psychiatric residents with opportunities to learn from experiences like my Chelsea rotation is necessary for acquiring first-hand knowledge of clinical problems. Providing such experiences without concomitant didactic and supervisory sessions can be significantly frustrating and may serve to discourage many residents from any further consideration of work in these areas. Cohen (1974) describes this potential difficulty as follows:

> When the therapist is not exposed to "training cases" of different sociocultural backgrounds, he has less opportunity to integrate the issues created by different cultures. He will not know how to cope with either the objective differences — the meanings of symbols, behavior patterns, use of speech, and expression of disorganized behavior — or his own gut reaction to patients' verbal and nonverbal expressions and his defensiveness that guards against a feeling of inability to understand, integrate, and interpret unfamiliar signals. The therapist in this situation becomes rigid and controlling, and projects the cause for lack of success onto the patient. This is one of the underlying rationalizations that labels the patient as "not motivated," "not fitting within the cultural framework of psychotherapy," "unable to use therapy." It generally points to the

therapist's frustration that he cannot become invested in this type of patient because he is not receiving feedback that the patient is progressing in comprehension of emotional conflicts.

Cohen has systematically identified a number of transcultural variables that are relevant to the training of psychiatrists to work with individuals of different ethnic and cultural backgrounds. Cultural attitudes influence the definition of mental illness for both the patient and doctor as well as the expression of dysfunction, which has a major impact on the patient-doctor interaction. A resident's life experience causes him or her to bring predetermined concepts of child rearing, feminine and masculine roles, disease and health to the process of diagnosis and treatment. These concepts undergo considerable revision as the residents develop their theoretical framework of understanding mental health and illness throughout their training. Cultural reactions to the dependent position of being a patient, as well as stereotypic perceptions of physicians from cultural backgrounds the minority patients will most likely have, are other patient-related variables, both for the initial establishment of a therapeutic alliance and throughout the psychotherapeutic process.

> As a psychotherapeutic intervention moves into areas which generally create increasing emotional reactions, issues of intimacy, status, sexuality, and other personal and narcissistic relationships, [they] trigger in patients associations and feelings which are colored by cultural modalities and in some cases are manifested as "acting out." If the therapist cannot himself understand and relate this to the cultural background of his patient, he will be misunderstanding and mislabeling the patient's perception of the real world and reality testing.

Independent of a patient's particular background factors such as race, ethnicity, social class, and religion contribute in major ways to a person's value system: his or her assumptive intrapsychic world. Wilder (1969) distinguishes four kinds of value systems as he describes how conflicts may arise between or within each realm: 1) conscious values, 2) preconscious, never verbalized, values, 3) repressed values, 4) unattended or ignored values. Numerous authors emphasize (Bernard 1953, Boyer 1964, Calnek 1970, Schacter and Butts 1968, Wilder 1969, Wittkower 1974) that a therapist's thorough analysis or self-analysis of his or her own value system is a necessary prerequisite for successfully helping patients with these types of conflicts. Writing in the late 1960s, Wilder sums up this important aspect of psychotherapeutic work as follows:

> Take a typical example of present-day psychotherapeutic practice: The college student who may be diagnosed as psychoneurotic, schizophrenic or just going through an "identity crisis;" His value conflicts may even be the presenting symptom or it may not take long to uncover them. How-

ever, to understand the case we must not only know all about his social milieu, past and present (for example, the hippie milieu), we must understand the language of the milieu, in many respects different from our own; we must be able to understand and evaluate the conflicting value systems which may be partly quite new to us. In order to do this, we must become very conscious of our own value systems and their conflicts and not take them for granted.

Studying the cultural attitudes of different minority groups can provide a major stimulus for resident psychiatrists to begin considering their own cultural values, which may not otherwise be subject to conscious reflection. Review of the predominant attitudes of our middle-class American culture with its Protestant and western European roots can be facilitated by learning the comparative and contrasting attitudes of other cultures. Consideration can then be more readily given to how prevailing American cultural values influence current psychiatric evaluation and treatment, as well as the influence of such values on the manifestation of psychic distress and dysfunction of white Americans (Draquns 1974).

Attempting to work with patients from different cultural backgrounds also provides invaluable experience for therapists in their effort to learn to listen to patients from a nonprojective, empathic frame of mind and to explore inevitable countertransference reactions that can occur between patient and therapist of different cultural backgrounds. Fischer (1971) provides an excellent example of the multiple layers of unconscious meaning that can be expressed through manifest interracial issues. Ticho's description (1971) of countertransference difficulties with a Latin male patient, based in part on her inadequate knowledge of the patient's cultural background, provides further emphasis for the importance of both self-awareness and education. Bradshaw (1978) notes that therapists' countertransference reactions can include a "potpourri of overidentification, overcompensation, condescension and flight, all linked together by countertransference involving warded-off aggression and compensatory mechanisms against feelings of inferiority and badness."

Inattention to racial stereotypes can lead to premature exclusion of patients from insight-oriented therapy. It also can bring about the establishment of patterns of racist behavior within psychotherapy groups (Ruffin 1973). Overemphasis on the effects of minority group membership can be experienced by the patient as a painful personal rejection, possibly reinforce unhealthy narcissistic satisfaction in being special, definitely reinforce the patient's own tendency to stereotype racial responses, and ultimately deprive the patients of a thorough uncovering and working through of their particular difficulties. In therapy, global denial or avoidance of race by a therapist or the immediate definition of all references to race as defensive can greatly compromise patient efforts to distinguish their own internal conflicts from the external realities they are responding to and can severely jeopardize the working alliance. Appreciating the importance of countertransference reactions and gaining a capacity to consider the roots of these reactions within oneself is a major aspect of the training of all psychotherapists. It is clear that this can also be a most critical variable in a psychiatrist's attempt to work with individuals from different cultural backgrounds.

Though much skepticism remains in the literature regarding the feasibility of effective psychotherapy across potential cultural barriers, Boyer's work with Apache Indians beautifully demonstrates the extent of meaningful interaction that can be accomplished (Boyer 1964). As Boyer describes, he and his wife approached their work with the assumption that ignorance and prejudice were major obstacles to establishing meaningful interaction between members of dissimilar ethnic groups. They thus learned the Apache language and studied available literature describing aboriginal Indian culture. As they began their work it was necessary for them to modify their frame of reference considerably when they learned from their interactions how the older cultural values and attitudes had been subject to considerable modification secondary to the influence of modern society. They commented also on the value of their personal analysis and the importance of keeping a consistent focus on the intended goal of their interactions. With these efforts it apparently did not take long for Boyer to be accepted in the role of a healer (a Shaman) and for the Indian patients he interacted with to gain significant benefit from his essentially unmodified, interpretative, psychotherapeutic technique. Boyer concludes the report of his work as follows:

> I am convinced that a principal source of difficulty in giving therapeutic treatment consists in the therapist's injecting his own personal problems into the therapeutic dyad. Members of cross-ethnic groups confront us with special problems because of the prejudices inculcated in us throughout our lives, because of our ignorance, and because of our tendency to think of them as children and their tendency to think of us as authoritarians. In dealing with our clients, we must be on guard against imposing our own problems on them or distorting the goals of the therapeutic relationship. It behooves us to examine our reactions and behavior carefully and to take steps to rectify them when we have hints that they may have been determined by countertransference phenomena.

RACISM

Perhaps the single most important fact for educators, trainees, and practitioners alike to realize is that the processes that determine the perpetuation of conscious and unconscious racist behavior are longstanding and profoundly resistant to change. Racism is defined by the United

States Commission on Civil Rights as "any attitude, action or institutional structure which subordinates a person or group because of his or her color" (Shapiro 1974). It is emphasized that this is an "operational" definition. It addresses how individuals actually behave, not how they consciously perceive their behavior. Implicit in this is the awareness that racism persists in the United States despite considerable conscious efforts to understand and change it. Numerous theories have been developed by behavioral scientists (Allport 1954, J.M. Jones 1972, R.L. Jones 1972, Kovel 1970, Pettigrew 1964, Pinderhughes 1970, Willie et al 1973) as possible explanations of the determinants of racism. The number of these theories, in part, reflects the complexity of the issue and also indicates the urgent need for a more integrated systematic approach to the problem. Hauser (1973) summarizes the current status of these clinical and research dilemmas as follows:

> The question of which forces underlie racist ideology and behavior and their varying degrees of importance is an empirical one....On the basis of studies of ideology and behavior we would suspect that generating and supporting racist behavior and thought are many levels of determinants which range from the intrapsychic to the abstract empirical systems of cultural symbols and beliefs. The type of explanation which will clarify the nature of racism will likely be one that formulates interactions of variables from several levels of complexities.

Hauser's review of the dilemmas involved in approaching questions about racism and psychiatry was prompted by his reading of Thomas and Sillen (1972). He identifies and recognizes the evidence outlined earlier that demonstrates ethnocentric influences on current mental health care and research efforts. He also notes the danger of reductionism, oversimplification, and selective attention that can compromise further attempts to understand and ratify the existing problems. The psychologic dimensions he considers relevant to the understanding of racism "include the group's or individual's level of awareness, the interplay between personal ideology and the group's cultural history, conscious and unconscious individual fantasies and the symbolic meanings held by individuals." The major task facing behavioral scientists in the decades to come will be efforts to correlate vast amounts of data from clinical psychosocial work, psychologic research, anthropologic studies, knowledge of animal behavior, and economic forces into more comprehensive hypotheses that can eventually be subjected to systematic, scientific evaluation.

Of particular note in terms of current theories regarding the origins of ethocentricity is the recognition that denigration of minority groups and simultaneous aggrandizement of the white majority within the United States is but one example of a ubiquitous pattern of human behavior

(Bion 1961, Frank 1967, Pinderhughes 1964, 1969a, 1969b, 1970, 1974; Poussaint 1969). As Person (1969) describes:

> History as the story of mankind chronicles largely the resolution and nonresolution of group conflicts. The group may be defined by a distinction of race, religion, language, culture, class or geographical boundaries, but the distinction is jealously guarded and is usually prized at about the value of common humanity. Prejudice, national supremacy, manifest destinies, wars and genocide on behalf of such group distinctions span the centuries and continents and seem almost universal.

Efforts to understand the dynamics of group behavior and the complex interface between individual personality structure and social processes lend themselves to a working hypothesis regarding the origins of racism. Pinderhughes (1964, 1969a, 1969b, 1970, 1971, 1974, 1979) has written extensively on his observations of interactions of individuals in groups. He describes a process of nonpathologic paranoia that has its beginnings in very early stages of intrapsychic development. As an infant attempts to maintain a sense of object constancy in its relationship with principal objects in its environment, ambivalent, intense, primitive, sexual and aggressive feelings are split; aggressive, potentially destructive affects are projected onto external bad objects while affiliative, positive, libidinal affects are projected and introjected in relation to good objects. As he describes, "In childhood idealization of familiar persons and fear of strange ones develops at an early age. Positive attributes are projected upon the known and negative on the unknown within the first year of life" (1970).

Pinderhughes is one of many authors who had noted that adult experiences in groups reactivate these early paranoid patterns of perception and relating (Bion 1961, Colman 1975, Jacques 1955, Miller and Rice 1964, Rice 1965). Winnicott's (1953) description of how cultural value systems are substituted for earlier transitional objects and allow for gradual decreased attachment to parental figures is an important conceptual link. It also adds considerable understanding to the reason why such phenomena are resistant to change. Again, as Pinderhughes summarizes:

> There is a need in the child part of human personality for constancy in relationship to the principal object relied on, whether this be a mother, a transitional object, a family or social group, or some component of a culture. Attachments to parents and to transitional objects weaken as cultural attachments develop. Whether they be adaptive or not and whether developing within one's group or imposed by outsiders, important cultural elements are clung to by adults with the intensity with which children cling to mothers, lollipops and teddy bears.

Jacques (1955) refers to Melanie Klein's work as he similarly postulates that adult individuals unconsciously use their interactions in institutions (or any group) to reinforce defenses against the early infantile experiences of persecutory (paranoid) and depressive anxiety. Klein in fact first described how a small infant defends against the anxiety and depression aroused by an inconstant parenting figure by splitting off and projecting the painful and potentially destructive ambivalent feelings onto some external object. Introjective, positive identification with members of the same societal subgroup provides individuals with a sense of security, which further reinforces the collusion to believe their projected fantasies. The minority subgroups acquiesce, again unconsciously, to the societal fantasies of inferiority because of the guilt that accompanies such affects.

Two examples from Pinderhughes' writings serve to highlight the actualization of such group dynamics within American culture. His 1964 article describes the historical realities of de facto segregation that was defined as a rigidly closed system within which Black individuals, families, and groups have been forced to develop. The sense of bondage and the need to behave in a docile, compliant manner while facing constant devaluation, have contributed significantly to internalizations of feelings of inferiority associated with being Black. These internalized self-representations further perpetuate the process of denigration and devaluation among minority group members. Black teachers in ghetto schools as well as Black parents have had to educate their children (both consciously and unconsciously) according to existing cultural norms.

In his 1970 article, Pinderhughes describes how the mass media served to perpetuate racist beliefs. During the civil rights movement of the 1960s, both Martin Luther King and Malcolm X were prominent Black leaders. The media rarely reported the activities and teachings of Dr. King except when he marshalled impressive major demonstrations. His teachings were based on the highest avowed national and religious ideals of this country, stressing mutual consideration, respect, sharing, and equality. Malcolm X supported the development of a more separate constructive self-rehabilitative and self-developing Black cultural identity. What the news media predominantly presented during the integration movement, however, was an image of Malcolm X's teachings as threatening, dangerous, destructive attacks on the white established majority's lives and institutions. The media's representation of his teaching with regard to whites portrayed them as unable to change, untrustworthy, exploitative, and "destructive to black men, as some kind of devils who had altered them, destroyed their families, group, culture, morality and basic humanity." Thus, the repressed primitive aggressive fantasies of both subgroups were presented by the media, offering further "validation" of the false, unconscious beliefs and greatly increasing resistance to substantive change.

When such deep-seated psychologic factors are identified as major determinants of human behavior, there is often a pessimistic response to any hopes for altering such phenomena. However, as with our work as individual psychotherapists, raising to conscious awareness previously unconscious motivation for behavior can stimulate further rational consideration and create problem-solving efforts. My own awareness of the existence of these unconscious forces came initially from participating in the A.K. Rice Institution Residential Conference on Group Process (Rice 1965). Rice developed the framework for these conferences from Bion's (1961) descriptions of groups. Bion's observation of group process included the primitive patterns of psychic defense mechanisms. He further described a constant tension within any group between a "work group mentality," where members of the group utilized their intellectual and other resources to address the group task, and a "basic assumption group mentality," which is dominated by shared group fantasies. Scapegoating and polarization of groups into minority and majority factions are part of the "fight/flight" basic assumption group mentality. The other two basic assumption group mentalities Bion described are the pairing and dependent groups. The A.K. Rice Institution Conferences are educational experiences designed to make manifest many of the unconscious processes that collectively affect individuals working in groups. As the racial, sexual, and educational backgrounds of the staff and membership of these conferences are intentionally diverse, many stereotypic attitudes are vividly acted out as conference members try to deal with the stressful tasks presented to them. Certainly, awareness of such dynamic processes can help educators and trainees alike in their endeavors to learn about ethnocentric attitudes within psychiatry without unconsciously neglecting these issues or reenacting the patterns in clinical, education and research settings.

OTHER AREAS OF PSYCHIATRIC EDUCATION

Understanding the patient's cultural (psychosocial) background is clearly needed in the areas of medical consultation, and medical student education, and primary care physician education. In addition, a number of authors (Brown 1976, Frank 1967, 1977, Lifton 1975, Wedge 1967) have written about the potential contributions a psychiatrist can make to efforts to resolve larger social issues including sought-for peaceful resolutions of international conflicts. If in fact such conflicts stem from the type of group-related dynamics described here, further research into these processes can have far-reaching applications.

BIBLIOGRAPHY

Allport GW: *The Nature of Prejudice: A Psychohistory.* Reading, Mass, Addison-Wesley, 1954.

Bernard VW: Psychoanalysis and members of minority groups. *J American Psychoanal Assoc* 1:256–257, 1953.

Bion WR: *Experiences in Groups and Other Papers.* New York, Ballantine, 1961.

Boyer B: Psychoanalytic insights in working with ethnic minorities. *Soc Casework* 519–526, Nov, 1964.

Bradshaw WH: Training psychiatrists for working with blacks in basic residency programs. *Am J Psychiatry* 135(12):1520–1523, 1978.

Brown BS: The life of psychiatry. *Am J Psychiatry* 133: 489–495, 1976.

Calnek M: Racial factors in the countertransferences: The black therapist and the black client. *Am J Orthopsychiatry* 40(1):39–40, 1970.

Cohen RE: Borderline conditions: Transcultural perspective. *Psychiatr Ann* 4(9):7–20, 1974.

Colman AD: Group consciousness as a developmental phase, in Colman AD, Bexton WH (eds): *Group Relations Reader.* San Francisco, Associated Printing and Publishing, 1975.

Draquns JG: Values reflected on psychopathology: The case of the protestant ethic. *Ethos* 2:115–136, 1974.

Fiman BG, Nordlie PG, Witten DL, et al: *Development of Quantitative Indices of Institutional Change with Regard to Racial Minorities and Women in NIMH External Programs.* McLean, Va, Human Sciences Research, 1975.

Fischer N: An interracial analysis: Transference and countertransference significance. *J Am Psychoanal Assoc* 19(4):736–745, 1971.

Frank J: *Sanity and Survival: The Psychological Aspects of War and Peace.* New York, Vintage, 1967.

Frank J: Psychiatry, the healthy invalid. *Am J Psychiatry* 134:1349–1355, 1977.

Gross H, Herbert MR, Khatterud GL, et al: The effect of race and sex on the variation of diagnosis and disposition in a psychiatric emergency room. *J Nerv Ment Dis* 48(6):638–642, 1969.

Hauser ST: Racism and psychiatry. Thinking about race and racism: Clinical and research dilemmas. *Int J Group Psychother* 23(2):242–259, 1973.

Jackson AM: Race as a variable affecting the treatment involvement of children. *J Am Acad Child Psychiatry* 13(1):20–31, 1974.

Jacques E: Social systems as a defense against persecutory and depressive anxiety, in Klein M, Heimann P, Morey-Kyrly RF (eds): *New Directions in Psychoanalysis.* New York, Basic Books, 1955, pp 478–498.

Jones BE, Lightfoot OB, Palmer D, et al: Psychiatric residents in white training institutions. *Am J Psychiatry* 127:798–803, 1970.

Jones JM: *Prejudice and Racism.* Reading, Mass, Addison-Wesley, 1972.

Jones RL (ed): *Black Psychology.* New York, Harper & Row, 1972.

Kerner O, Lindsay JV, Harris FR, et al: *Report of the National Advisory Commission on Civil Disorders.* Washington, DC, U.S. Government Printing Office, 1968.

King LM: Social and cultural influences on psychopathology. *Ann Rev Psychol* 29:405–433, 1978.

Kovel J: *White Racism: A Psychohistory.* New York, Pantheon, 1970.

Lifton RJ: Advocacy and corruption in the healing professions. *Conn Med* 39:803–813, 1975.

Miller EJ, Rice AK: *Systems of Organization*. London, Tavistock, 1964.

Pardes H: Academic psychiatry and national issues: An address. *J Operational Psychiatry* 9(2):5–10, 1978.

Person ES: Racism: Evil or ill. *Int J Psychiatry* 8:929–933, 1969.

Pettigrew TF: *A Profile of the Negro American*. Princeton, Van Nostrand, 1964.

Pinderhughes CA: Effects of ethnic group concentration upon educational process, personality formation and mental health. *J Natl Med Assoc* 56(5):407–414, 1964.

Pinderhughes CA: The origins of racism. *Int J Psychiatry* 8:934–941, 1969a.

Pinderhughes CA: Understanding black power: Processes and prospects. *Am J Psychiatry* 125(11):106–111, 1969b.

Pinderhughes CA: The universal resolution of ambivalence by paranoia with an example in black and white. *Am J Psychother* 24:597, 1970.

Pinderhughes CA: Psychological and physiological origins of racism and other social discrimination. *J Natl Med Assoc* 63(1):25–29, 1971.

Pinderhughes CA: Ego development and cultural differences. *Am J Psychiatry* 131(2):171–175, 1974.

Pinderhughes CA: Differential bonding: Toward a psychophysiological theory of stereotyping. *Am J Psychiatry* 136(1): 33–38, 1979.

Poussaint AF: Racism and psychiatry. *Int J Psychiatry* 8:942–944, 1969.

President's Commission on Mental Health: Report. *ADAMHA News* 4(7):47, Apr 28, 1978.

Rice AK: *Learning for Leadership*. London, Tavistock, 1965.

Rosenfeld AH (ed): *Psychiatric Education: Prologue to the 1980s*. Baltimore, Garamond/Pridemark, 1976.

Ruffin JE: Racism as countertransference in psychotherapy groups. *Perspect Psychiatr Care* 11(4):172–178, 1973.

Senate Bill 2373: Minority Mental Health Program Act of 1977, December 15, 1977 (introduced by Senators Inouye and Matsunaga).

Sabshin M, Diensenhaus H, Wilkeson R: Dimensions of institutional racism in psychiatry. *Am J Psychiatry* 127:787–793, 1970.

Schacter J, Butts HF: Transference and countertransference in inter-racial analysis. *J Am Psychoanal Assoc* 16:792–808, 1968.

Semrad EV, Van Buskirk D: *Teaching Psychotherapy of Psychotic Patients: Supervision of Beginning Residents in the "Clinical Approach."* New York, Grune & Stratton, 1969.

Shapiro RM: Racism and community mental health. Unpublished paper, 1974. (Available through author: Assistant Chief for Racism and Mental Health, NIMH, Rockville, Maryland.)

Stanley S: Community mental health services to minority groups. *Am Psychol* 32(3):616–624, 1977.

Steadman HJ: The psychiatrist as a conservation agent of social control. *Soc Probl* 20:263–271, 1978.

Thomas A, Sillen S: *Racism and Psychiatry*. New York, Brunner/Mazel, 1972.

Ticho GR: Cultural aspects of transference and countertransference. *Bull Menninger Clin* 35(5):313–334, 1971.

Wedge B: Psychiatry and international affairs. *Science* 157:281–285, 1967.

Wilder J: Value and psychotherapy. *Am J Psychother* 23(3):405–414, 1969.

Willie V, Kramer BM, Brown BS (eds): *Racism and Mental Health: Essays*. Pittsburgh, University of Pittsburgh Press, 1973.

Winnicott DW: Transitional objects and transitional phenomena. *Int J Psychoanal* 34:89–97, 1953.

Wittkower ED: Cultural aspects of psychotherapy. *Am J Psychother* 28:566–573, 1974.

Yamamoto J: Cultural problems in psychiatric therapy. *Arch Gen Psychiatry* 19:45–49, 1968.

18 Discussion: Cultural Issues in Psychiatric Training: Perspectives of Training Directors and Residents

Lindbergh S. Sata, MD

Dr. Wilkeson's astute and sensitive presentation reinforces the principle that people learn when they are ready to learn and conversely tend not to learn if they are not open to learning. Wilkeson has suggested in her presentation there was insufficient attention to cultural relevance in her psychiatric training, that such is the norm rather than the exception in most training programs, that institutional racism still pervades much of academia, and that, despite good intentions of faculties, their behaviors suggest either gross stupidity or cultural insensitivity or both. I doubt that one would seriously contest such a statement. At the same time, there is an aspect of myself responding with a twinge of amusement while carrying on a parallel conversation with myself and asking the question, "Who is this person who says she has been attended to poorly?" As I examine her paper I am struck with the inclusion of 55 references in her bibliography, the vast majority of which are current and within the past 4 to 5 years. If her paper reflects inadequate attention to cultural issues alluded to earlier or is a product of self-correction to offset a deprived educational experience, perhaps she has not done badly in her psychiatric training.

Her comments bring back comparable questions I raised during my training regarding inaccessibility of mental health services for minority populations. At that time there were several standard references provided which included Allport's text, *The Nature of Prejudice,* an article by Viola Bernard, and several studies from within the field of sociology. My continuing to raise questions regarding nonuse of mental health services by Mexican Americans led eventually to a 4-year project of attempting to establish an exchange training program between Latin American countries and the United States. While that experience was extremely educational and valuable for me, nothing substantive was accomplished to improve the plight of Mexican American patients seeking mental health services.

To place things into proper perspective, my generation of psychiatric residents were of a different time from Wilkeson's generation, and we were also of a different psychologic set. To begin with, rapid transportation was still being introduced in the late 1950s, television and mass media communication were still not completely developed, and most minority populations were oppressed, persecuted, and preoccupied with their own survival with little awareness, interest, or desire to engage with other persons of color. The concept of identification with the aggressor was well ingrained as evidenced by my first name or the names of four ethnic brothers among my acquaintances whose first names were Grant, McKinley, Lincoln, and Hoover. Such an orientation reinforced preexistent ethnocentric biases as well as justifying more recently acquired prejudices regarding less fortunate minority groupings.

As I think about it, my early interactions were clumsy and characterized by learning through trial and error. As a child, along with other children, I threw racial slurs at anyone and everyone at the border of my neighborhood, which was a ghetto. My community was adjacent to skid row and sandwiched between the Chinese, Black, and Filipino communities. As children we resembled vocal butterflies fluttering around strangers and throwing racial epithets only so long as our victims were moving away, but we would rapidly retreat if they stopped or returned. Our belief systems regarding others were simple, racist, and constantly associated with fantasies of violence as we truly believed Chinese used hatchets, whites their hands, Blacks razors, and Filipinos guns, and all were to be avoided. The world as we experienced it was constantly hostile, and we fervently believed the only ones who truly practiced fairness, democracy, and patriotism were we. It was unquestionably bigotry in its finest hour.

The disruptive impact of World War II, while clearly outside the scope of this discussion, placed me in peculiar occupational roles, each associated with specific cultural learnings. As a migratory farmworker, I worked with German and Italian POWs before attending the University.

In my premedical years I worked as a houseboy, waiter, dishwasher, delivery boy, bellboy, and postal worker with other minority coworkers. In medical school I tended bar for several years in a private Black club and was further exposed to similarities and differences in still another fascinating learning setting. All during these experiences I recurrently found myself confronting myself with my racism as I gradually came to appreciate persons of other cultures.

Wilkeson's paper evoked recollections catapulting me back through time to residency training. It brings into sharp relief my first encounter with a person of color in psychiatry whose response to my question, "Are there other Japanese psychiatrists in the United States?" brought out a thoughtful and reflective response, "Not many." The truth of the matter was that the dyad, namely Joe Yamamoto and I, constituted one-seventh of all Japanese American psychiatrists in the United States at that time. We had little knowledge of other Asian psychiatrists and, in fact, we were still experiencing isolation from our non-Japanese Asian colleagues as a result of enmity growing out of World War II. The *1963 APA Directory,* which was the earliest reference I could readily obtain, identified a total of 63 Asian psychiatrists composed of 7 Filipinos, 30 Chinese, 3 Koreans, 5 Indian, 14 Japanese, 3 Pakistani, and 1 Ceylonese. In the half which followed we have experienced a phenomenal expansion of Asian psychiatric resources from a total of 63 in 1963 to 1486 in 1978. While on the one hand we have had a phenomenal growth spurt, the vast majority of Asian psychiatrists are foreign medical graduate physicians. During the 15 years since the *1963 APA Directory* finding, United States medical graduate Asian psychiatrists have grown from 21 to approximately 80, while foreign medical graduate psychiatrists have grown from 42 in 1963 to approximately 1400 in 1979.

Given the recent influx of major numbers of Asian foreign medical graduate psychiatrists, any consideration for incorporating culturally relevant training must simultaneously address sensitizing and educating foreign medical graduate psychiatrists if they are to contribute to the treatment of minority populations. We have a responsibility for developing stratagems to prevent foreign medical graduate psychiatrists from being scapegoated since, like it or not, they do constitute a primary group of psychiatrists providing mental health services to minority populations. This development places the least culturally knowledgeable psychiatrists with the responsibility of treating diverse patient groupings that require the greatest degree of cultural sensitivity and understanding.

Charles and Elaine Pinderhughes' chapter is carefully and thoughtfully developed and, indeed, reflects ongoing efforts to address cultural perspectives within psychiatric training. While I both applaud and envy what has been possible in the Boston area, there are some nagging problems pertaining to implementation of such a program in other settings.

There are some givens that need to be stated explicitly if we are to be successful. Training programs must have minority faculty to be successful. While didactic seminars and readings may not necessarily require persons of color as resources, clinical training and the development of a working knowledge of cultural influences is probably not possible without the sensitivity of having experienced how it is to be a minority group member and a person of color. In this regard, foreign medical graduate Asian psychiatrists may not fully appreciate minority status since their origins are from countries in which they enjoyed majority rather than minority status.

There are other limitations needing to be further recognized. In the absence of sufficient numbers of minority groupings, culturally relevant training may be harder to implement. Certainly without faculty who are sensitive and committed, it may be difficult to mobilize local teaching personnel who might theoretically support such training.

And lastly, without adequate numbers of residents there may be lessened opportunities to develop small-group discussions and the sharing of new information. The current pool of incoming residents into psychiatry has shrunk from 12% of graduating seniors to less than 4% of graduating seniors currently electing psychiatry as their specialty. There is nothing to indicate a reversal of this trend, particularly in the face of increasing popularity of family medicine as a newly emerging specialty discipline.

Cultural sensitivity requires curiosity, interest in others, and the willingness to expend time and energy to identify, monitor, and synthesize complex verbal and nonverbal communications. One needs to be reflective as well as responsive to the intent of the communication before a meaningful interactive mode can be developed. Since cultural sensitivity is learned behavior, it can be momentarily forgotten, overlooked, overprescribed, or avoided and therefore may be identified by others as inconsistent, insincere, bigoted, insensitive, or racist. What is less appreciated is the recognition that many psychiatric professionals with commitments for humanism may lose their more recently acquired culturally sensitive behaviors in the presence of stress. Many colleagues in the face of heavy clinical demands appear incapable of sustaining intellectually agreeable, culturally responsive behaviors, and such inconsistencies trigger racial conflicts among staff. This would occur most commonly when the workload exceeded the psychologic and physical capabilities of staff.

Problems would manifest themselves as staff members act out their discomfort of working with excessive numbers of acutely psychotic patients. An expression of such acting out could entail selective inattention for patients of color or disproportionate assignment of minority patients to minority staff. Staff members, whether minority or majority, might appear able to intellectualize and appreciate sociocultural factors, including societal oppression as partial explanations for paranoid and aggressive responses of minority patients. But when stressed with increased clinical responsibilities, staff might respond to such aggressive behaviors with rejection or fear or both, with a resultant inability to work with the patient with a sense of compassion and understanding. Furthermore, aggressive behaviors by majority and minority patients might receive differential responses; majority patients being dealt with appropriately while minority patients are frequently avoided, ignored, or transferred to long-term care institutions. Trainees, including medical students and psychiatric residents, might not only be exposed to confusing and contradictory views but also be coopted by staff factions needlessly.

The inability to incorporate concepts such as culture-bound syndromes is on a higher level of conceptualization as contrasted to the continuing tendency to identify all Asiatic patients as chronic schizophrenics. This error takes place in spite of repeated demonstrations by the patients themselves of successfully resolving psychotic symptoms within the first several days of hospitalization. Despite such occurrences, diagnoses are rarely altered, and the chronicity label becomes immutably established.

In implementing training programs with attention to cultural relevance, certain ingredients are required and may be quickly worth reviewing. Certainly, an appropriate mix of minority-majority patients is needed. A city such as Boston is unusual because of its Asian, Black and Hispanic populations as well as easily identifiable multiethnic communities. In some cities a training program may address only a narrow socioeconomic majority population segment, in which case cultural relevance appears moot and academic.

I have the peculiar sense that culturally relevant training has some of the same problems of implementation as the equal rights movement. In a short statement by Palmer four stages have been described in the enlightenment of people to the equal rights movement: 1) the introductory phase of curiosity and exploration; 2) a period of identification associated with the sharing of a common language and interacting with other women in a collaborative mode in the definition of their position in relation to others; 3) one of affective change stemming from the recognition of past transgressions and of the role of women in the process of victimization; and 4) consolidation with a shifting of a sense of helplessness to a problem-solving orientation. Whether one talks of cultural relevance in training or the equal rights movement, the principal obstacles appear to be tied to phase 3, in which individuals and programs appear incapable of completing the affective crossover. From my experience this tends not to occur for psychiatrists unless they are individuals who have worked extensively with people of different cultures.

While progress is slow, there appears to be the continued accumulation of culturally relevant data and an accumulation of resource individuals. The recently highly publicized work by Alex Haley has popularized and legitimized the concept of examining one's origins. In another development, even closer to the profession of psychiatry, is the recent creation of a task force within the American Psychiatric Association on ethnicity and chaired by Dr. John Spiegel.

In closing, the road we have been exploring is a familiar one with many renowned past travelers. The opportunities to interact with and share views with the Alexander Leightons, the Paul Lemkaus, and the Eugene Brodys have opened up new vistas of understanding across many cultures. I am also aware of the relatively modest impact we have had in incorporating culturally relevant training in psychiatric residency training programs. Perhaps the gradual acceptance of culturally relevant training within psychiatry will occur as Tsung-yi Lin has suggested: when we legitimize our collective activities with research and develop investigative models to captivate the interest of our academic colleagues. Perhaps on another level, as minority populations continue to grow in numbers, our profession, albeit belatedly, will address these issues collectively.

APPENDIX A

THE FUNCTIONAL PREREQUISITES OF A SOCIETY

D.F. Aberle, A.K. Cohen, A.K. Davis, M.J. Levy, Jr., F.X. Sutton

A comparative social science requires a generalized system of concepts which will enable the scientific observer to compare and contrast large bodies of concretely different social phenomena in consistent terms. A promising step in furthering the development[1] of systematic social analysis is a tentative formulation of the functional prerequisites of a society. Functional prerequisites refer broadly to the things that must get done in any society if it is to continue as a going concern, ie, the generalized conditions necessary for the maintenance of the system concerned. The specific structural arrangements for meeting the functional prerequisites differ, of course, from one society to another and, in the course of time, change in any given society.[2]

This paper offers 1) a definition of a society on the most general level; 2) a statement of four generalized conditions, the complete realization of any one of which would terminate the existence of a society as defined; 3) a list of the functional prerequisites of a society. It seeks to justify the inclusion of each prerequisite by the demonstration that in its hypothetical absence the society could not survive, since at least one of the four conditions terminating a society would occur. There is no reason to believe that the list of functional prerequisites offered here is definitive. It is subject to revision with the growth of general theory and with experience in its application to concrete situations.

Any formation of functional prerequisites depends for its categories on the theory of action employed. Our theory of action uses the concept of an actor whose orientation to his situation is threefold: cognitive, affective, and goal-directed. The actor is an abstraction from the total

---

Reprinted with permission of author and University of Chicago Press. From *Ethics*, 60 (January 1960), 100–111.

[1]Already well under way. Cf. Talcott Parsons, "The Position of Sociological Theory," *American Sociological Review, XIII (1948),* 156–64, and the references cited therein, esp. the "Discussion" by Robert K. Merton, *ibid.,* pp. 164–68.

[2]Thus all societies must allocate goods and services somehow. A particular society may change from one method, say business enterprise, to another, say a centrally planned economy, without the destruction of the society as a society but merely with a change in its concrete structures.

We seek to avoid the limitation inherent in defining the function of a social element solely in terms of its contribution to the survival or maintenance of the particular system of which it is a component. Structural analysis, which has recently undergone notable development, is prone to focus attention on static equilibriums. We consider *what* must be done in *any* society and hope our effort may be of use in considering the alterations that take place in *how* things are done in a society while that society persists.

human being. Many of the qualities of the human being constitute part of the situation, the set of means and conditions, within which the actor operates.[3]

Though the definition of the functional prerequisites of a society logically precedes the development of a scheme of structural prerequisites — which tell *how* the functional prerequisites may be met — in actuality the theoretic development of the two approaches is indivisible.

A DEFINITION OF A SOCIETY

The unit we have selected for analysis is a *society,* such as a nation, tribe, or band, and not any social system in general. The statement of the functional prerequisites of *any social system* — a monastery, a church, or a town, for example — would be on two general a level for the present discussion, though it may be an important task. Furthermore, once the functional prerequisites of a society are outlined, it becomes easier to state those of other types of social systems, often by dropping certain prerequisites from the list, since most of these other types of systems are parts of a society (or result from the interrelations of two or more societies) and depend for their perpetuation on the existence of a society.

A society is a group of human beings sharing a self-sufficient system of action which is capable of existing longer than the life-span of an individual, the group being recruited at least in part by the sexual reproduction of the members.

The identity and continuity of a society inhere in the persistence of the system of action in which the actors participate rather than in the particular set of actors themselves. There may be a complete turnover of individuals, but the society may survive. The individuals may survive, but the society may disintegrate. A system may persist in a situation while its component relationships change. Its persistence inheres in the fact that it maintains its separation from the situation, ie, it inheres in the *integrity* of the organism, not in its fixity or unalterable character.

A system of action always exists in a situation. In the case of a society this situation includes the nonhuman environment and, in almost every case, it includes other societies. The viability of a social system and its recognition as a society within the terms of this definition depend upon the particular set of conditions in which it functions. Study of the system itself cannot alone determine whether the system meets the criteria of the definition. What is crucial is that a social system contain successful

---

[3]Neither the nature of the dependence of our formulation on this theory of action nor the theory of action itself can be further elaborated here. The theory of action is outlined briefly in Talcott Parsons, *Essays in Sociological Theory* (Glencoe: Free Press, 1949), pp. 32–33.

arrangements for meeting the chronic and recurrent features of its milieu.[4]

"Longer than the life-span of an individual" reminds us that a society must be able to replace its members with effectively socialized individuals from the maturing generation. The requirement of sexual reproduction excludes from consideration such groups (monasteries, cliques) as depend *solely* on types of recruitment other than sexual. But a society may be recruited in part by non-sexual means, eg, by immigration and conquest.

The heart of the definition is "self-sufficient system of action."[5] Its full meaning will be developed in the exposition of the functional prerequisites and in the next paragraphs.

A number of questions are bound to arise in the reader's mind as to the application of the definition to particular social systems and as to the basis on which the decision is to be made as to whether such systems fall within the definition of a society. We emphasize that the definition is an ideal type. *A concrete aggregate is a society in so far as it approaches the generalized model.* The following examples, though not definitive, suggest the way in which the definition may be applied.

A society is not a culture. Culture is socially transmitted behavior conceived as an abstraction from concrete social groups. Two or more *societies* may have the same *culture* or similar cultures. Though the Greek city-states shared similar culture patterns, each possessed a self-sufficient structure of action and is hence to be considered a separate society. One society may be composed of groups with some marked differences in culture. The union of agricultural, industrial, and pastoral groups in a single structure of action is an example. We discuss below the limits as to the amount of diversity possible and the conditions under which such diversity may occur without the disintegration of the society.

To some degree two different societies may possess overlapping personnel and even structural elements without losing their identity as distinct societies. The fact that Englishmen live in the United States as diplomats and traders and function, in effect, as actors in both systems, does not destroy the identity or the self-sufficiency of the United States or of Great Britian as action-systems.

To be considered a society, a group need not be self-sufficient with

---

[4]This point receives further treatment below. A social system need not be copperplated to meet the definition of a society. Natural catastrophe may terminate a concrete society. Such an event does not represent a failure to meet the functional prerequisites but is rather to be considered the result of a change in the nonhuman environment beyond the limits assumed here as the setting of a society. Many concrete societies have been assimilated by the expansions of groups with which these societies had had little or no previous contact. This, too, represents an alteration in the situation of the society beyond the limits within which it had been meeting its functional prerequisites.

[5]"System" and "structure" will be used interchangeably throughout the remainder of this treatment.

respect to resources. It is the structure of action that must be self-sufficient. Thus, the United States is a society. While imports and exports are necessary to its maintenance, arrangements for foreign trade are part of its self-sufficient structure of action. It is this, and not the group of individuals, that is self-sufficient. Hence Chinese-American trade does not make China and America parts of a larger society. Trade relationships are limited and relatively unstable. Their existence does not involve the two aggregates in the same self-sufficient structure of action. For parallel reasons the British Empire and the United Nations are not societies but associations.

A series of difficult decisions about the relationships of various social systems can be resolved by the introduction of a point of crucial differentiation. When a social aggregate is not capable of providing a structure, structures, or parts of structures which can meet the functional prerequisites in question, it is not to be considered a society. Thus, occupied Japan does not constitute part of American society, since in the absence of American forces Japan would seem to be able to continue control and the legitimized use of force. A group of American Indians governed by the United States for a sufficient length of time may lack the crucial structures necessary for continued existence as an independent entity and therefore be considered part of American society, in spite of an important cultural variation. An American town does not constitute a society because of its thorough participation in American political, economic, value, and other structures. The early Mormon settlement in Utah, however, did constitute a society.[6]

Under what circumstances do considerations of social change lead us to speak of a "new" society? Whenever social change results in a change of social structure on the most general level under consideration, we shall speak of a "new society" having been brought about. Such transitions may be gradual (evolutionary) or sudden and chaotic (revolutionary). The determination of the exact point of change may be extremely complex but is in theory possible. This criterion for a "new society" will not ordinarily enter the study of comparative institutions unless the developmental picture of some particular society (or societies) is under consideration.

We assume that social change characterizes all societies. Change may be gradual and peaceful or characterized by severe conflicts. In either case there may be profound structural changes. Societies may split or merge

---

[6]There is no intention of making the political variable the sole criterion for the decision as to what constitutes a society. The nature of economic ties, the degree to which value-systems are shared, and the like are also crucial in making the differentiation between two systems of action.

Thus the decision as to the distinctness of two or more aggregates as societies rests on the analysis of all aspects of the systems of action, and not merely of a single variable, in their consequences for the self-sufficient character of the systems of action. Borderline cases undoubtedly exist, but the treatment made here is sufficiently refined for the purposes at hand.

peacefully or violently. In all these instances a society of some sort exists. Whether it is considered the same society or a new one depends on the relation between the level of the stuctural change and the level of analysis. The changes in question may be analyzed in terms of this frame of reference. We may examine the way in which a society meets its functional prerequisites, the points of tension (those functional prerequisites least effectively met), and the responses to those strains. We do not assume the perfect integration of any society.

We have omitted from our definition any statements regarding territoriality. Action, it has been pointed out, always takes place in a situation, one feature of which is a spatial dimension. The existence of two societies intermingled during a civil war, or any such example, does not negate considerations of spatiality, which are always an essential background feature of any society.

FOUR CONDITIONS TERMINATING THE EXISTENCE OF A SOCIETY

The realization of any of the following conditions terminates the existence of a society — the existence of the structure of action, though not necessarily of the members.

A. *The biological extinction or dispersion of the members.* — To arrive at this condition, a society need not lose all its members but need only suffer such losses as to make inoperative its structure of action. Analyses of such conditions may be made at this level in terms of fertility, morbidity, and migration rates, without reference to the highly complex factors underlying them.[7]

B. *Apathy of the members.* — Apathy means the cessation of individual motivation. This condition affects some individuals to some extent in all societies and large numbers in a few societies. That migrant Polynesian laborers have died of nostalgia is well known. It is claimed that whole societies in Melanesia have withered away from ennui. In these cases, physical extinction is merely an extreme consequence of the cessation of motivation.

C. *The war of all against all.* — This condition appears if the members of an aggregate pursue their ends by means selected only on the basis of instrumental efficiency. Though the choice of means on this basis may result at times in co-operative combinations, these combinations are by definition subject to immediate dissolution if, for example, exploita-

---

[7]In this regard certain catastrophic occurrences deriving from marked alterations in the situation are excluded from consideration in accordance with the line of reasoning previously outlined.

tion or annihilation becomes more advantageous for any one member. Hence a state of indeterminate flux, rather than a system of action, exists. The use of force is efficient only for limited purposes. Force is a sanction, but never the essence, of a society. A society based solely on force is a contradiction in terms that raises the classical question, *Quis custodiet ipsos custodes?*

D. *The absorption of the society into another society.* — This entails the partial loss of identity and self-sufficiency of the total action-system but not necessarily the extinction of the members.[8]

The more fully these four conditions are realized, the more indeterminate is the structure of action, a condition also induced when the rate of social change is very rapid. Hence we may hypothesize that fluctuations in the vital indices, in apathy, and in coercion are to some extent functions of the rate of social change. In fact, revolutions (extreme social change) are characterized by increases in mortality, morbidity, apathy, force, and fraud. The faster the change, the greater the stress, two manifestations of which are force and/or apathy. Viewing coercion as a response to stress should help us to put the discussion of the role of force in social systems on a nonideological basis.

THE FUNCTIONAL PREREQUISITES OF A SOCIETY

The performance of a given function is prerequisite to a society if in its absence one or more of the four conditions dissolving a society results. This can be demonstrated clearly in some cases. Less clearly, but still convincingly, the nonfulfillment of certain other functions can be shown at least to foster one or more of the conditions negating a society. No specific action-pattern is prerequisite to the existence of our ideal-typical society. We are concerned with *what* must get done in a society, not with *how* it is done.

A. *Provision for adequate relationship to the environment and for sexual recruitment.* — This includes modes of adapting to, manipulating, and altering the environment in such a way as (a) to maintain a sufficient number and kind of members of the society at an adequate level of functioning; (b) to deal with the existence of other societies in a manner which permits the persistence of the system of action; and (c) to pattern heterosexual relationships to insure opportunities and motivation for a

---

[8] It is worth re-emphasizing that a given society may at one time contain arrangements for maintaining its distinctness from other societies that form part of its situation, but that an alteration of that situation (the arrival of a numerically and technically superior group bent on conquest) may render these arrangements ineffective. We would not, therefore, say that the society thus absorbed had never *been* a society, but that in a *new* situation it showed a relative inadequacy of one of its functional prerequisites that resulted in its absorption.

sufficient rate of reproduction. In the absence of these provisions, the group will suffer biological extinction through the death of the members or failure to reproduce or it will suffer absorption into another social system.

A society, however, need not provide equally for the physiological needs of all its members. Infanticide, geronticide, limitation of marriage, and birth control may be necessary to maintain certain societies. Which members, and in what proportions, are most important for the functioning of a society depends on its social organization. Every society needs enough adult members to insure reproduction and to man the essential status-positions.

A society must adapt to, manipulate, and alter its situation. Among the features thus dealt with may be chronically threatening aspects of the situation. In a dry region a society may employ techniques of food storage, irrigation, nomadic migration. If neighboring societies are hostile, an army may be essential and the society thus dependent on the deliberate hazarding of some of its members' lives. The existence of Murngin society depends partly on the destruction of a portion of its adult males by chronic warfare. Resistance is only one possible response to hostile neighbors. Certain "men-o-bush" tribes of New Guinea make but little resistance to raids. These raids, however, do not threaten to extinguish the society. Only if they do can such a passive adaptation be said to be inadequate to meet the functional prerequisite.

The inclusion of such apparently disparate features as maintenance of the organism, defense, and provision for sexual reproduction under one heading is by no means arbitrary. From the point of view of a social system, the nonhuman environment, the biological nature of man, and the existence of other societies are all part of the situation of action. To none of these aspects of the situation is passive adaptation the only mode of adequate relationship. Thus the biological basis of society itself is molded. Individuals have constitutional differences, but the latter are variously evaluated and dealt with by societies. The biological birth-growth-death cycle is a dynamic process in its own right, yet societies both adapt to it and modify it in a number of ways. In noting the necessity for a society to meet certain biological prerequisites, we remark also upon the great plasticity of individuals. It is scarcely necessary to remark that, concretely, societies alter their modes of relationship to their situations; that technological changes occur, sometimes through loss, more often by invention and diffusion.

B. *Role differentiation and role assignment.* — This signifies the systematic and stable division of activities. We will treat under other headings role-learning and the sanctions perpetuating the role structure.

In any society there are activities which must be regularly performed if the society is to persist. If they are to be done dependably, these extensive and varied activities must be broken down and assigned to capable individuals trained and motivated to carry them out. Otherwise everyone would be doing everything or nothing – a state of indeterminacy which is the antithesis of a society and which precludes getting essential activities carried out. The universal problems of scarcity and order are insoluble without legitimized allocation of property rights and authority, and these, in turn, are unattainable without reasonably integrated role-differentiation. While a given individual is often the locus of several roles, he can never combine all the roles of his society in himself. Age and sex differences impose a degree of role-differentiation everywhere; in some societies class and occupation are additional bases of differentiation. Arguments for specialization based on differential ability, while of great force in complex societies, have no clear bearing on societies so simple that any technique can be learned by any individual who is not feeble-minded. Whatever the society, activities necessary to its survival must be worked out in predictable, determinate ways, or else apathy or the war of each against all must prevail. Without reliable provision for child-rearing activities and without their assignment to specific persons or groups, the society invites extinction, since children at birth are helpless. The absence of role-differentiation and of role-assignment thus makes for three of the conditions negating a society. A system of role-differentiation alone is useless without a system of selection for assigning individuals to those roles.

Mention should be made of one particular type of role-differentiation that is a requirement for any society, namely, stratification. Stratification is that particular type of role-differentiation which discriminates between higher and lower standings in terms of one or more criteria. Given the universality of scarcity, some system of differential allocation of the scarce values of a society is essential. These values may consist of such desiderata as wealth, power, magic, women and ceremonial precedence. That conflict over scarce values may destroy a society will be shown in another connection below. Our present point is that the rank order must be legitimized and accepted by most of the members – at least by the important ones – of a society if stability is to be attained. Allocation of ranks may be on the basis of ascribed or achieved qualities or both.

Role-differentiation implies organization. Precedence in specialized activities must be correlated to some extent with rank order. Coercive sanctions and initiative must be vested in specified status-positions. Some individuals will thus receive more than others. These privileges are usually made acceptable to the rank and file by joining to the greater rights of the elite a larger share of responsibilities. The Brahmins stand closer to other-worldly nonexistence than do the members of any other Hindu caste, but they also have to observe the most elaborate ritual obligations. The

Trobriand chief enjoys a multiple share of wealth and wives; he must also finance community enterprises and exhibit at all times more generosity than anyone else.

Even the simplest societies have hierarchical sex and age grading. Modern societies are much more elaborately stratified. Symbolic activities or ritual must be carefully organized to effect successfully their latent functions of allaying anxiety and recreating allegorically the basic meanings and affirmations of the society. In group enterprises some roles tend to rank others, though the individuals filling the roles may rotate freely, as in the case of the citizens of the Greek city-state. Regardless of the type of stratification and authority-system, a normative scale of priorities for allocating scarce values (precedence, property rights, power, etc.) is always a vital portion of the differntiation of roles in any society.

C. *Communication.* — Evidence from deaf-mutes, "wolf children," and bilinguals shows that speech, the basic form of communication, is learned and that only rudimentary communication is possible in the absence of shared, learned linguistic symbols. Without learned symbolic communication only a few highly general emotional states — eg, anger, sexual passion — in one individual can evoke an appropriate response in another; only a few skills may be conveyed by imitation.

No society, however simple, can exist without shared, learned symbolic modes of communication, because without them it cannot maintain the common-value structure or the protective sanctions which hold back the war of each against all. Communication is indispensable if socialization and role-differentiation are to function effectively. That each functional prerequisite thus depends in part on other functional prerequisites does not vitiate our argument so long as the functional prerequisites are logically separable. But they need not be empirically distinct activities, since any action-system may contribute to several functional prerequisites.

In a simple society, where relationships are exclusively face-to-face, shared speech forms suffice. In complex societies, other than oral communication is necessary for the system as a whole, though not for sub-systems. Thus, in China, writing facilitates the survival of the society despite local dialect differences too great to permit oral communication without bilingual intermediaries. Clearly, no modern society could survive without writing. Thus, communication requires language, a medium of communication, and channels.

D. *Shared cognitive orientations.* — In any society the members must share a body of cognitive orientations which (a) make possible adaptation to and manipulation of the situation; (b) make stable, meaningful, and predictable the social situations in which they are engaged; and (c) account for those significant aspects of the situation over which they do not have adequate prediction and control in such a way as to sustain and not to destroy motivation.

If the first criterion were not met, biological existence would be impossible. If the second were not, interpersonal and intergroup relations could not exist. Private definitions of social situations or the absence of such definitions could lead only to mutually incompatible actions and the war of each against all. In no society are all conditions predictable and controllable; so the frustration of expectations is a chronic feature of social life. Without a reasonably determinate explanation of such areas of existence, the individual would exist in an unstructured world and could not avoid psychological disorganization. In the absence of shared orientations, serious clashes would ensue.

Cognitive orientations must be shared, but only in so far as the actors are involved in the same situation of action. A housewife may not distinguish a colonel from a corporal; a solider may not appreciate that he is using his hostess' "wedding silver." They must agree, however, that a foot is "so long" and that that gentleman is a "policeman." But though a farmer may pray for rain and an aviator rub a rabbit's foot for good weather with no resultant difficulties between them both must define the American political system in a roughly similar fashion if they are to vote.

E. *A shared, articulated set of goals.* — To phrase this prerequisite in terms of ultimate ends of action produces a vague and not very useful formulation like Thomas' four wishes. It is equally difficult to operate in terms of motivations, since these are exceedingly diverse and are intricately articulated with the social structure. Our statement in terms of goals seeks a middle ground and is couched in the terms most suitable for considering a system of action.

Because there is role-differentiation in every society, we must consider a set of goals rather than a common goal. The facts of scarcity and of differential individual endowment, features of all societies, also make it necessary to speak of a set of goals. It is the range of goals, however narrow, that provides alternatives for individuals and thus reduces one serious source of conflict in societies. (The possibility of universally sought goals in a society is not ruled out.)

The goals must be sufficiently articulated to insure the performance of socially necessary activities. They must not include too much action which threatens the existence of a society. A cult of sexual abstinence, if universalized, would terminate the society. The goals must be shared to some degree, though this will vary with the differentiation of the society. Finally, the goals of one individual must be meaningful to another in so far as they share a common structure of action.

There will be both empirical and nonempirical goals. Some goals may be mutually incompatible without being destructive to the society. Without an articulated set of goals the society would invite extinction, apathy, or the war of all against all.

F. *The normative regulation of means.* — This functional prerequisite is the precription of means for attaining the socially formulated goals of a society and its subsystems. It complements but does not overlap the functional prerequisite of "effective control of disruptive behavior." The "normative regulation of means" defines positively the means (mostly noncoercive) to the society's goals.

That these means must be stated clearly for the sake of order and the effective functioning of the society follows from (a) the nature of other functional prerequisites and (b) the *anomie* that must result from the lack of recognized legitimized means. First, role-differentiation specifies *who* is to act, while the common articulated set of goals defines *what* is to be done. The normative regulation of means tells *how* those goals may be won. Second, the absence of normative regulation of means invites apathy or the war of each against all. Without socially precribed means, a goal must be either devalued or forcibly seized. As the loss of a bolt may cause a great machine to beat itself to pieces, so the absence of normatively regulated means operates cumulatively to destroy the social structure.

Especially in ritual and initiatory activities must procedures be normatively specified. The content of prescriptions may vary greatly among societies; what is indispensable is simply that socially accepted directives for ceremonial and symbolic action exist. This point emphasizes the necessity for the category of normative regulation of means, in addition to the effective control of disruptive behavior. Moreover, there are often alternative, noncoercive ways of realizing goals, and they must be differentially evaluated for the sake of order, or else some must be ruled out.

G. *The regulation of affective expression.* — In any society the affective states of the members must be mutually communicable and comprehensible. Furthermore, not every affect can be expressed in every situation. Some must be suppressed or repressed. Lastly, there are affects which must be produced in the members if the social structure is to survive. All these aspects are included in the regulation of affective expression.

In the absence of the first of these conditions, stability of expectations between individuals is destroyed, and apathetic or destructive reactions will occur. This is true alike of states of anger and of affection, of love, lust and the like.[9] Without comprehensibility and communicability, mutually inappropriate responses in affectively charged situations can only result in the destruction of the relationship. In a love affair, if one member's expression of affection has the intended meaning of a flirtation, while to the other it signifies willingness to consummate the affair, the relationship is headed for a crisis. The same state of affairs with respect to the expression of affect in an entire society is clearly incompatible with the

---

[9]It may be that gross affective states are mutually communicable in the absence of regulation, but such communication is not sufficient to obviate all the problems dealt with here.

continuation of that society. This is not a matter of a lack of a shared cognitive frame of reference; rather, the conflicts are potentially explosive because of the emotional involvement. The cues that make affective expression comprehensible range from obvious and subtle linguistic behavior to posture, facial expression, gesture, and tone of voice. Many of these cues are not consciously recognized by the actors themselves.

In the face of regulated competitive, co-operative, and authority relationships, some of which are entailed in any conceivable system of role-allocation, taken together with disturbances of expectation and scarcity situations, no society can survive if it permits complete latitude of affective expression in all situations. The ungoverned expression of lust and rage leads to the disruption of relationships and ultimately to the war of all against all.

Finally, a society must not only structure the way in which affects are expressed and restrict certain forms of emotional expression; it must actively foster some affects. Unless we adopt the view that all relationships in all societies can be rational and contractual in character, we must take the position that some relationships depend on regulated affects for their perpetuation.[10] In the absence of the production of appropriate affects, the family, for example, would not survive. The question of what affects must regularly be produced in any society is closely related to the way other functional prerequisites are fulfilled. In American society the urban middle-class conjugal family depends heavily on the establishment of strong affective ties between spouses. The American family system in meeting the demands of a highly mobile society is deprived of certain bases of stability which other family systems possess, and the mutual affection of spouses becomes of correspondingly greater importance.

H. *Socialization.* — A problem is posed for any society by the fact that its structure of action must be learned by new members. To each individual must be transmitted so much of the modes of dealing with the total situation — the modes of communication, the shared cognitive frame of reference, goal-system, attitudes involved in the regulation of means, modes of expression, and the like — as will render him capable of adequate performance in his several roles throughout life, both as respects skills and as respects attitudes. Socialization thus is a different concept from the maintenance of the child in a state of biological well-being.

Furthermore, socialization includes both the development of new adult members from infants and the induction of an individual of any age into any role of the society or its subsystems where new learning is required.

---

[10]This arguement is an example of the dependence of our system of functional prerequisites on a theory of action. A theory which includes an affective aspect in the actor's orientation can and must include this functional prerequisite.

A society cannot persist unless it perpetuates a self-sufficient system of action — whether in changed or traditional form — through the socialization of new members, drawn, in part, from the maturing generation. Whatever the defects of any particular mode of socialization, a universal failure of socialization means the extinction of the society, through a combination of all four of the terminating conditions mentioned previously.[11]

One indivdual cannot become equally familiar with all aspects of his society; indeed, he may remain completely ignorant of some. But he must acquire a working knowledge of the behavior and attitudes relevant to his various roles and identify to some degree with such values as are shared by the whole society or segments thereof wherever his behavior articulates with that of other members of the society. A Brahmin and an Untouchable learn some skills and attitudes unknown to each other. Both, however, must learn that the Hindu world is made up of castes and that this is the way things should be.

I. *The effective control of disruptive forms of behavior.* — Prominent among disruptive modes of behavior are force and fraud. The extent to which such behavior will occur is dependent on the way that various other functional prerequisites are met: role-allocation, goal-system, regulation of means and of expression, and socialization being the more obvious cases in point. All these functional prerequisites, it is clear from the preceding argument, tend to prevent the occurrence of disruptive behavior. In addition to, and separate from, these is the effective control of such behavior when it occurs. To understand why this functional prerequisite is necessary, we must ask: Why would not a perfectly integrated society exist in its absence?

The answer lies in three conditions inherent in any society: scarcity of means, frustrations of expectations, and imperfections of socialization. That many of the desiderata of life are ultimately scarce needs no emphasis. Since sexual objects are differentially evaluated by a society, those few at the top of the scale tend to be sought by a large number of the opposite sex. Wealth, however defined, is basically scarce for the mass of individuals everywhere. Force and fraud are often the most efficient methods of acquiring scarce values. Indeed, only scarce values can be objects of rationally directed coercive effort. To argue that society without coercion and deceit can exist, one must first demonstrate the absence of scarcity. Frustration of expectations is inevitable for many individuals in

---

[11]The complexities of personality development arising from the interaction of individuals of varying constitutional endowment with the modes of child care and socialization and various other aspects of the social situation, as well as with more random situations, cannot be dealt with in any way here. It is sufficient to say that no socialization system is ideally efficient, ie, in no society are all individuals equally well socialized nor is any one individual perfectly socialized.

any society so long as there are such universal realities as unexpected consequences of purposive behavior, scarcity, and uncertainty.

Imperfect socialization results, among other things, in evasions of the normatively prescribed paths of action. Together with frustrations of expectations, it results in explosive outbursts of anger and violence.[12] Thus, both rationally directed exercise of force and fraud and less rational outbursts of emotion continually press to disrupt stable social relationships. If resort to these disruptive behaviors is restricted only by opportunity, the war of all against all will ultimately result. (Some disruptive action may also tend in the direction of an apathetic breakdown. This does not alter the nature of the argument.)

The system of goals tells *what* must be done; the normative regulation of means prescribes *how*. It also includes pre- and proscriptions regarding the use of force and fraud. In addition, however, the society must have techniques for handling those who, for reasons outlined, use these disruptive means or are subject to these outbreaks. The form of control and the degree of efficiency may vary greatly. What type of action is directly destructive of a society depends on the nature of the society: patricide in a society founded on patriarchal clans, violation of property rights in a property-emphasizing society, and so on. Conversely, some societies can tolerate forms of these behaviors that others cannot. Chuckchee social structure, for example, withstands a high homicide rate.

CONCLUSION

This treatment makes no claim to be final. Our list of functional prerequisites can be elaborated and altered by the reader by making explicit the elements we have left implicit. At present, a statement of the functional prerequisites of a society is primarily useful as a contribution to general social theory rather than as a tool for analyzing individual societies. It should be especially useful for constructing a general system of structural prerequisites that will tell us how the functional prerequisites may be met, and this in turn may lead to a more comprehensive and precise comparative sociology.

Even at the present stage, however, the authors have found this approach useful as a point of reference for analyses of societies and their subsystems, and for suggesting inadequacies in the analysis of given societies and in the empirical data available. It directs attention to features of social systems, relationships among institutional structures, and implications for social change which might otherwise be overlooked.

---

[12]Other distruptive modes of behavior, including apathy, also may occur. But a refined analysis of the problem of deviancy is beyond the scope of this book.

STEEL AXES FOR STONE AGE AUSTRALIANS*

Lauriston Sharp

1. In 1623 a Dutch expedition landed on the coasts now occupied by the Yir Yoront. All cultural items (although few in number) recorded in the Dutch log for the aboriginals they encountered were still in use among the Yir Yoront in 1935. To this inventory the Dutch added pieces of iron and beads in an effort to attract the frightened "Indians." They remained at this spot for two days, during which they were able to kidnap one and shoot another of a group of some hundred males. Today metal and beads have disappeared, as has any memory of this first encounter with whites.

2. The next recorded contact in this area occurred in 1864, and here there is more positive assurance that the natives concerned were the immediate ancestors of the Yir Yoront community. These aboriginals had the temerity to attack a party of cattlemen who were driving a small herd from southern Queensland through the whole length of the then unknown Cape York Peninsula to a newly established government station at the Peninsula's northern tip. As a result there occurred what became known as the "Battle of the Mitchell River," one of the rare instances in which Australian aboriginals stood up to European gunfire for any length of time. A diary kept by the cattlemen records the incident: "...ten carbines poured volley after volley into them from all directions, killing and wounding with every shot with very little return, nearly all their spears having already been expended....About thirty being killed, the leader thought it prudent to hold his hand, and let the rest escape. Many more must have been wounded and probably drowned, for fifty-nine rounds were counted as discharged." The European party was in the Yir Yoront area for three days, then disappeared over the horizon to the north, not to return.

During the anthropological investigation some seventy years later, lasting almost three years, there was not one reference to this shocking contact with Europeans, nor anything that could be interpreted as a reference to it, in all the material of hundreds of free association interviews, in hundreds of dreams and myths, in genealogies, and eventually in hundreds of answers to direct and indirect questioning on just this particular matter.

3. The aboriginal accounts of their first remembered contact with whites begin with references to persons known to have had sporadic but

---

*Reprinted from Spicer EH (ed): *Human Problems in Technological Change*. New York: Russell Sage Foundation, Publishers, 1952, pp 70–90. By permission, Basic Books, Inc.

lethal encounters with them beginning about 1900, and it may be noted that from that time on whites continued to remain on the southern periphery of Yir Yoront territory. With the establishment of cattle stations or ranches to the south, occasional excursions among the "wild blackfellows" were made by cattlemen wishing to inspect the country and abduct natives to be trained as cattle boys and "house girls." At least one such expedition reached the Coleman River, where a number of Yir Yoront men and women were shot, apparently on general principles. A stick of trade tobacco, the natives now claim, was left with each body; but this kindness was evidently unappreciated, for the leader of the excursion was eventually speared to death by a native fighting party.

4. It was about this time that the government was persuaded to sponsor the establishment of three mission stations along the seven hundred mile western coast of the Peninsula as an aid in regulating the treatment of natives. To further this purpose a strip of coastal territory was set aside as an aboriginal reserve and closed to further white settlement.

In 1915 an Anglican mission station was established near the mouth of the Mitchell River in the territory of a tribe neighboring the Yir Yoront on the south and about three days' march from the heart of the Yir Yoront country. Some of the Yir Yoront refused to have anything to do with the mission or to go near it, others visited it on occasion, while a few eventually settled more or less permanently in one of the three "villages" at the mission.

5. Thus, the majority of the Yir Yoront continued to live their old self-supporting life in the bush, protected until 1942 by the government reserve and the intervening mission from the cruder realities of the encroaching new order which had come up from the south. To the east was poor country, uninhabited. To the north were other bush tribes extending on along the coast to the distant Archer River Presbyterian mission with which the Yir Yoront had no contact. Westward was the expanse of the shallow Gulf of Carpentaria, on which the natives saw only a mission lugger making its infrequent dry-season trips to the Mitchell River. In this protected environment for over a generation the Yir Yoront were able to recuperate from former shocks received at the hands of civilized society. During the 1930s their raiding and fighting, their trading and stealing of women, their evisceration and two- to three-year care of their dead, their totemic ceremonies continued apparently uninhibited by western influence. In 1931 they killed a European who wandered into their territory from the east, but the investigating police never approached the group whose members were responsible for the act. In 1934 the anthropologist observed a case of extra-tribal revenge cannibalism. The visitor among the bush Yir Yoront at this time found himself in the presence of times past, in an essentially paleolithic society which had been changed, to the casual eye, chiefly by the addition of oddments of European implements and goods put to a variety of uses.

6. As a direct result of the work of the Mitchell River mission, all Yir Yoront received a great many more western artifacts of all kinds than they ever had obtained before, As part of their plan for raising native living standards, the missionaries made it possible for aboriginals at the mission to earn some western goods, many of which were then given or traded out to natives still living under bush conditions; or they handed out gratis both to mission and to bush aboriginals certain useful articles which were in demand. They prevented guns, liquor, and damaging narcotics, as well as decimating diseases, from reaching the tribes of this area, while encouraging the introduction of goods they considered "improving." As has been noted, no item of western technology that was available, with the possible exception of trade tobacco, was in greater demand among all groups of aboriginals than the short-handled steel axe. A good supply of this type of axe was therefore always kept in stock at the mission for sale; and at Christmas parties or other mission festivals steel axes were given away to mission or visiting aboriginals indiscriminately and in considerable numbers. In addition, some steel axes, as well as other European goods, were still traded in to the Yir Yoront by natives in contact with cattle stations established south of the missions. Indeed, such axes had probably come to the Yir Yoront along established lines of aboriginal trade long before any regular contact with whites had occurred.

RELEVANT FACTORS

If we concentrate our attention on Yir Yoront behavior centering about the original stone age, rather than on the axe—the thing—we should get some conception of the role this implement played in aboriginal culture. This conception, in turn, should permit us to foresee with considerable accuracy some of the results of the displacement of stone axes by steel axes acquired directly or indirectly from Europeans by the Yir Yoront.

The production of a stone axe required a number of simple skills. With the idea of the axe in its various details well in mind, the adult men—and only the adult men—could set about producing it, a task not considered appropriate for women or children. First of all, a man had to know the location and properties of several natural resources found in his immediate environment: pliable wood, which could be doubled or bent over the axe head and bound tightly to form a handle; bark, which could be rolled into cord for the binding; and gum, with which the stone head could be firmly fixed in the haft. These materials had to be correctly gathered, stored, prepared, cut to size, and applied or manipulated. They were plentifully supplied by nature, and could be taken by a man from anyone's property without special permission. Postponing consideration of the stone head of the axe, we see that a simple knowledge of nature and of the technological skills involved, together with the possession of fire (for heating the gum) and a few simple cutting tools, which might be nothing more than the sharp shells of plentiful bivalves, all of which were available to everyone, were sufficient to enable any normal man to make a stone axe.

The use of the stone axe as a piece of capital equipment for the production of other goods indicates its very great importance in the subsistence economy of the aboriginal. Anyone—man, woman, or child—could use the axe; indeed, it was used more by women, for theirs was the onerous, daily task of obtaining sufficient wood to keep the campfire of each family burning all day for cooking or other purposes and all night against mosquitoes and cold (in July, winter temperature might drop below forty degrees). In a normal lifetime any woman would use the axe to cut or knock down literally tons of firewood. Men and women, and sometimes children, needed the axe to make other tools, or weapons, or a variety of material equipment required by the aboriginal in his daily life. The stone axe was essential in making the wet-season domed huts, which keep out some rain and some insects; or platforms, which provide dry storage; or shelters, which give shade when days are bright and hot. In hunting and fishing and in gathering vegetable or animal food the axe was also a necessary tool; and in this tropical culture without preservatives or other means of storage, the native spends more time obtaining food than in any other occupation except sleeping.

In only two instances was the use of the stone axe strictly limited to adult men: Wild honey, the most prized food known to the Yir Yoront, was gathered only by men who usually used the axe to get it; and only men could make the secret paraphernalia for ceremonies, an activity often requiring use of the axe. From this brief listing of some of the activities in which the axe was used, it is easy to understand why there was at least one stone axe in every camp, in every hunting or fighting party, in every group out on a "walk-about" in the bush.

While the stone axe helped relate men and women and often children to nature in technological behavior, in the transformation of natural into cultural equipment, it also was prominent in that aspect of behavior which may be called conduct, primarily directed toward persons. Yir Yoront men were dependent upon interpersonal relations for their stone axe heads, since the flat, geologically recent alluvial country over which they range, provides no stone from which axe heads can be made. The stone they used comes from known quarries four hundred miles to the south. It reached the Yir Yoront through long lines of male trading partners, some of these chains terminating with the Yir Yoront men, while others extended on farther north to other groups, having utilized Yir Yoront men as links. Almost every older adult man had one or more regular trading partners, some to the north and some to the south. His partner or partners in the south he provided with surplus spears, and particularly fighting spears tipped with the barbed spines of sting ray which snap into vicious fragments when they penetrate human flesh. For a dozen spears, some of which he may have obtained from a partner to the north, he would receive from a southern partner one stone axe head. Studies have shown that the sting ray spears become more and more valuable as they move south farther from the sea, being passed on in recent times from a native on one cattle station to a native on another where they are used during the wet season, when almost all aboriginal employees are thrust into the bush to shift for themselves until the next cattle-working dry season is at hand. A hundred and fifty miles south of the Yir Yoront one such spear may be exchanged for one stone axe head. Although actual investigations could not be made, presumably still farther south and nearer the quarries, one sting ray spear would bring several stone axe heads. It is apparent that links in the middle of the chain who make neither spears nor axe heads receive both as a middleman's profit simply for passing them back and forth. While many other objects may move along these chains of trading partners, they are still characterized by both bush and station aboriginals as lines along which spears move south and axes move north. Thus trading relations, which may extend the individual's personal relationships out beyond the boundaries of his own group, are associated with two of the most important items in a man's equipment, spears and axes, whether the latter are of stone or steel. Finally, most of the exchanges between partners take place during the dry season at times when the great aboriginal fiestas occur, which center about initiation rites or other totemic ceremonials that attract hundreds and are the occasion for much exciting activity besides trading.

Returning to the Yir Yoront, we find that not only was it adult men alone who obtained axe heads and produced finished axes, but it was adult males who retained the axes, keeping them with other parts of their equipment in camp, or carrying them at the back slipped through a human hair belt when traveling. Thus, every woman or child who wanted to use an axe — and this might be frequently during the day — must get one from some man, use it promptly, and return it to the man in good condition. While a man might speak of "my axe," a woman or child could not; for them it was always "your axe," addressing a male, or "his axe."

This necessary and constant borrowing of axes from older men by women and children was done according to regular patterns of kinship behavior. A woman on good terms with her husband would expect to use his axe unless he were using it; a husband on good terms with his wives would let any one of them use his axe without question. If a woman was unmarried or her husband was absent, she would go first to her older brother or to her father for an axe. Only in extraordinary circumstances would she seek a stone axe from a mother's brother or certain other male kin with whom she had to be most circumspect. A girl, a boy, or a young man would look to a father or an older brother to provide an axe for her or his use, but would never approach a mother's brother, who would be at the same time a potential father-in-law, with such a request. Older men, too, would follow similar rules if they had to borrow an axe.

It will be noted that these social relationships in which the stone axe had a place are all pair relationships and that the use of the axe helped define and maintain the character of the relationships and the roles of the two individual participants. Every active relationship among the Yir Yoront involved a definite and accepted status of superordination or subordination. A person could have no dealings with any other on exactly equal terms. Women and children were dependent on, or subordinate to, older males in every action in which the axe entered. Among the men, the younger was dependent on the older or on certain kinds of kin. The nearest approach to equality was between brothers, although the older was always superordinate to the younger. Since the exchange of goods in a trading relationship involved a mutual reciprocity, trading partners were usually a kind of brother to each other or stood in a brotherly type of relationship, although one was always classified as older than the other and would have some advantage in case of dispute. It can be seen that repeated and widespread conduct centering on the axe helped to generalize and standardize throughout the society these sex, age, and kinship roles, both in their normal benevolent and in exceptional malevolent aspects, and helped to build up expectancies regarding the conduct of others defined as having a particular status.

The status of any individual Yir Yoront was determined not only by sex, age, and extended kin relationships, but also by membership in one of two dozen patrilineal totemic clans into which the entire community was divided. A person's names, rights in particular areas of land, and, in the case of a man, his roles in the totemic ceremonies (from which women are excluded) were all a function of belonging to one clan rather than another. Each clan had literally hundreds of totems, one or two of which gave the clan its name, and from any of which the personal names of clan members were derived. These totems included not only natural species or phenomena like the sun, stars, and daybreak, but also cultural "species": imagined ghosts, rainbow serpents, heroic ancesters; such eternal cultural verities as fires, spears, huts; and such human activities, conditions, or attributes as eating, vomiting, swimming, fighting, babies and corpses, milk and blood, lips and loins. While individual members of such totemic classes or species might disappear or be destroyed, the class itself was obviously ever present and indestructible. The totems therefore lent permanence and stability to the clans, to the groupings of human individuals who generation after generation were each associated with one set of totems that distinguished one clan from another.

Among the many totems of the Sunlit Cloud Iguana clan, and important among them, was the stone axe. The names of many members of this clan referred to the axe itself, or to activities like trading or wild honey gathering in which the axe played a vital part, or to the clan's mythical ancestors with whom the axe was prominently associated. When it was necessary to represent the stone axe in totemic ceremonies, it was only men of this clan who exhibited it or pantomimed its use. In secular life the axe could be made by any man and used by all; but in the sacred realm of the totems it belonged exclusively to the Sunlit Cloud Iguana people.

Supporting those aspects of cultural behavior which we have called technology and conduct is a third area of culture, including ideas, sentiments, and values. These are most difficult to deal with, for they are latent and covert or even unconscious and must be deduced from overt actions and language or other communicating behavior. In this aspect of the culture lies the "meaning" of the stone axe, its significance to the Yir Yoront and to their cultural way of life. The ideal conception of the axe, the knowledge of how to produce it (apart from the purely muscular habits used in its production) are part of the Yir Yoront adult masculine role, just as ideas regarding its technical use are included in the feminine role. These technical ideas constitute a kind of "science" regarding the axe which may be more important in relation to behavioral change than are the neurophysiological patterns drilled into the body by years of practice. Similarly there are normative ideas regarding the part played by the axe in conduct which constitute a kind of "morality" of the axe, and which again may be more important than the overt habits of social interaction in determining the role of the axe in social relationships. More than ideas regarding technology, ideas regarding conduct are likely to be closely associated, or "charged," with sentiment or value. Ideas and sentiments help guide and inform overt behavior; in turn, overt behavior helps support and validate ideas and sentiments.

The stone axe was an important symbol of masculinity among the Yir Yoront (just as pants or pipes are among ourselves). By a complicated set of ideas which we would label "ownership" the axe was defined as "belonging" to males. Everyone in the society (except untrained infants) accepted these ideas. Similarly spears, spear throwers, and fire-making sticks were associated with males, were owned only by them, and were symbols of masculinity. But the masculine values represented by the stone axe were constantly being impressed on all members of society by the fact that non-males had to use the axe and had to go to males for it, whereas they never borrowed other masculine artifacts. Thus, the axe stood for an important theme that ran all through Yir Yoront culture: the superiority and rightful dominance of the male, and the greater value of his concerns and of all things associated with him. We should call this androcentrism rather than patriarchy, or paternal rule. It is the recognition by all that the values of the man *(andros)* take precedence over feminine values, an idea backed by very strong sentiments among the Yir Yoront. Since the axe had to be borrowed also by the younger from the older, it also represented the prestige of age, another important theme running all through Yir Yoront behavior.

Important for an understanding of the Yir Yoront culture is a system of ideas, which may be called their totemic ideology. A fundamental belief of the aboriginal divided time into two great epochs, a distant and sacred period at the beginning of the world, when the earth was peopled by mildly marvelous ancestral beings or culture heroes who in a special sense are the forebears of the clans; and a second period, when the old was succeeded by a new order that includes the present. Originally there was no anticipation of another era supplanting the present; the future would simply be an eternal continuation and reproduction of the present, which itself had remained unchanged since the epochal revolution of ancestral times.

The mythical sacred world of the ancestors with which time began turns out on investigation to be a detailed reproduction of the present aboriginal world of nature, man, and culture altered by phantasy. In short, the idea system expressed in the mythology regarding the ancestral epoch was directly derived from Yir Yoront behavior patterns—normal and abnormal, actual and ideal, conscious and unconscious. The important thing to note, however, is that the native believed it was just the other way around, that the present world, as a natural and cultural environment, was and should be simply a detailed reproduction of the world of the ancestors. He believed that the entire universe "is now as it was in the beginning" when it was established and left by the ancestors. The ordinary cultural life of the ancestors became the daily life of the Yir Yoront camps, and the extraordinary life of the ancestors remained extant in the recurring symbolic pantomimes and paraphernalia found only in the most sacred atmosphere of the totemic rites.

Such beliefs, accordingly, opened up the way for ideas of what *should be* (because it supposedly *was*) to influence or help determine what actually *is*. Dog-chases-iguana-up-a-tree-and-barks-at-him-all-night had that and other names because, so he believed, his ancestral alter ego had these same names; he was a member of the Sunlit Cloud Iguana clan because his ancestor was; he was associated with particular countries and totems of this same ancester; during an initiation he played the role of a dog and symbolically attacked and killed certain members of other clans because his ancester (conveniently either anthropomorphic or kynomorphic) really did the same to the ancestral alter egos of these men; and he would avoid his mother-in-law, joke with a distant mother's brother, and make spears in a certain way because his and other people's ancestors did these things. His behavior in these rather than in other ways was outlined for him, and to that extent determined, by a set of ideas concerning the past and the relation of the present to the past.

But when we are informed that Dog-chases...had two wives from the Spear Black Duck clan and one from the Native Companion clan with such and such names, one of them being blind; that he had four children with such and such names; that he had a broken wrist and was left-handed, all because his ancestor had exactly these same attributes, then we know (though he apparently did not) that the present has influenced the past, that the mythical world has been somewhat adjusted to meet the exigencies and accidents of the inescapably real present.

There was thus in Yir Yoront ideology a nice balance in which the mythical world was adjusted in part to the real world, and real world in part to the ideal preexisting mythical world, the adjustments occurring to maintain a fundamental tenet of native faith that the present must be a mirror of the past. Thus, the stone axe in all its aspects, uses, and associations was integrated into the context of Yir Yoront technology and conduct because a myth, a set of ideas, had put it there.

ANALYSIS

The introduction of the steel axe indiscriminately and in large numbers into the Yir Yoront technology was only one of many changes occurring at the same time. It is therefore impossible to factor out all the results of this single innovation alone. Nevertheless, a number of specific effects of the change from stone axes to steel axes may be noted; and the steel axe may be used as an epitome of the European goods and implements received by the aboriginals in increasing quantity and of their general influence on the native culture. The use of the steel axe to illustrate such influences would seem to be justified, for it was one of the first European artifacts to be adopted for regular use by the Yir Yoront; and the axe, whether of stone or steel, was clearly one of the most important items of cultural equipment they possessed.

The shift from stone to steel axes provided no major technological difficulties. While the aboriginals themselves could not manufacture steel axe heads, a steady supply from outside continued; and broken wooden axe handles could easily be replaced from bush timbers with aboriginal tools. Among the Yir Yoront the new axe never acquired all the uses it had on mission or cattle stations (carpentry work, pounding tent pegs, use as a hammer, and so on); and, indeed, it was used for little more than the stone axe had been, so that it had no practical effect in improving the native standard of living. It did some jobs better, and could be used longer without breakage; and these factors were sufficient to make it of value to the native. But the assumption of the white man (based in part on a realization that a shift from steel to stone axe in his case would be a definite regression) that his axe was much more efficient, that its use would save time, and that it therefore represented technical "progress" toward goals which he had set for the native was hardly borne out in aboriginal practice. Any leisure time the Yir Yoront might gain by using steel axes or other western tools was invested, not in "improving the conditions of life," and certainly not in developing aesthetic activities, but in sleep, an art they had thoroughly mastered.

Having acquired an axe head through regular trading partners of whom he knew what to expect, a man wanting a stone axe was then dependent solely upon a known and an adequate nature and upon his own skills or easily acquired techniques. A man wanting a steel axe, however, was in no such self-reliant position. While he might acquire one through trade, he now had the new alternative of dispensing with technological behavior in relation with a predictable nature and conduct in relation with a predictable trading partner and of turning instead to conduct alone in relation with a highly erratic missionary. If he attended one of the mission festivals when steel axes were handed out as gifts, he might receive one simply by chance or if he had happened somehow to impress upon the mission staff that he was one of the "better' bush aboriginals (their definition of "better" being quite different from that of his bush fellows). Or he might — but again almost by pure chance — be given some brief job in connection with the mission which would enable him to earn a steel axe. In either case, for older men a preference for the steel axe helped create a situation of dependence in place of a situation of self-reliance and a behavior shift from situations in technology or conduct which were well structured or defined to situations in conduct alone which were ill defined. It was particularly the older ones among the men, whose earlier experience or knowledge of the white man's harshness in any event made them suspicious, who would avoid having any relations with the mission at all, and who thus excluded themselves from acquiring steel axes directly from that source.

The steel axe was the root of psychological stress among the Yir Yoront even more significantly in other aspects of social relations. This was the result of new factors which the missionary considered all to the good: the simple numerical increase in axes per capita as a result of mission distribution; and distribution from the mission directly to younger men, women, and even children. By winning the favor of the mission staff, a woman might be given a steel axe. This was clearly intended to be hers. The situation was quite different from that involved in borrowing an axe from a male relative, with the result that a woman called such an axe "my" steel axe, a possessive form she never used for a stone axe. (Lexically, the steel axe was differentiated from the stone by an adjectival suffix signifying "metal," the element "axe" remaining identical.) Furtheremore, young men or even boys might also obtain steel axes directly from the mission. A result was that older men no longer had a complete monopoly of all the axes in the bush community. Indeed, an old man might have only a stone axe, while his wives and sons had steel axes which they considered their own and which he might even desire to borrow. All this led to a revolutionary confusion of sex, age, and kinship roles, with a major gain in independence and loss of subordination on the part of those able now to acquire steel axes when they had been unable to possess stone axes before.

The trading partner relationship was also affected by the new situation. A Yir Yoront might have a trading partner in a tribe to the south whom he defined as a younger brother, and on whom as an older brother he would therefore have an edge. But if the partner were in contact with the mission or had other easier access to steel axes, his subordination to his bush colleague was obviously decreased. Indeed, under the new dispensation he might prefer to give his axe to a bush "sweetheart" in return for favors or otherwise dispose of it outside regular trade channels, since many steel axes were so distributed between natives in new ways. Among other things, this took some of the excitement away from the fiesta-like tribal gatherings centering around initiations during the dry season. These had traditionally been the climactic annual occasions for exchanges between trading partners, when a man might seek to acquire a whole year's supply of stone axe heads. Now he might find himself prostituting his wife to almost total strangers in return for steel axes or other white men's goods. With trading partnerships weakened, there was less reason to attend the fiestas, and less fun for those who did. A decline in one of the important social activities which had symbolized these great gatherings created a lessening interest in the other social aspects of these events.

Not only did an increase in steel axes and their distribution to women change the character of the relations between individual and individual, the paired relationships that have been noted, but a new type of relationship, hitherto practically unknown among the Yir Yoront, was created in their axe-acquiring conduct with whites. In the aboriginal society there were almost no occasions outside the immediate family when one individual would initiate action to several other people at once. For in any average group, while a person in accordance with the kinship system might be superordinate to several people to whom he could suggest or command action, at the same time he was also subordinate to several others, in relation with whom such behavior would be tabu. There was thus no over-all chieftainship or authoritarian leadership of any kind. Such complicated operations as grassburning, animal drives, or totemic ceremonies could be carried out smoothly because each person knew his roles both in technology and conduct.

On both mission and cattle stations, however, the whites imposed upon the aboriginals their conception of leadership roles, with one person in a controlling relationship with a subordinate group. Aboriginals called together to receive gifts, including axes, at a mission Christmas party found themselves facing one or two whites who sought to control their behavior for the occasion, who disregarded the age, sex, and kinship variables among them of which they were so conscious, and who considered them all at one subordinate level. Or the white might impose similar patterns on a working party. (But if he placed an aboriginal in charge of a mixed group of post hole diggers, for example, half of the group, those subordinate to the "boss," would work while the other half, who were superordinate to him, would sleep.) The steel axe, together, of course, with other European goods, came to symbolize for the aboriginal this new and uncomfortable form of social organization, the leader-group relationship.

The most disturbing effects of the steel axe, operating in conjunction with other elements also being introduced from the white man's several subcultures, developed in the realm of traditional ideas, sentiments, and values. These were undermined at a rapidly mounting rate, without new conceptions being defined to replace them. The result was a mental and moral void which foreshadowed the collapse and destruction of all Yir Yoront culture, if not, indeed, the extinction of the biological group itself.

From what has been said it should be clear how changes in overt behavior, in technology and conduct, weakened the values inherent in a reliance on nature, in androcentrism or the prestige of masculinity, in age prestige, and in the various kinship relations. A scene was set in which a wife or young son, his initiation perhaps not even yet completed, need no longer bow to the husband or father, who was left confused and insecure as he asked to borrow a steel axe from them. For the woman and boy the steel axe helped establish a new degree of freedom which was accepted readily as an escape from the unconscious stress of the old patterns, but which left them also confused and insecure. Ownership became less well defined, so that stealing and treaspass were introduced into technology and conduct. Some of the excitement surrounding the great ceremonies evaporated, so that the only fiestas the people had became less festive, less interesting. Indeed, life itself became less interesting, although this did not lead the Yir Yoront to invent suicide, a concept foreign to them.

The whole process may be most specifically illustrated in terms of the totemic system, and this will also illustrate the significant role which a system of ideas, in this case a totemic ideology, may play in the breakdown of a culture.

In the first place, under pre-European aboriginal conditions in which the native culture has become adjusted to a relatively stable environment in which there can occur few, if any, unheard of or catastrophic crises, it is clear that the totemic system must serve very effectively to inhibit radical cultural changes. The closed system of totemic ideas, explaining and categorizing a well-known universe as it was fixed at the beginning of time, presents a considerable obstacle to the adoption of new or the dropping of old culture traits. The obstacle is not insurmountable and the system allows for the minor variations which occur about the norms of daily life, but the inception of major changes cannot easily take place.

Among the bush Yir Yoront the only means of water transport is a light wood log, to which they cling in their constant swimming of rivers, salt creeks, and tidal inlets. These natives know that forty-five miles north of them are tribes who have a bark canoe. They know these northern tribes can thus fish from midstream or out at sea, instead of clinging to the river banks and beaches, and can cross coastal waters infested with crocodiles, sharks, sting rays, and Portuguese-men-or-war without the recurring mortality, pain, or anxiety to which they themselves are constantly subjected. They know they lack any magic to do for them what the canoe could do. They know of the materials of which the canoe is made are present in their own environment. But they also know, as they say, that their own mythical ancestors lack the canoe, and therefore they lack it, while they assume that the canoe was part of the ancestral universe of the northern tribes. For them, then, the adoption of the canoe would not be simply a matter of learning a number of new behavioral skills for its manufacture and use. The adoption would require at the same time a much more difficult procedure, the acceptance by the entire society of a myth, either locally developed or borrowed, which would explain the presence of the canoe, associate it with some one or more of the several hundred mythical ancestors (and how decide which?), and thus establish it as an accepted totem of one of the clans ready to be used by the whole community. The Yir Yoront have not made this adjustment, and in this case we can only say that ideas have for the time being at least won out over very real pressures for technological change. In the elaborateness and explicitness of the totemic ideologies we seem to have one explanation for the notorious stability of Australian cultures under aboriginal conditions, an explanation which gives due weight to the importance of ideas in determining human behavior.

At a later stage of the contact situation, as has been indicated, phenomena unaccounted for by the totemic ideological system began to appear with regularity and frequency and remain within the range of native experience. Accordingly, they cannot be ignored (as the "Battle of the Mitchell River" was apparently ignored), and an attempt is made to assimilate them and account for them along the lines of principles inherent in the ideology. The bush Yir Yoront of the mid-1930s represent this stage of the acculturation process. Still trying to maintain their aboriginal definition of the situation, they accept European artifacts and behavior patterns, but fit them into their totemic system, assigning them as totems to various clans on a par with original totems. There is an attempt to have the myth-making process keep up with these cultural changes so that the idea system can continue to support the rest of the culture. But analysis of overt behavior, of dreams, and of some of the new myths indicates that this arrangement is not entirely satisfactory; that the native clings to his totemic system with intellectual loyalty, lacking any substitute ideology; but that associated sentiments and values are weakened. His attitudes toward his own and toward European culture are found to be highly ambivalent.

All ghosts are totems of the Head-to-the-East Corpse clan. They are thought of as white, and are, of course, closely associated with death. The white man, too, is white and was closely associated with death, so that he and all things pertaining to him are naturally assigned to the Corpse clan as totems. The steel axe, as a totem, was thus associated with the Corpse clan. But it is an "axe," and is clearly linked with the stone axe, which is a totem of the Sunlit Cloud Iguana clan. Moreover, the steel axe, like most European goods, has no distinctive origin myth, nor are mythical ancestors associated with it. Can anyone, sitting of an afternoon in the shade of a ti tree, create a myth to resolve this confusion? No one has, and the horrid suspicion arises that perhaps the origin myths are wrong, which took into account so little of this vast new universe of the white man. The steel axe, shifting hopelessly between one clan and the other, is not only replacing the stone axe physically, but is hacking at the supports of the entire cultural system.

The aboriginals to the south of the Yir Yoront have clearly passed beyond this stage. They are engulfed by European culture, in this area by either the mission or cattle station subcultures, or for some natives a baffling, paradoxical combination of both incongruent varieties. The totemic ideology can no longer support the inrushing mass of foreign culture traits and the myth-making process in its native form breaks down completely. Both intellectually and emotionally a saturation point is reached, so that the myriad new traits which can neither be ignored nor any longer assimilated simply force the aboriginal to abandon his totemic system. With the collapse of this system of ideas, which is so closely related with so many other aspects of the native culture, there follows an appallingly sudden and complete cultural disintegration and a demoralization of the individual such as has seldom been recorded for areas other than Australia. Without the support of a system of ideas well devised to provide cultural stability in a stable environment but admittedly too rigid for the new realities pressing in from outside, native behavior and native sentiments and values are simply dead. Apathy reigns. The aboriginal has passed beyond the reach of any outsider who might wish to do him well or ill.

Returning from the broken natives huddled on cattle stations or on the fringes of frontier towns to the ambivalent but still lively aboriginals settled on the Mitchell River mission, we note one further devious result of the introduction of European artifacts. During a wet season stay at the mission, the anthropologist discovered that his supply of tooth paste was being depleted at an alarming rate. Investigation showed that it was being taken by old men for use in a new tooth paste cult. Old materials of magic having failed, new materials were being tried out in a malevolent magic directed toward the mission staff and some of the younger aboriginal men. Old males, largely ignored by the missionaries, were seeking to regain some of their lost power and prestige. This mild aggression proved hardly effective, but perhaps only because confidence in any kind of magic on the mission was by this time at a low ebb.

For the Yir Yoront still in the bush a time could be predicted when personal deprivation and frustration in a confused culture would produce an overload of anxiety. The mythical past of the totemic ancestors would disappear as a guarantee of a present of which the future was supposed to be a stable continuation. Without the past, the present would be meaningless and the future unstructured and uncertain. Insecurities would be inevitable. Reaction to this stress might be some form of symbolic aggression, or withdrawal and apathy, or some more realistic approach. In such a situation the missionary with understanding of the processes going on about him would find his opportunity to introduce religion and to help create the constitution of a new cultural universe.

THERAPEUTIC PROCESS IN CULTURAL PERSPECTIVE*

Alexander H. Leighton

The following abbreviated account is based on observations made when I was living among the Navaho Indians of New Mexico in 1940. It also draws on the insights and knowledge of the late Clyde Kluckholn.

Picture a Navaho hut or hogan amid the sage and pinyon pines characteristic of the high table lands at the southern end of the Rocky Mountains. It is spring, and one of the family has been "off his feed" for some months — anxious and depressed, "feels bad all over," as he puts it. Arrangements have been made to summon a well known Singer (medicine man), and all the relatives have gathered. The ceremonial is to last nine days and nights.

On the first day at dawn the hogan is swept out, the materials of daily living put away, and the fire removed from the center of the floor. The doorway is covered with blankets. The Singer and his helpers light a new fire. They use a fire drill instead of matches, powdered lightning-struck rock, charcoal from the scar of a struck tree, and they sing lightning songs. The patient and others who wish to join in the treatment undress outside. Four pokers are laid on the ground, radiating from the fire toward the cardinal points of the compass, the homes of the gods. The pokers are made of carefully selected lightning-struck pinyon and cedar and represent men who chase evil away.

The patient and the other participants enter the hogan and sit around the fire at specified spots. The heat grows intense. At the fire is a pot which contains an emetic composed of buckthorne, limberpine, bearberry, wild currant, juniper, and Colorado blue spruce. Each person gets a portion of it and washes himself from the feet up, then drinks and vomits. The Singer takes a brush made of wing and tail feathers from an eagle and an owl feather that fell out while the bird was flying. He brushes the patient, the others present, and then the whole hut, making motions that sweep evil toward the door. The ends of the pokers are warmed and applied to the patient's body by the Singer. Then the others apply them to themselves, rubbing the warm wood on any part that hurts. The patient and the other participants walk around the fire sunwise, stepping over the pokers. Evil cannot cross the pokers and thus they leave evil behind. The live coals represent lightning. Songs and prayers accompany each stage of the ritual. The heat is continuously very intense and all sweat profusely.

At the end, the door blanket is lifted with one of the pokers and the

*Reprinted from the *American Journal of Psychiatry* 124:8–10, March 1968. By permission of the American Psychiatric Association.

patient steps out, followed by the others. After fire, ashes, and vomitus have been disposed of, all return and the Singer, using the eagle feathers, sprinkles participants and hut with a fragrant lotion made of mint, horse-mint, windodor, and penny-royal, kept in an abalone shell. Glowing coals are placed before each participant and on these is sprinkled a fumigant made of a plant root, sulphur, corn meal, down from chickadee, tit-mouse, woodpecker, bluebird, and yellow warbler. These have been previously ground together by a virgin while the Singer sang songs. Every one breathes the fumes and rubs them into his body. After this the coals are thrown out the smoke hole, taking evil with them.

This description passes over many details of importance but ex-emplifies the other movements in the ceremonial. At all phases the singer pours out songs that reflect the significance of what is being done.

On the last night of nine, about two hours after supper, the final movement of the ceremonial begins and continues all night. The hut is jammed with spectators; the firelight flickers on their faces and makes deep and moving shadows. The Singer and the patient sit on the west side facing east. All the women present sit on the north side and the men on the south. The Singer sings a verse and then the crowd takes it up with increasing volume. The more who sing, the sooner the patient will get well. The songs deal with the legends, things the gods have done, and the origin of the ceremonial. It is repeated and repeated that the patient is identified with the gods. It is said, in regard to the spirit of the mountain, that his feet are the patient's feet, the patient walks in his tracks and wears his moccasins. The blue horse spirit belongs to the patient, the turquoise horse with lightning feet, with a mane like distant rain, black star for an eye and white shells for teeth, the horse spirit who feeds only on the pollen of flowers.

There are songs that take up the patient's health directly, asking, "His feet restore for him, his mind restore for him, his voice restore for him." There are repetitions of thoughts that proclaim that all is well: thus, "My feet are getting better, my head is feeling better, I am better all over." Finally, it is said over and over again that all is being made beautiful and harmonious. The songs come in groups that form patterned relationships with each other. The effect of repetition, rhythm, and the antiphonal chorus is very impressive.

Before the first streak of dawn the Singer smears meal across the faces of the patient, himself, and those who have performed well. This is to mark them so the gods will know them. When dawn begins the patient walks around the fire four times, preceded by one of the Singer's assistants who sprinkles the fragrant lotion. The patient goes out alone and faces the dawn. Inside, the Singer closes the ceremonial with a prayer; he asks protection from the consequences of any mistake he may have made, then prays for everybody.

Outside the patient stands facing the east, breathing in the dawn four times.

> In beauty I walk.
> With beauty before me, may I walk.
> With beauty behind me, may I walk.
> With beauty all around me, may I walk.
> In old age wandering on a trail of beauty, lively, may I walk.
> In old age wandering on a trail of beauty, living again, may I walk.
> It is finished in beauty. It is finished in beauty.

One of the aspects of interest in this ceremonial is the contrast it presents to the report of Prince, just given. Yet when one assembles and compares many forms of treatment across many cultures it seems evident that there are a number of recurrent underlying characteristics:

1. Every individual is prepared during the course of his life by a set of expectancies regarding illness and treatment which are part of his culture. These are inculcated long before his own condition as a patient comes about. They are heightened, however, as he approaches being a patient and increase the suggestive power of many of the experiences he undergoes.

2. There is always at least one healer who has prestige and mystique. The patient achieves some measure of the healer's distinction when he emerges as one who has been successfully treated. In many places, becoming a healer involves first being a patient.

3. At some point, usually early, the patient experiences a profound emotional shakeup. This is obtained in one or more of the following ways:

    a) By the application of external and internal medications;

    b) By physical pain or psychological discomfort, eg, in being made to confess his iniquities or inadequacies;

    c) By having to perform in front of other people;

    d) By the drama of a ritual that builds to a climax; or

    e) By esthetic appeal through poetry, song, music (especially rhythm), and color.

There is often a period of heightened fear, followed by a release from fear, and there is generally a terminal period of euphoria or ecstatic state. It is as if the whole procedure brought about a situation in which the structure of the patient's personality becomes soft, and then, after the emotional crisis, resets in a new form.

4. Concomitant with all of the above, there is, as the treatment progresses, an increasing dependency on the healer by the patient, and with this goes an increasing susceptibility to suggestion.

5. Underlying the treatment procedure is a dramatic myth with the following functions and characteristics:

   a) It provides a general orientation with regard to the phenomena of life, the characteristics of illness, and the rationale of treatment.

   b) It is worked over during the course of the treatment, producing an increased acquaintance on the part of the patient with this explanatory framework.

   c) The ceremonial itself, or some parts of it, constitutes a symbolic reenactment of something which went wrong in the past and which is now being set right, and which is comprehensible in the setting of the myth. The "what went wrong" is revealed in some part of the ceremonial and then must be corrected. There is usually a battle of anthropormorphic entities which may take place inside or outside the patient's psyche. The ritual of the ceremonial or other therapeutic activity is concerned with making this battle come out on the side of the patient. The patient does it over again symbolically without the mistake, and so through the mediation of the healer comes into harmony with great and mysterious forces within and without himself. Profound belief in the myth by both healer and patient heightens the force of suggestion and the influence of the matrix of subtle cues which are only partly realized by either.

6. In many ceremonials, typified by the Navaho, there is strong enhancement by the expectation of group members. Thus, family members and sometimes whole communities are involved, sharing in the sense of benefit, contributing material, work, and prayers to the outcome. Group forces are thus linked on the side of the patient's treatment, and the people with whom he has most of his interactions become committed to accepting a state of change. Hence, if the patient's personality does get set in a new pattern, the group in which he is enmeshed are prepared for it, emotionally as well as cognitively.

7. The culture generally prescribes post-treatment sentiments for patient, healer, and persons in the community. This cultural set constitutes strong motivation to play the role of the successfully treated patient.

To sum up, I would suggest that the myth is central—that is, the belief in a doctrine—but its function seems the point of interest rather than its content. The content varies widely from one cultural group to another and from one time to another, but there is always a myth and it always has a feature role in the induction of the change. The participants always believe the content and stress its importance, but to the comparative observer this seems less important than the existence of the belief and the manner in which it functions.

THE EROSION OF NORMS*

Alexander H. Leighton

This paper is concerned with explaining one aspect of life today as a consequence of interplay among certain social and psychological processes. The central thesis is that social disintegration tends to perpetuate and increase itself through the psychological responses it evokes in the individuals it affects. In part, these psychological responses consist in behavior and feelings frequently designated and treated as mental illness.

The interplay is maladaptive because progressive social disintegration is life threatening. Ultimately, progressive disintegration is progressive annihilation. Fortunately disintegration also evokes counteracting social and psychological responses. Thus one of the requirements before mankind at the present time is that of understanding and fostering these countercurrents.

The theoretical basis of the discussion to be presented is derived from several decades of research in psychatric epidemiology known as the "Stirling County Study" (Leighton 1959, 1971). This work has focused on elucidating the relationships between mental health and mental illness on the one hand, and social and cultural factors on the other. Although the central investigations have been in rural and urban North America, numbers of cross-cultural studies have also been conducted in Africa and among Eskimos in Alaska. It would be a mistake, however, to claim that the theory has been established by the studies. The position is rather, that it has been suggested by them, and constitutes a stimulus to new work. It should also be acknowledged that we draw heavily on theories of Emil Durkheim, Bronislaw Malinowski, Robert Merton and Adolf Meyer.

In what follows I shall attempt to apply integration-disintegration theory to a recent movement among young people – "the Counter Culture." It can be argued that the tag is now out of date because the Counter Culture movement has faded. I shall use the term nonetheless since it is convenient and relevant to the ideas and trends that will be discussed and because these still are problems of youth. Furthermore, it is my impression that if the Counter Culture has faded, this is because it has, as a network of ideas and feelings become more diffuse, affecting larger numbers

*Presented at the 10th Annual Congress, Australian and New Zealand College of Psychiatrists; Sydney, October 1973.
Reprinted from the *Australian and New Zealand Journal of Psychiatry* 8:223-227, 1974. By permission of the publisher.

and kinds of people and hence more rather than less influential. Whatever the name, the process is still with us.

As a point of departure, let us take that feature of the Counter Culture which is implied by its name: opposition to the culture of the West.

In essence, the Counter Culture is against the way of life that has been exemplified by the Commonwealth of Nations, the United States, Europe and much of the rest of the world where industrialization, technological development and material wealth are either aspiration or accomplishment. The members of the Counter Culture say that the net effect of these approaches to life result in such evils as the rich-poor dichotomy; pollution of the good earth, the wide seas and the free air; the degradation of human values by a machine dominated technology; fires of battle around the world that never die out; the strangling grip of bureaucracy on individual freedom; the exploitive immorality of advertising and industrial management; the use of the big lie in politics; and much else, but overall and finally the hovering, inextinguishable threat of nuclear destruction, a supreme achievement of science.

Associated with these negative views is another: disbelief that the evils of Western Culture can be mended from within.

It would be naive to suppose that the manifest content of the criticisms levelled at Western Culture is sufficient to explain the Counter Culture. There are obviously other factors of major importance including the psychodynamics of adolescence. On the other hand, the criticisms are realistic and they have meaning as shared symbols that affect group behaviour. It is, therefore, justifiable to keep them in the foreground of this discussion.

A wide variety of behaviours are associated with the negative views just outlined, but they can be roughly grouped into three main types. One is to seek detachment from the web of worldly interaction by withdrawal to an inner life, as in yoga. Drugs and music (especially listening) can help in pursuing this kind of subjective freedom, as aids to disengagement and making inner being all in all. The pursuit of freedom as an individualistic experience can also take the more active form of intoxication with excitement through roving (as exemplified in the writings of Jack Kerouac) and through sex, committing crimes for thrill, and genrally living on kicks, with and without the aid of drugs and music. An extreme of this is the "Manson Family" in California who practiced ritual torture and murder and employed Counter Culture rhetoric. As Camus pointed out years ago, if you really believe in the hopelessness of the human condition, then the Marquis de Sade offers a cogent, and logically justifiable philosophy. Dostoevski, albeit in very differnt terms, has repeatedly raised the question "Why not murder?"

A second trend is one directed, not so much toward the evolvement of inner-self, as against existing society. This can surface in attacks on various institutions, as for instance universities and banks, and in acts of disruption and terror. Counter Culture behaviour of this kind is to be distinguished from similar acts by militant minorities such as the I.R.A., who are seeking to make political gains by a species of blackmail. The radical activist in the Counter culture is more anarchist than this and aims at the destruction of the "whole system." His claim is that when all of society and culture as they now exist, have been swept away, real freedom and a far, far better way of life for all mankind will emerge. With this justification, he subjects us to his experiments.

These two extremes have between them many mixtures and middle grounds tinged with varying degrees of hope and despair. One such constitutes my third category; namely, the effort to build a new society, with a new culture, outside the framework of the old. This aim seeks to create a true participant democracy, not just of mind, but of soul. Thus there emerge groups such as communes that try to live amid the major culture without being of it.

What has been said thus far can be summed up by observing that the features of the Counter Culture selected for attention here are its rejection of Western Culture and its action patterns of withdrawal, attack and Utopia formation.

There is another component, however, that runs through the other features; namely, devotion to an ideal of individual freedom. Love of freedom for individual self-expression, and hatred of Western Culture because it is oppressive, can be regarded as a unitary feeling — a love-hate axis about which nearly everything else turns.

In considering all this it should be kept in mind that in all likelihood the total number of young people who have ever filled the extreme categories is small. On the other hand these ideas and beliefs are widely promoted in one form or another by numbers of spokesmen such as Norman Brown, Allen Ginsberg, Paul Goodman, Herbert Marcuse, and Theodore Rozak, and have what seems to be expanding influence. While the disciples may be relatively few, the bemused are many.

At this point, I would like to set aside the Counter Culture and turn to describing certain features of the societal process which constitute the setting of the Counter Culture, and which place limits on its potentialities.

The most elemental proposition is that human life is only possible within the framework of a social system of some sort. This assertion is based on the biological fact that human beings cannot otherwise survive. The facts of human child dependency and slow growth require some kind of family if there is to be continuation of the species. But families in turn must give rise to other families, and to make such unions possible, there must be networks of communication among people across family lines. Thus, at its most stark and simplistic level the perpetuation of the human creature is inextricably bound to the existence of social systems. How elemental and prehuman this is, can be seen in the work with primates of DeVore, Goodall and others. It follows, therefore, that the struggles of the extreme proponents of freedom in the Counter Culture are toward impossible goals.

All this does not gainsay, of course, the possibility of seeking a better societal system, nor of achieving radical alterations. It does say, however, that individual freedom is a relative matter and a question of arrangements within a system.

It says further that detachment pushed too far is suicidal, and that efforts to destroy society are not only short term violence, but would become long term mass murder should they succeed in destroying the network of interrelationships upon which we all depend.

If societal systems are necessary to life, do they have properties that are transcultural? Having in mind as a model for discussion a geographically localized community, one can say that in many ways a society is like an organism; it is in the business of survival in a world full of dangers. It girds itself to obtain subsistence, to create new members and introduce them into the system so there will be continuity, to store up experience as knowledge, to make divisions of labour and to defend itself against the Four Horsemen of the Apocalypse. These properties have been called the "functional prerequisites of a society" in cultural anthropology (Appendix A).

If the social system is to exist at all, its functions have to be laid out in terms of sub-systems. Schools for example constitute one subsystem, the family is another, the government of the community is still another and so on.

Just as the total system of the community is composed of subsystems, so too the sub-systems have others within them. A basic unit in the total structure is the "role" and out of roles the rest are built. Roles can be illustrated by such words as father, wife, lawyer, storekeeper, psychiatrist, community council member, mayor, etc., and obviously the functioning of the social system depends on there being people who are both motivated and capable of filling the roles.

For system, sub-systems and roles to work in the interests of the functional prerequisites upon which survival depends, communication and coordination are essential. Coordination and communication, in turn, require shared values, commonly accepted symbols and agreed upon patterns of interaction among people.

The word-symbols that make up language exemplify this. It may be, as an extreme member of the Counter Culture might say, that no one has the right to tell me what the sounds I utter shall mean; it may be my inalienable right to choose the meanings I wish, or to have no meaning at all; and I can exercise these rights if I live alone. But if I live in a community and choose to have right mean left and stop mean go, I am apt to create a traffic snarl and may end in causing injury and death to myself and others.

The functioning of a social system can be conceptualized as dynamic equilibrium. The word "dynamic" means that work is involved, that is to say, the patterning of community systems and sub-systems is maintained through the expenditure of energy against a multitude of forces both within and external to the system which tend to dissolve and dissipate it. Thus, new events that interfere with the functioning of the system are met with counter-actions which restore functioning and establish equilibrium.

Objections have been made to the application of dynamic equilibrium to human affairs on the ground that the concept does not allow for growth and change. This is no more true, however, in social systems than it is in ecological systems or other living systems. Restoration of balance and the maintenance of functioning does not necessarily mean return to the *status quo ante*. On the contrary, one of the characteristics of dynamic equilibria is that change can be met by establishing a new pattern of equilibrium. The vital matter is that this be accomplished in such a way as to maintain the functions upon which the group's survival depends. This is generally achieved through adjustments of roles, sub-systems and eventually of the community as a whole. New values, symbols and patterns of interaction emerge.

To sum up dynamic equilibrium with an oversimplification: the community can be regarded as composed of two major sets of forces, one centripetal, concerned with self-maintenance and one centrifugal tending toward dissolution — a struggle, in short, between life and lifelessness.

The nature of the dissoliving, centrifugal forces is not a mystery. We have touched on some of them already in mentioning the Four Horsemen and the functional prerequisites of social systems. One not yet mentioned, and one that is of great importance, is the disharmony between individual desires and the demands of the roles essential to keeping a social system going. The problem of this tension has rarely been adequately solved by mankind, and much of the history of the West is a see-saw between extremes of dominance by the social system (Sparta, Rome) and extremes of individualistic assertion (the Dark Ages). Indeed, one can speculate that there is a cyclical pattern such that after a Louis XIV comes a French Revolution; and after a French Revolution comes a Napoleon.

In noting that social systems have great capacities for growth and change, it must also be observed that there are two major limitations. One is that the functional prerequisites must be fulfilled.

The other is that rate of adaptation and adjustment is tied to the neurophysiological properties of the human organism. Learning is time-bound. Thus there is an irreducible minimum of time necessary for people to acquire new shared values, new symbols, and new habits of interaction.

When events demanding adaptation come in torrents and continuously, process failures begin to occur, at first in patches and then cumulatively. Centrifugal forces prevail and the whole social system moves in the direction of disintegration. As this happens, the failures of the system themselves become increments to the dissolution, and hence there is a spiralling tendency.

The picture in mind here is perhaps familiar in terms of the effects of Western technology on peoples of the Third World. It occurs, too, however, within Western society, manifest at present in the hearts of many large cities. In milder forms, which are perhaps just early phases, it is found over much of the earth, among the rich as well as the poor. It is the social process aspect of what Alvin Toffler has called "Future Shock."

What are these events that are too many and too large for handling by the world's communities? Some of the answer is provided in the criticisms made by the Counter Culture. Technology *has* confronted social systems with repeated accelerating jumps without intervals of assimilation: Computers, mass communication facilities, the pill, mood altering drugs and organ transplants that require a new definition of death—to name but a few of the innovations that have come trailing clouds of secondary consequences. Population changes constitute another source of difficulty for social systems. There is evidently an almost worldwide trend away from the country into urban areas, urban areas that are usually ill prepared to handle the influx. There is also a circulating kind of migration in which people shift from community to community in search of jobs, or in search of themselves. It is easy to see that if this turnover is great, instability may be introduced into role performance within community systems.

Values and ideologies must also be reckoned among the factors that impinge on communities, factors which can strike deeply into the symbols and beliefs upon which social systems depend for coordination and the achievement of the functional prerequisites. This brings us to the erosion of norms, for the change is not so much from old values to new as to a state approaching chaos. Traditional orientations exemplified in the great religions have in many instances been replaced by vast numbers of small groups with competing patterns of belief that range from what one might properly call a religion to those that can better be described as superstitions, and both are often manipulated by exploiters.

These multiple mystical trends mean, of course, that the traditions of science and scholarship are faring no better than the great religions. It is ironic that having for over a century played its part in chipping away at the creeds, science now finds itself cast by many into the same rubbish heap.

The rejection of rationality serves, of course, to protect mystical and intuitive beliefs from in-roads by evidence and reason. One expression of this drift is the attacks on psychiatry in recent years of which we have all become aware. For the mystic, a discipline which takes reality testing as a criterion of health is necessarily an enemy.

Beyond this is the rejection of the whole notion of mental illness. If inner being is all in all, and truth is a matter of subjective conviction, who has the right to make such distinctions? After all, it may be that the so-called "insane" are the very ones who have the best grasp of truth, and the label "psychotic" may be merely the work of an oppressive society. Don Quixote re-emerges as "The Man from La Mancha."

Nihilistic beliefs are also part of the disarray. For over a century, European and American writers have been telling mankind in a rising chorus of derisive voices that the human condition is one of injustice and horror. According to this, man is born to slavery, misery and death and there is no escape. A derivative of this view is that it is impossible to have a set of values that both integrates a community and has a basis in truth. If reality is bitter and meaningless, what possible motivation can there be for people to play the roles necessary for community functioning? Any ideology to the contrary is a lie that serves to hold men more firmly in their slavery. Believers are like Becket's idiots who sit about waiting for Godot.

I would like now to offer in Figure D-1 a schematic representation of the disintegration process.

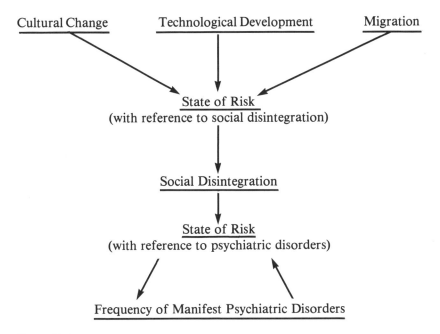

Figure D-1

The top-line refers to the kinds of topics about which I have just been writing: technological, population and ideational changes. The words that you see there are only indicators of a larger array of possibilities. The theory with which we are concerned is that these events create a state of risk in the social system in which they occur—risk of disintegration. Whether the disintegration occurs or not, and whether it progresses to a serious stage, depends on such factors as the rapidity and magnitude of the events and the pre-existing state and adaptive resources of the social system. Thus, there is no one-to-one relationship between cultural change and disintegration, or technological change and disintegration, etc., but rather an interplay of degree, and of available compensations.

If the social system moves into a state of disintegration, then our theory holds that this constitutes a state of risk with regard to increased frequency of manifest psychiatric disorders in the population. This is because disintegration imposes a variety of psychological stresses on the members of the affected social system. Whether or not the actual frequency of disorders will increase depends on such other factors as the distribution of genetic endowment, and the availability of psychological supports of various sorts with which to neutralize the stress. By and large, however, the greater the disintegration, the greater the prevalence of psychiatric disorder.

This scheme offers a way of explaining why such social environment conditions as cultural change, technological change and migration sometimes are and sometimes are not associated with increased frequencies of psychiatric disorders. The key notion is that they are associated with mental illness if the cultural change, migration, etc. leads to disintegration, but are not associated if the social system manages to avoid disintegration.

When disintegration does occur, the resultant rise in the frequency of psychiatric disorders—that is to say, anxieties, apathies, resentments, depressions, emotional instabilities, acting out, delusions, etc.—these have a tendency to increase the disintegration, and thus they constitute a sort of vicious spiral. The bottom arrow at the right of the schematic diagram is intended to indicate this.

It should be said that our emphasis on disintegration is not to be construed as meaning that this is the only set of social factors responsible for increased mental symptoms in a population. Indeed, I believe there are noxious conditions that are due to overintegration and rigidity of systems. These are however, less relevant to the present discussion.

One final point about the scheme: as noted earlier the trend toward disintegration (represented downwardly in the top half) is not conceived to be a smooth progression toward the dissolution of all patterning. There is pulling backward and forward and one intermediate stage is characterized by the appearance of multiple semi-detached clumps of roles for which I suggest the term "flocculation." Derived from sub-systems in the original community, these flocculants struggle to re-establish the functional prerequisites for their members. Thus, we see in some urban areas that unions, church groups, minority organizational and "liberation armies" begin to cohere more strongly and to attempt carrying out functional prerequisites for members that were formerly managed by the community. This can appear as protection, providing jobs and creating roles in the flocculant that give people a sense of identity and belonging. Unfortunately flocculation is sometimes far from suc-cessful in creating functionally adequate social systems because of the paralyzing conflict that may develop among them, like Balkan wars.

Nonetheless, there are here the seeds of renewal. Some flocculants may have a potential for developing into social systems that can survive, and can better meet the demands of the times.

Putting all this together with the Counter Culture, I would like to suggest as the first of three concluding points that the Counter Culture is in part an expression of cultural change and in part a manifestation of social disintegration.

It is one aspect of the response of an over-stressed system, and it is carried forward by individuals trying desperately to escape from the fear and pain caused by societal malfunctioning. Hence the withdrawal, attack, and utopia-formation, and the rocket bursts of new beliefs and efforts at finding new life styles. It has been primarily a response of the young who have strong emotions, great impatience and only a few years of experience. Like numerous other responses of disintegrating social systems, it is in many respects maladaptive and tends to accelerate rather than counteract the dissolution. It is in part joined with the centrifugal forces.

My second point is that some of the behavior characteristic of the Counter Culture is an expression of manifest psychiatric disorder, the response of individuals to the stress of the disintegration. This is particularly true of people who exhibit the more extreme tendencies. Con-sidering that this behavior increases disintegration and societal malfunc-tion and that this malfunction threatens eventual annihilation there is perhaps some literal truth in the saying that those whom the gods would destroy they first make mad.

The final point is to suggest that the communes and related efforts to create new societies is an exceedingly important kind of flocculation. Most communes will probably not last, but it is possible that somewhere among them they contain the germs of remedy to our problems and the beginning of reconstruction. At the very least, they are experiments and opportunities to learn by trying. They are one place where there is whole hearted effort to control the rate of change regardless of how much that may be at variance with material values. This is a central matter in reversing and preventing social disintegration and hence, if our theories are correct, a vital concern to the mental health field.

BIBLIOGRAPHY

Leighton AH: *My Name is Legion: Foundations for a Theory of Man in Relation to Culture.* vol 1, The Stirling County Study of Psychiatric Disorder and Sociocultural Environment. New York, Basic Books, 1959.

Leighton AH: Cosmos in the Gallup City dump, in Kaplan BH (ed) in collaboration with Leighton AH, Murphy JM and Freydberg N: *Psychiatric Disorder and the Urban Environment.* New York, Behavioral Publications, 1971.